BEETHOVEN IN PERSON

BEETHOVEN IN PERSON

His Deafness, Illnesses, and Death

PETER J. DAVIES

Contributions to the Study of Music and Dance, Number 59

GREENWOOD PRESS
Westport, Connecticut • London

Library of Congress Cataloging-in-Publication Data

Davies, Peter J., 1937–
  Beethoven in person : his deafness, illnesses, and death / by Peter J. Davies.
    p. cm.—(Contributions to the study of music and dance, ISSN 0193–9041 ; no. 59)
  Includes bibliographical references (p.) and indexes.
  ISBN 0–313–31587–6 (alk. paper)
  1. Beethoven, Ludwig van, 1770–1827—Health. 2. Composers—Austria—Biography. I.
Title. II. Series.
ML410.B4D28   2001
780'.92—dc21   00–042655
  [B]

British Library Cataloguing in Publication Data is available.

Library of Congress Catalog Card Number: 00–042655
ISBN: 0–313–31587–6
ISSN: 0193–9041

First published in 2001

Greenwood Press, 88 Post Road West, Westport, CT 06881
An imprint of Greenwood Publishing Group, Inc.
www.greenwood.com

Printed in the United States of America

The paper used in this book complies with the
Permanent Paper Standard issued by the National
Information Standards Organization (Z39.48–1984).

10 9 8 7 6 5 4 3 2 1

Copyright Acknowledgments

The author and publisher are grateful to the following for granting permission to reprint from their materials:

Peter J. Davies, "Beethoven's Nephropathy and Death: Discussion Paper," *Journal of the Royal Society of Medicine* 86 (March 1993): 159–161, courtesy of the *Journal of the Royal Society of Medicine.*

Peter J. Davies, "Was Beethoven's Cirrhosis Due to Hemochromatosis?" *Renal Failure* 17, no. 1 (1995), pp. 77–86, courtesy of Marcel Dekker, Inc.

Brenton Broadstock et al., eds., "The Cause of Beethoven's Deafness," in *Aflame with Music: 100 Years of Music at the University of Melbourne,* 143–151 (Parkville: University of Melbourne, Centre for Studies in Australian Music, 1996).

Davies, P. J. "Beethoven's Deafness: A New Theory." MJA 1988; 149: 644–649. © Copyright 1988. *The Medical Journal of Australia*—reproduced with permission.

Emily Anderson, ed., *The Letters of Beethoven,* 3 vols. (London: Macmillan, 1961), reprinted by permission of Macmillan Press, Ltd.

Oscar G. Sonneck, ed., *Beethoven: Impressions by His Contemporaries* (New York: Dover, 1967), courtesy of Dover Publications, Inc.

Contents

14   Eye Disorder   200

15   The Cause of Beethoven's Death   207

Appendix 1: Beethoven's Conversation with Herr Sandra   217

Appendix 2: Beethoven's Compositions   219

Glossary of Medical Terms   233

Select Bibliography   243

General Index   253

Index of Beethoven's Works in This Volume   261

Photo essay follows p. 120

Tables

Preface

Beethoven's greatness, not only as an artist, but also as a human being, was emphasized by Johann Aloys Schlosser in his first biography. Indeed, Beethoven's transformation of his many sufferings into so much of the greatest music ever composed is a masterstroke of human achievement. I. von Seyfried's *Beethoven Studies*, published in 1832 by Haslinger in Vienna, conveyed, in the *Heiligenstadt Testament*, this sublime composer's reaction to the suffering caused by his deafness. Seyfried's translation of Dr. Wagner's autopsy report into German also attracted the curiosity of the medical profession.

Following the publication by Ludwig Nohl of Beethoven's letters in 1876, the wide diversity of his medical complaints, other than his deafness and depression, became apparent. His letters detailed his abdominal pain, constipation alternating with diarrhea, liver disease, respiratory catarrhs, rheumatic complaints, an eye disorder, and recurrent headaches.

The broad diversity of systems tempted physicians to diagnose a multisystem disorder. After making a study of Seyfried's autopsy report, Sir George Grove's friend, Dr. Lauder Brunton, made a diagnosis of syphilis, which was then quite prevalent.

The hypothesis of syphilis remained well accepted until it was thoroughly repudiated in Waldemar Schweisheimer's inaugural medical study. The following year, in the first monograph on Beethoven's deafness, the Italian ear specialist G. Bilancioni favored otosclerosis as the cause.

In his distinguished little volume (1956), Walther Forster included a concise review of the medical literature up to the mid-1950s. Over the past thirty years, alternative multisystem disorders, including systemic lupus erythematosis or some such related autoimmune disorder, sarcoidosis, Whipple's Disease, amyloidosis, and Paget's disease of bone, have been proposed.

The rediscovery in 1970 of Wagner's original autopsy report in Latin, as well as a study of three fragments of Beethoven's skull that had been confiscated during the first exhumation, paved the way for a third German medical biography written by H. Bankl and H. Jesserer (1987). Recent reports of elevated lead levels in Beethoven's hair has raised the question of plumbism.

It has been an exciting story. With the hindsight of the astonishing advances made in medicine during the last fifty years of the twentieth century, it is now appropriate to make a thorough reevaluation of Beethoven's health in this first English monograph.

It should be emphasized that I have taken meticulous care to select only reputable source material after detailed critical analysis. Dr. Sieghard Brandenburg's comprehensive updating of Beethoven's letters (1996–1998) has been incorporated into these studies.

During the two decades between 1840 and 1860, Anton Schindler made deliberate falsifications to conceal certain defects in Beethoven's character, as well as detrimental remarks about himself. Schindler's inaccuracies have permeated not only the biographical reminiscences of F. Wegeler and F. Ries (1987) and Gerhard von Breuning (1992), but nearly all subsequent biographies.

I have carefully scrutinized Schindler's first and third editions, detected and noted further errors, and excluded unsubstantiated material from these studies. In particular I have criticized Schindler's defamation of Dr. Wawruch's character. The conversation-book entries of Dr. Braunhofer and Dr. Wawruch offer fascinating insights into Brunonianism, homeopathy, and the spa cures. Beethoven's conversations with a deaf man, Herr Sandra, are most illuminating.

The accounts of Beethoven's illnesses, by himself and by his contemporaries, do not permit expression in free-flowing narrative. I therefore have grouped his illnesses, other than his deafness, into anatomical areas. Two chapters are devoted to the accounts of, and the cause of, his deafness.

While most of Beethoven's letters quoted in this volume were taken from Emily Anderson's translation (1961), other editions by Nohl, A. C. Kalischer (1909), O. G. Sonneck (1927), D. W. MacArdle and L. Misch (1957), Theodore Albrecht (1996), and Sieghard Brandenburg (1996–1998) were also consulted.

Other essential source documents included the editions of the conversation-books by G. Schünemann (1941–1943) and the Deutscher Verlag für Musik in Leipzig, Beethoven's Tagebuch, and the accounts of contemporaries by Nohl, Sonneck, Gerhard von Breuning, Wegeler and Ries, and others in the biographies of A. W. Thayer, M. Solomon (1978), and the documentary study of H.C.R. Landon (1970). The vast medical literature was also consulted, although it was not possible to trace all the articles published in Eastern Europe. A glossary of medical terms is included to assist the reader, as well as a list of abbreviations frequently used.

Beethoven's mental health, as reflected in his music, is discussed in an analogous companion volume, *Beethoven in Person: The Character of a Genius*, which includes a detailed discussion of his paranoia, personality traits, bipolar tendencies, hypochondriasis, mental sufferings, religious beliefs and attitudes, youth, work, habits, pastimes, stresses, crises, and creativity.

Acknowledgments

During the twelve years of researching these studies I have been assisted by many talented people.

Erna Schwerin again provided numerous translations of German source materials, and I am also grateful for her contribution to Beethovenian psychodynamics.

My gratitude also goes to other translators: Bruce Cooper Clarke, Andrew C. Newell, Sheila Krysz, Aldo Rebeschini, Henri Coutanceau, and Monika Windsor.

Professor Jack Martin read the entire manuscript and offered many helpful suggestions.

I thank Mario Cotela for the photographs.

At the Beethoven Archiv, in Bonn, Sieghard Brandenburg, Hans-Werner Küthen, and Michael Ladenburger assisted me graciously on many occasions.

I also thank Otto Biba at the Gesellschaft der Musikfreunde in Vienna, and William Meredith at the Ira F. Brilliant Center for Beethoven Studies in San Jose, California.

Alan Tyson supplied much invaluable help and advice prior to his illness.

I also thank the Beethoven Museums in Vienna and Baden bei Wien, Austria.

The generous assistance of Karl Portele and Beatrix Patzak at the Federal Pathologic-Anatomy Museum in Vienna was much appreciated.

My thanks to the following libraries in Melbourne: St. Vincent's Hospital, the Brownless, the Eye and Ear Hospital, the Royal Australasian College of Surgeons, and the State Library of Victoria.

I am grateful also to the Royal Australasian College of Physicians Library in Sydney, the library of the Royal Society of Medicine in London, and the Wellcome Institute of the History of Medicine in London.

My thanks also to the British Library, the Bodleian Library at Oxford, and the Cambridge University Library.

My special gratitude is expressed to Ted Albrecht, Professor Harold Attwood, G. Dean Beaumont, Ira F. Brilliant, Margaret Cavello, Hugh Cobbe, Barry Cooper, Yves F. Cudennec, Professor J. S. Dooley, Professor O. H. Drummer, Michael E. Fish, June Halliday, Brenda Heagney, J. Keith Henderson, John Horan, Gerald Little, Leonard Murphy, Desmond O'Shaughnessy, John G. O'Shea, Robin Price, Professor Guenter Risse, Professor J. Rode, Stanley Sadie, Joe Santamaria, Professor Peter Scheuer, Heidi Sequenzia, Maynard Solomon, W. E. Thomas, Augustin Watson, and Hilary Weaver.

I thank Professor Brenton Broadstock for permission to repeat extracts of my essay "The Cause of Beethoven's Deafness" in *Aflame with Music: 100 Years of Music at the University of Melbourne* (1996).

My gratitude is also extended to the editors of the following journals, for permission to reprint material from my previously published articles:

The Medical Journal of Australia, "Beethoven's Deafness: A New Theory" 149 (1988): 644–49; *The Journal of the Royal Society of Medicine*, "Beethoven's Nephropathy and Death: A Discussion Paper" 86 (1993): 159–61; and *Renal Failure*, "Was Beethoven's Cirrhosis due to Hemochromatosis?" 17 (1995): 77–86.

On a personal note I would like to pay a special tribute to my wife Clare, who typed the manuscript, and who was always available to offer sound advice.

This book is dedicated to my teachers.

Abbreviations

AMZ	*Allgemeine Musikalische Zeitung*
Albrecht Letters-	No. of the letter in Albrecht's edition
A-	No. of the letter in Anderson's edition
BE	Beethoven Essays
BJ	*Beethoven Journal* (vols. 10–; 1995–)
BN	*Beethoven Newsletter* (vols. 1–9; 1986–1994)
BS	*Beethoven Studies*
B-	No. of the letter in Brandenburg's edition
FRHB	T. Frimmel, ed. *Beethoven Handbuch*, 2 vols. Leipzig: Breitkopf and Härtel, 1926
JAMS	*Journal of the American Musicological Society*
JM	*Journal of Musicology*
JTW	D. Johnson, A. Tyson, and R. Winter. *The Beethoven Sketchbooks*. Oxford: Clarendon Press, 1985
Kerst	F. Kerst, ed. *Die Erinnerungen an Beethoven*, 2 vols. Stuttgart: J. Hoffmann, 1913, reprinted, 1925
KHV	G. Kinsky and H. Halm, eds. *Das Werk Beethovens Thematisch-Bibliographisches Verzeichnis*. Munich: G. Henle, 1955.
LvBCB	K. H. Köhler, G. Herre, and D. Beck, eds. *Ludwig van Beethovens Konversationshefte*, 9 vols. Leipzig: VEB Deutscher Verlag für Musik, 1968–1988
MT	*Musical Times*

Schindler-   D. W. MacArdle, ed. *Beethoven As I Knew Him: A Biography*
MacArdle   *by Anton Felix Schindler*. Translated by Constance S. Jolly.
                      London: Faber and Faber, 1966

Schindler-   Ignace Moscheles, ed. *Anton Schindler's The Life of Beethoven*.
Moscheles   2 vols. London: Henry Colburn, 1841

Tagebuch-   No. of entry in Beethoven's *Tagebuch* (1812–1818) in A. Ty-
                      son, BS3, 1982, 193–288; and M. Solomon, BE, 233–95.

TDR   Alexander Wheelock Thayer. *Ludwig van Beethovens Leben*,
                      continued Hermann Deiters, completed Hugo Riemann, re-
                      printed Hildesheim: Georg Olms, 1970–1972, 5 vols.

TF   Elliot Forbes, ed. *Thayer's Life of Beethoven*. Princeton, N.J.:
                      Princeton University Press, 1967

TK   Henry Edward Krehbiel, ed. *Alexander Wheelock Thayer's The
                      Life of van Beethoven*. 3 vols. London: Centaur Press, 1960

Medical Chronological Calendar

1740	Early January?	Birth of Johann van Beethoven (father)
1746	19 December	Birth of Maria Magdalena Keverich (mother)
1769	2 April	Baptism of older brother, Ludwig Maria
	8 April	Death of Ludwig Maria
1770	16 December	Probable date of Beethoven's birth
	17 December	Beethoven christened Ludovicus
1773	24 December	Death of grandfather, Louis
1774	8 April	Baptism of brother, Caspar Anton Carl
1775	30 September	Death of grandmother, Maria Josepha
1776	2 October	Baptism of brother, Nikolaus Johann
1779	23 February	Baptism of sister, Anna Maria Franziska
	27 February	Death of Anna Maria Franziska
1781	17 January	Baptism of brother, Franz Georg
1783	16 August	Death of Franz Georg
?	?	Smallpox during childhood
1786	5 May	Baptism of sister, Maria Margarete Josepha
1787	May–September	Asthma and depression in Bonn
	17 July	Death of mother
	25 November	Death of sister, Maria Margarete Josepha
1789	20 November	Father's dismissal from job
1790 or 1791		First bouts of gastrointestinal disorder
1791	5 December	Death of Wolfgang Amadeus Mozart

1792	October	French troops invade Rhinelands
	Early November	Departs Bonn and arrives in Vienna about 10 November
	18 December	Death of father
1796	May–July	In Berlin
	Summer	Serious illness
1798		Initial mention of persistent hearing loss
1800	Autumn	Takes cold baths
1801	June	Consults Dr. Vering
	Summer	Declaration of deafness to Wegeler and Amenda
		Worsening of gastrointestinal disorder
1802		Consults Dr. J. A. Schmidt
	6 October	Writes *Heiligenstadt Testament* with a postscript on 10 October
1803	April	Violent fever
1804	May–early November	Relapsing fever
1805	Spring	Heavy cold
	November	Abdominal pains
1806	4 September	Birth of nephew, Carl
1807	June–September	Dental abscess and headache
1808	February	Finger abscess
1809	19 February	Death of Dr. Schmidt; succeeded by Dr. Malfatti
	11 May	Takes refuge in a cellar during the third siege of Vienna by the French army
	31 May	Death of Franz Joseph Haydn
	December	Febrile illness
1810	January–May	Relapsing abdominal complaint
	November–December	Sore foot and headache
1811	Spring	Fever and headache
	Summer	Mention of ringing in his ears in the "Petter" Sketchbook
1812	Winter	"Fierce attacks"
	Summer	Takes the spas at Teplitz, Carlsbad, and Franzensbrunn
	July	Meets Dr. Staudenheim in Teplitz
	September	Further abdominal problems in Teplitz
1813		Depression
	April	Fever and Fainting; an injured foot
	September	Bad cold

1814	April	Heavy cold
	20 or 21 May	Dines with Dr. Bertolini at the Roman Emperor tavern
	Summer	At Baden spa for abdominal complaint
1814–1815		Mälzel's ear trumpets
	18 September–9 June	Congress of Vienna
1815	Summer	Illness and depression
	15 November	Death of brother, Caspar Carl
1816		Recurrent abdominal pain
	April–May	Chest complaint and depression
	18 September	Nephew Carl's hernia operation
	October–November	Feverish catarrh
1816–1817		Recurrent headache
1817	January–February	Lingering bronchial catarrh
	April–October	Consults Dr. Staudenheim who treats him with powders, tea, a tincture, rubs with a volatile ointment, and spa cures
	May–June	Spa at Heiligenstadt
	Late June–October	Spa at Nussdorf
	7 July	Requests a louder piano from Streicher
	Autumn	Frightful attack of rheumatism
	27 December	Broadwood piano is dispatched from London but is damaged in transit
		Suffers a bad chill
1818	January	Severe pain; violent cold and cough
	24 January	Carl leaves boarding school and lives with Beethoven under a private tutor
	February	Begins using conversation-books
	21 May	Takes his first bath at Mödling
	18 June	Stomach trouble
	3 December	Carl runs away to his mother
1819	20 March	"I am never in good health"
	12 May	In Mödling to take the baths
1820	March	Consults Dr. Braunhofer about his headaches
	4 March	Composes a song for Dr. Braunhofer
	May–October	Takes the baths at Mödling
	September	Catches a chill after a drenching rain

1821	January–March	Confined to bed with a violent bout of rheumatism
	Mid-July–end of August	Jaundice at Unterdöbling
	September–October	At Baden spa where suffers from diarrhea
1822	January–April	Respiratory infection; "gout on the chest"
	11 February	Earache
	May	In Oberdöbling for the cure of baths, mineral water, and powders
	September–October	Takes thirty baths at Baden
1823	January	Recurrence of diarrhea
	April	Conversations with Herr Sandra
		Consults Dr. Smetana about his diarrhea and a burning irritation in his throat
	Early-May	Onset of eye disorder
	July	Relapse of diarrhea
	13 August	In Baden with catarrh
	17 September	Eye disorder clearing up
1824	March	Resolution of the eye disorder
		Troublesome hemorrhoids
	Late May	Short stay at Penzing
	Late May–November	At the Baden spa
	1 August	Has a premonition of his death
	November	Confined indoors with a chill
	Winter	Ominous nose bleeds
1825	Mid-April	Illness: abdominal pain, belching, constipation, weakness, yellowish complexion, weight loss, passage of dark urine; treated by Dr. Braunhofer
	April	Carl enters the Polytechnic Institute
	May	At the Baden spa
	13 May	Composes witty canon (WoO 189) for Dr. Braunhofer
	Mid-May	Composes the *Heiliger Dankgesang* of the Op. 132 String Quartet to celebrate his recovery from illness
	18 May	Suffers from diarrhea after eating asparagus
	15 October	Removal to Schwarzspanierhaus
1826	January–February	Bowel trouble, rheumatic pains, and backache; Dr. Braunhofer diagnoses gout

	6 August	Carl's suicide attempt
	October	Diarrhea at Gneixendorf
	November	Abdominal swelling, swollen feet, excessive thirst, weight loss, and weakness
		Total deafness
	1 December	Hasty departure from Gneixendorf
	2 December	Final return to Schwarzspanierhaus and onset of final illness
	5 December	Dr. Wawruch's first visit
	10 December	Violent abdominal pain and jaundice
	Mid-December	Arrival of George Frideric Handel's works
	19 December	Visit from Johann Baptist Jenger
	20 December	First operation
1827	2 January	Carl leaves to join his regiment
	3 January	Will drafted
	8 January	Second operation
	11 January	Council of physicians
	19 January	Reconciled with Dr. Malfatti
	Late January	Hayseed vapor bath
	3 February	Third operation
	Mid-February	Receives a lithograph of Haydn's birthplace
	22 February	Extreme emaciation
	27 February	Fourth operation
	March	Visit from Franz Schubert?
	8 March	First visit of J. N. Hummel and F. Hiller
	10 March	Arrival of fine Rhine wines from Schott's Sons
	13 March	Second visit of Hummel and Hiller
	23 March	Third visit of Hummel with his wife
		Signs a codicil to his will
	24 March	Arrival of fine wines from Schott's
		Anointed and receives Holy Viaticum
		Lapses into a coma in the evening
	26 March	Dies at 5:45 P.M., aged fifty-six years
	27 March	Dr. Wagner performs an autopsy
	29 March	Funeral
	April	Publication of *Missa solemnis* by Schott's Sons
	May	Publication of Op. 130 String Quartet by Artaria
		Publication of Op. 133 Fugue by Artaria

	4 June	Death of Dr. Stephan von Breuning
	June	Publication of Op. 131 String Quartet by Schott's Sons
	September	Publication of Op. 132 String Quartet by Schlesinger
		Publication of Op. 135 String Quartet by Schlesinger
	5 November	Auction of estate
1863	12 October	First exhumation
1888	21 June	Second exhumation

BEETHOVEN IN PERSON

1

Beethoven's Physicians and Their Treatments

The physicians who attended Beethoven have been granted fame by posterity, although five of them had earned outstanding reputations in Vienna during their own lifetimes. There is no record of the medical treatment of Beethoven's smallpox in his childhood, his chest ailment and melancholia in 1787, or his "terrible typhus" in 1796.

Two of Beethoven's most intimate friends in Bonn, Franz Gerhard Wegeler and Lorenz von Breuning, became medical graduates. On 1 October 1792 his other medical friend in Bonn, Dr. Johann Heinrich Crevelt (1751–1818), wrote verses in his album.[1] In Bonn, Beethoven was also acquainted with Dr. Ferdinand Johann Wurzer (1765–1844) and both Drs. Rovantini from the family of his grandmother.[2]

VIENNESE MEDICINE DURING BEETHOVEN'S LIFE

In Vienna Beethoven tasted and took a vivid interest in the changing art of medical practice. The traditional humoral-pathological system, perpetuated by Hippocrates,[3] Boerhaave,[4] and Stoll,[5] underwent challenges from Brunonianism, phrenology, galvanism or the therapeutic use of direct electrical current, homeopathy, natural philosophy, and the emerging vitalistic concepts of Romantic medicine.

Christian Wilhelm Hufeland's book about the German spas was in Beethoven's library. A leading physician of Berlin and an early opponent of Brunonianism, Hufeland (1762–1836) practiced the method of rational empiricism. Aware of the absence of knowledge of causation of most diseases, he advocated a cautious approach to treatment, with avoidance of excesses, and guidance by cognizable facts. For example, he advocated the use of mercury for the treatment of syphilis[6] and fruit juices for the cure of scurvy.[7] In 1853 his book *The Art of Prolonging Human Life* was translated into English.[8]

THE SPAS

The humoral physicians gave advice to their patients about diet and the taking of exercise, although in internal disorders they relied heavily on purging the corrupted humors with purgatives and enemas. Especially in febrile disorders, they resorted to bloodletting, cupping, various blistering techniques, and the application of leeches to expel the "noxious humours."

They also regularly sent their patients to various spa resorts for the consumption of medicinal waters and the taking of baths. From the classical times of Pliny, Hippocrates, Asclepiades, Celsus, and others, it was held that the taking of the waters promoted good health by regulating the humoral balance. Spa cures were also promoted for various acute and chronic disorders of the joints, skin, chest, abdomen, and head.

The consumption of the medicinal waters was guided by their thermal effects or the potency of their chemical constitution in sulphur, salt, alkali, calcium, iron, arsenic, or other minerals. Cold baths varied from 32° to 77°F (0° to 25°C), tepid baths ranged from 77° to 95°F (25° to 35°C), warm baths ranged from 95° to 100.4°F (35° to 38°C), and hot baths varied from 100.4° to 107.6°F (38° to 42°C).[9]

Typically, while the patient was immersed in the bath up to the neck, various methods of douching were employed, together with massage, or the application of peat, fango (clay mud), or mud. Some of the spas were effervescent. The application was, according to need, altered to gargling, or inhaling vapors, or injecting them into the rectum or vagina. Poultices of bran or linseed, with mustard, were sometimes applied over an ailing organ, such as the liver, for a cure.[10] Dr. Johann Malfatti von Montereggio ordered a hayseed vapor bath for Beethoven during his final illness.

Detailed chemical analyses of the spas were undertaken, and hydrotherapy gained prestige as a therapeutic art. During the summer of 1858, soon after gaining his doctorate of medicine, the outstanding composer and chemist Alexander Borodin studied the chemical and medicinal properties of the spas at Soligalich in Russia.[11] In 1862 Wilhelm Winternitz (1835–1917), whose research provided a physiological basis for balneology, or the science of the therapeutic use of baths, opened a clinic and institute of hydrotherapy near Vienna. His many international students included Dr. J. H. Kellogg of the Battle Creek Sanatorium, in Michigan, who invented and manufactured his now famous cornflakes as a health food.[12]

Teplitz

During the summers of 1811 and 1812, Dr. Malfatti ordered Beethoven to take the spa cure at Teplitz in Czechoslovakia. His second visit there was celebrated not only by his writing the letters to the "Immortal Beloved" and his meetings with Johann Wolfgang von Goethe, but also by the unprecedented influx of notables that year, in the wake of Napoléon Bonaparte's catastrophic invasion of Russia.[13] Beethoven also met Dr. Jakob Staudenheim, who advised him to take the waters at Carlsbad and Franzensbrunn.

Teplitz, which means spa in the Slavonic language, is situated at the base of the Mittelgebirge at an altitude of 730 feet. The thermal waters there reach temperatures from 83° to 114°F (28.3° to 45.6°C). Sodium bicarbonate accounts for 57 percent of the total solids, which are low at 0.7 per thousand; the radium emanation is 28.72 millimicrocuries per liter. The surrounding moor supplied an excellent peat which was used for the baths. The season lasted from May until Michaelmas, or September 29. The Teplitz springs were considered to be beneficial especially for rheumatic disorders and chronic skin diseases.[14] It also attracted patients with gout, headaches, and ear disorders.

Carlsbad

This famous Czech alkaline spa is situated in a natural amphitheatre at an altitude of 1,230 feet. The hot springs rise at varied temperatures from 122° to 197°F (50° to 91.7°C). The celebrated gushing Sprudel contains sodium sulphate of 2.4 parts per thousand, sodium bicarbonate of 1.3 parts per thousand, sodium chloride of 1.0 parts per thousand; free carbonic acid gas, 100 cubic centimeters per liter, together with carbonates of lime and magnesia and traces of iron, manganese, strontium, phosphate of lime, iodine, and bromine, with a radioactivity of 19.8 millimicrocuries per liter.

The season here lasts from May until October. When taken by mouth, these waters have a mild cathartic and diuretic effect, and it was held that this cleansing of the digestive tract and kidneys was beneficial for liver disorders, gallstones, dyspepsia, constipation, diarrhea, mucous colitis, hemorrhoids, recurrent headaches, and such metabolic disorders as gout and diabetes. The combination of aperient waters, peat baths, and a strict diet were also beneficial for obesity. Peat packs were applied to the abdomen or joints for their local effect.[15]

At the best spas, there was always an emphasis on the importance of appropriate dieting and regular exercise. Dr. Lauder Brunton described the patients' mode of life at Carlsbad:

They get up about 6 o'clock in the morning, and they go out without any food to the Sprudel, which is the large well where the hot saline springs bubble up, and here they fill their glasses, and walk round and round the promenade for nearly an hour, and at every two or three steps they take a sip of hot Carlsbad water. In this way they get through three to four tumblers in the course of the promenade; then they go to the confectioner's and have a small cup of coffee, and on the way there they buy a small roll or two, and this they eat without butter along with their coffee. Then they will rest for awhile, and after midday, perhaps, go for another walk, and probably take some more water, after which they will have an evening meal, and then go to bed. The food eaten at meals is also regulated. One day I went into a restaurant in Carlsbad, and looking through the bill of fare, I said: "I would like this." The waiter said: "Are you under treatment, sir? The doctors here do not usually allow it, and if you are under treatment you cannot have it without special leave from your doctor." In most other places you simply have what you like, but in Carlsbad you cannot have it. Patients go there for the purpose of getting well, and so they willingly go back to Carlsbad, because they feel the benefit of it, although they would be unwilling to be kept so strictly at home. It is almost impossible to treat them in the same way as at Carlsbad, so we send our patients there.[16]

Franzensbrunn

The twelve cold alkaline springs at Franzensbrunn (Franzensbad) in Czechoslovakia are situated at an altitude of 1,600 feet. The temperature of the Franzenquelle spring was 51°F (10.6°C), and the constituents were 3.2 parts per thousand of sodium sulphate, 1.2 of sodium chloride, 0.7 of sodium bicarbonate, 0.2 of calcium carbonate, and 0.03 of bicarbonate of iron; 1,460 cubic centimeters per liter of free carbonic acid gas; and a radioactivity of 0.491 millimicrocuries per liter. These waters were considered beneficial especially for disorders of the stomach and liver.[17]

In the summer of 1812 Beethoven spent a month with Franz and Antonie Brentano at Franzensbrunn. Some two years earlier Dr. Poeschmann of Franzensbad had obtained dramatic relief from rheumatic complaints by immersing his patients in a peat bath. The addition of the iron-enriched moor peat produced a pultaceous consistency, allowing the patient to tolerate a higher bath temperature; for example, a peat bath of 102°F (38.9°C) was equivalent to a water bath of 90°F (32.2°C). When peat baths were discovered to allay the pain of pelvic inflammation, the Franzensbad spas became a famous center for the treatment of gynecological disorders. The season extended from May to Michaelmas.[18]

Baden bei Wien

Between 1804 and 1825, Beethoven visited Baden bei Wien in Austria frequently. The hot sulphur springs there, situated at an altitude of 760 feet, rose at a temperature of 93°F (33.9°C). These waters contained 0.02 parts per thousand of calcium sulphide, 0.6 of calcium sulphate, and 0.6 of hydrogen sulphide. Mud baths were available during the season from May to October. The Baden spa was especially beneficial for fibrositis, arthritis, chronic skin disorders, and hemorrhoids.[19] Various other additives to the baths included sand, seaweed, and aromatic substances such as pine needles.[20]

J. M. Gully (1851) claimed to have cured a forty-eight-year-old woman who was suffering from headache, tinnitus, and deafness owing to congestion of the brain at his Malvern clinic in 1845, after a two-month treatment with the following regime. Before breakfast she was packed in a wet sheet for an hour, or immersed in a shallow cold bath for four minutes, while being rubbed vigorously. Cold water was repeatedly poured over her head.

At noon she was immersed in a sitz bath at 70°F for fifteen minutes, which was repeated at 5:00 P.M. While she was subjected to foot baths of cold water and mustard twice daily, the nape of her neck was rubbed with the same mixture.

At bedtime hot fomentations were applied to her abdomen for an hour. The flannels were changed every ten minutes, and she consumed a wine glass of cold spa water.

Cold toast with a little butter sufficed for breakfast, and during the day three or four tumblers of water were sipped slowly. For dinner three times a week three ounces of meat was permitted; on the other days, a cup of cocoa was taken either with buttered cold toast or a lukewarm farinaceous pudding.

Exercise was encouraged during the afternoons. During the second month an emetic was taken to induce an internal crisis, which was manifested by repeated vomiting and the passage of blood from the bowel.[21]

It is now clear that many of the cures attributed to the spas were simply spontaneous recoveries induced by the substantial natural recuperative powers of the human condition.

MEDICAL LECTURES ON KANT IN VIENNA

Following the election of a collegium of professors in 1790 for the teaching of medicine, there were 410 medical practitioners in Vienna in 1800.[22] Throughout the Germanic universities then, the teaching of medicine was closely allied to a coherent philosophical system which was inspired in large part by the epistemology of German philosopher Immanuel Kant (1724–1804).

Private lectures on Kant were given in Vienna by such leading lights as J. N. Hunczowsky (1752–1798), J. A. Schmidt (1759–1809), Wilhelm Schmidt, the Imperial & Royal Physician, Dr Göffert, and several others. These lectures were attended by Wegeler, who tried in vain to persuade Beethoven to go to them.[23]

JOHANN NEPOMUK HUNCZOWSKY

This Czech-born medical practitioner was also a scholar and art connoisseur. He rose to become a professor of surgery and gynecology at the Josephinium Academy and the military hospital in the Gumpendorf suburb of Vienna.

As a freemason he belonged to the True Concord lodge, and he treated Constanze Mozart during the delivery of her fifth child, Anna, who died an hour after birth on 16 November 1789.

Beethoven first became acquainted with the music-loving Hunczowsky during his short first visit to Vienna in 1787. From 1794 the Hunczowskys had been regular attenders at the musical soirees of Stephan von Breuning. Furthermore, he was one of the teachers of Lenz von Breuning, who often attended his home for social and musical gatherings.[24]

A textbook of surgery; *Bibliothek der neuesten medizinisch-chirurgischen Literatur für die K. K. Feldchirurgen*, edited by J. Hunczowski and J. A. Schmidt, was published in two volumes, with copper-plated engravings, in 1791 by Joseph Stahel in Vienna.

THE STOLL-BROWN CONTROVERSY

On the third page of his letter of 13 May 1825 to Dr. Anton Braunhofer, Beethoven joked about the Stoll-Brown controversy: "D[octor]: I will help you, I will alternate Brown's method with that of Stoll. Pat[ient]: I should like to be able to sit at my writing-desk again and feel a little stronger."[25]

While Dr. Stoll favored the traditional methods of treatment by purging and bloodletting, John Brown prescribed controversial remedies with alcohol and opiates.

Maximilian Stoll (1742–1787), one of the leading physicians of the eighteenth century, was born in Erzingen, Germany, the son of a surgeon. After trying his hand as a lay teacher of classical languages in the Jesuit order, he studied medicine initially at Strasbourg, France, and then at Vienna, under Anton de Haen, whom he succeeded as the director of the Vienna Medical Clinic from 1776 until his premature death on 23 May 1787 from a stroke.

An outstanding clinician and teacher in the school of Dr. Hermann Boerhaave of Leyden, Stoll practiced and taught the art of percussion discovered by Leopold Auenbrugger and later popularized by Napoléon Bonaparte's physician, Corvisart. Keen to advance the accuracy of diagnosis by comparison of clinical findings with anatomical pathology, Stoll regularly performed autopsies. He believed that the seasons and the weather generated an important influence on the onset of illnesses and, contrary to Anton de Haen, he favored inoculation.

When Emperor Joseph II invited submissions for a competition for the design of a building plan for the Vienna General Hospital, Stoll's preference for hospital pavilions was discarded in favor of Quarin's ward system.[26]

One of Stoll's most influential patients was Prince Kaunitz,[27] whose librarian, Councillor Rücker, was succeeded by Johann Pezzl, now famous for his *Sketch of Vienna, 1786–90*.

In his letter, to an unknown friend, dated 1 May 1785, Stoll wrote: "You no doubt know, my friend, that this year tuition in all subjects must be paid for, but not to the teacher but the university." Stoll concluded with the following irony,

Everything has its order here, with system, monotony of method and matter. Whoever draws on other sources of knowledge, cannot make headway here, even if it were more productive and profitable. But I am not worried about the future of my children, because I rely on the ever-changing times and the ephemeral duration of our wise institutions.[28]

Joseph Ludwig Stoll

Stoll's son, Joseph (1778–1815), then aged seven, became a poet who died in poverty. In 1808 Joseph Stoll and Leo von Seckendorf edited the periodical *Prometheus*, which ceased publication after a year. Soon after that, Beethoven wrote to the distinguished orientalist Joseph Hammer (1774–1856), exhorting him to assist the poor unfortunate poet.[29]

Beethoven's first setting of Stoll's poem *An die Geliebte*, WoO 140, was presented to Antonie Brentano. A revised version was published in Vienna in 1814 in the journal *Friedensblätter*.[30]

In 1810 Beethoven agreed to act as a guarantor for a loan of four louis d'or to Stoll from the merchant firm Offenheimer and Herz, who employed Franz Oliva as a clerk.[31] Stoll was then in receipt of a yearly pension from Napoléon of 500 francs, and the story goes that the French emperor was under the false impression that he was supporting the famous physician Maximilian Stoll. Uhland's poem *Auf einem verhungerten Dichter* (On a starved poet) was dedicated to Joseph Stoll.[32]

Stoll and Frank

Maximilian Stoll supported Johann Peter Frank's appointment as professor of clinical medicine at the University of Pavia. On 26 July 1785, Stoll wrote to Frank,

I hope you are thriving in Italy among the learned masters, and away from the one [in Göttingen] who envied you and poisoned everything, so that you are now able to continue your splendid work with pleasure. I myself continue on my hurried path, like an honest citizen crossing the street in performance of his tasks, and who from time to time had to suffer the splatter of mud by a careless street urchin. This man cleans himself up as best he can, continuing on his way without looking back.[33]

In 1785 Stoll cured the poet Alois Blumauer (1755–1798), who suffered from dropsy. Two years later, Stoll himself was beset by a fever which improved somewhat after a venesection, or bloodletting. When Dr. Mertens was called following a deterioration, Stoll pointed his finger to his forehead, saying, "Apoplectic," and he died soon afterward.

Blumauer wrote a poem of lasting tribute[34] and edited Pezzl's biography.[35] At the time of his death only three of the seven parts of Stoll's treatise on the practice of medicine had been published.[36]

John Brown

The founder of the Brunonian system of medicine was born in Scotland in 1735 or 1736, of humble stock, in the village of Preston or Lintlaws in the parish of Buncle in Berwickshire.[37] He was a child prodigy who by the age of five had read all the Old Testament. Brown attended school at Dunse where the brilliant student was seldom seen without a book in his hand.

Following his father's death, his mother married again and apprenticed John to a weaver, but he was soon at grammar school under Mr. Cruickshank. Brown, a natural academic, remained at school in Dunse until his twentieth year. He trained for the ministry and excelled in Latin.

After his failure to qualify as a preacher or a teacher of the classics, he turned his ambition to the study of medicine, gained entrance to the campus of the University of Edinburgh as a medical "grinder," and assisted students in the preparation of their graduation theses in Latin.[38]

This charming, generous, jovial innovator, with a high Doric dialect, soon became a popular figure at the university. Indeed during the years from 1759 to 1764 he was granted free admittance to the lectures in anatomy, materia medica, chemistry, and the practice of medicine. A professor of chemistry, William Cullen (1710–1790), engaged Brown as a Latin tutor for his family.

In 1765 Brown married and opened a collegiate boardinghouse, which soon became the gathering place for medical students in Edinburgh. Many a lively discussion initiated there was concluded in the convivial atmosphere of a nearby tavern.

From 1766 to 1769 Brown attended lectures in physiology, pathology, botany, the practice of medicine, medical theory, materia medica, midwifery, and the practice of physic. In 1770 his study of rational philosophy was interrupted by a severe attack of gout. Despite adhering to a strict vegetarian diet, porridge, and drinking only water for a year, Brown was discouraged by the recurrence of the gout four times. He attempted to cure himself with the liberal consumption of meat and alcohol. A remission from gout for several years coincided with his treatment.

In 1773 Brown was elected president of the Medical Society of Edinburgh, while Cullen took the chair of practical medicine. After attending courses in anatomy and surgery in 1774 and 1775, he attended lectures in natural philosophy in 1775 and 1776 from the famous mathematician John Robinson (1739–1805).

In 1776 his relations with Cullen were strained when Brown failed in his bid to take the vacant chair of the Institutes of Medicine, Theoretical Physiology and Pathology. During the autumn he enjoyed himself while living in a tavern at Leyden, and he attended lectures in botany at the famous university there.

Returning to Edinburgh in February 1777, he was again frustrated in his bid for the vacant chair of natural history and botany, which was filled by Cullen's friend, Reverend John Walker. Brown himself treated a recurrence of gout with alcohol and laudanum, but in the process he became addicted to the laudanum.

Brown's breach with Cullen became permanent when not only was he refused admission to Edinburgh's distinguished Philosophical Society, but especially when his doctoral dissertation was rejected. In September 1779, Brown graduated with an M.D. from the nearby university of St. Andrews.

In his lectures after his return to Edinburgh, Brown attacked the teachings of Cullen, and following the publication in Latin of his *Elementa Medicinae* in 1780, Brunonian ideas and methods were banned at the university.

The following year, Brown was involved in a public scandal over the treatment of a university student named Isaacson. Although Brown's founding in 1785 of a Masonic lodge, the Roman Eagle, with ceremonies conducted in Latin, attracted loyal students and some of the aristocracy, living in Edinburgh was no longer viable for him, and in 1786 he moved to London.[39]

Brown's lectures given at his lodgings in Golden Square and at the Devil Tavern in Fleet Street were poorly attended. During his lectures he would sometimes take several draughts of as many as forty or fifty drops of laudanum in whisky. Unable to pay his debts he was imprisoned for a while in the King's Bench, until he was bailed out by his friendly book publishers, Mr. Murray and Mr. Maddison. He was paid fifty pounds by the firm of J. Johnson for the translation of his *Elementa Medicinae* into English.

Brown's prospects were looking brighter when he agreed to write a treatise on gout for 500 pounds; however, on 7 October 1788, he retired after his usual large dose of laudanum and died in his sleep, apparently from a stroke.[40]

BRUNONIANISM

In emulation of Isaac Newton (1643–1727), John Brown was very much influenced by Robinson's geometric reasoning in producing his simplistic quantified system of medicine. Brown's system of medicine was woven from the basic concepts of William Cullen and Robert Whytt (1714–1766), with additional input from Boerhaave and especially the hydrodynamic theories of Friedrich Hoffmann (1660–1742).[41]

Brown called the essential property of all living animal and vegetable matter "excitability." This vital excitability was associated with the capacity to perceive and the ability to respond to various internal and external agents or stimuli.[42] The external stimuli included heat, food, drink, other substances taken into the stomach, the blood, the fluids secreted from the blood, and the air. The internal stimuli consisted of such bodily functions as muscular contractions, sense of perception, and the energy used by the brain in thinking or in exciting emotion or passion. These external and internal stimuli were called "exciting powers." The effect of the exciting powers acting on the excitability was called "excitement." The stimuli could be universal or local.[43]

The quantitative changes in excitement could readily be subjected to mathematical analysis.[44] Health was for Brown a precarious state of balance between stimulation and excitability. A healthy state was dependent upon a moderate

Table 1.1
The Brunonian Scale of Excitability

Degrees	State of Health
0	Death
1–9	Indirect debility
10–25	Sthenic diseases*
26–39	Sthenic diathesis
40	Good health
41–54	Asthenic diathesis
55–70	Asthenic diseases**
71–79	Direct debility
80	Death

*Sthenic diseases: Most fevers, exanthemata (e.g., scarlet fever), smallpox, measles.
**Asthenic diseases: Mild: scabies, scurvy, rickets, hemorrhoids, menstrual disorders; moderate: gout, epilepsy, hysteria, hypochondriasis, asthma, dyspepsia, tetanus; severe: intermittent fevers, plague, confluent smallpox, dysentery.

amount of excitement induced by the exciting powers, so that the degree of excitability corresponded to a scale of 40 out of 80 (see Table 1.1).

When there occurred persistent excessive excitement, there was a gradual depletion of excitability with eventual death, unless there was an appropriate intervention by the physician. When the excitability was reduced by excessive stimulation to less than 25 degrees, the sthenic diathesis had already developed into a sthenic disease, characterized by evidence of excessive blood flow such as a hard full pulse, thirst, diminished perspiration, redness of the face, and muscular spasms.[45]

The aim of treatment of the sthenic disease was to restore excitability by the application of only weak stimuli. Only a vegetarian diet and watery drinks were permitted. Sweating was induced, as well as gentle emesis and purging. Moderate bleeding was restricted to the severest cases.[46] When, despite this treatment, the scale of excitability had fallen to 5 degrees, a moribund state of "indirect debility" was present.[47]

On the other hand, if the excitement was deficient, there was a buildup of excitability through the stages of asthenic diathesis, asthenic disease, direct debility, and death. Asthenic disease was characterized by a weak, soft pulse, facial pallor, and muscular hypotonia.[48]

The aim of treatment in asthenic disease was to reduce the excitability through the stimulation of excitement by way of stimulating foods, roasted meat, rich soups, wines, other alcoholic beverages, and the prescription of strong stimulants such as opium, musk, camphor, and ether. The taking of fresh air and gentle exercise were also encouraged.[49]

Brunonianism in Vienna

It is little wonder that Beethoven was conversant with John Brown's treatments, since Beethoven himself was personally acquainted with five of the leading Brunonians in Vienna: Joseph Frank, Johann Peter Frank, Gerhard von Vering, Johann Adam Schmidt, and Johann Malfatti.[50] Even so, its popularity in the Austrian capital was short lived, and by 1804 it had been eclipsed by Friedrich Schelling's *Naturphilosophie*.[51] The collapse of Brunonianism in Vienna was all the more remarkable given that senior statesman Clemens von Metternich, an attentive student of Johann Peter Frank, based his political system on the model of Brown's hypothesis concerning the equilibrium between stimuli and excitability.

JOSEPH FRANK

The eldest son of Johann Peter Frank was born on 23 December 1771.[52] Soon after his graduation in medicine, at the age of nineteen from the University of Parma in June 1791, Joseph traveled with his father to Switzerland, where he was influenced by enthusiastic reports about John Brown's system of medicine.

After returning to Pavia, Joseph Frank undertook an intensive investigation of Brown's methods starting, together with his friend Vincent Solenghi, with a study of the book written by Brown's pupil Robert Jones.[53] In 1795 Joseph Frank appended his own notes to an Italian translation of Jones' volume.

While working as a physician at the Ospedale di San Matteo in Pavia from 1792, Joseph Frank tested Brunonian principles at the bedside.[54] It must be emphasized that Brown himself was primarily a theoretician; he had relatively little experience in the practice of clinical medicine at the bedside. Brown had admitted that at times it was difficult, when confronted with a sick patient, to decide whether the diagnosis was asthenic or sthenic. In such cases, he recommended a therapeutic trial.

Joseph Frank soon found that while the majority of his patients suffered with an asthenic disorder, it was often difficult to decide which category in Brown's system was most appropriate. He prescribed much smaller doses than Brown of opium and such stimulants as Peruvian bark, camphor, and musk. However, like Brown, he prescribed liberal quantities of alcohol, for example up to a quart of white or red wine daily, or even up to four quarts of diluted wine soup in a day.

Malaga wine was popular, but, in the interest of economy, Frank invented his famous *potus excitans* which was prepared by mixing one part of concentrated distilled alcohol to one part of honey and two parts of water. Frank's popular egg nog consisted of a fortified wine mixed with sugar, eggs, and nutmeg.[55]

A Göttingen graduate, Dr. Adalbert Marcus, also practiced Brunonian therapeutics at the 120-bed Bamberg Hospital, which opened its doors on 11 November 1787.[56]

When, on 20 November 1795, Emperor Francis II appointed Dr. Johann Peter Frank as imperial court counsellor, director of the Vienna General Hospital, and full professor of the practice of medicine at the University of Vienna, on a salary of 5,000 gulden, exempt of all deductions, together with a fine residence and traveling expenses, his son Joseph Frank was appointed chief physician to the General Hospital. However the emperor ordered Joseph to remain in Pavia, as an associate professor in charge of the hospital clinics and chair of medicine, until his father's successor had been appointed.

Johann Peter Frank gave his first lecture in Latin on the practice of medicine at the university on 14 December 1795, and a few days later he opened the clinical section of the General Hospital.[57]

Joseph Frank joined his father in Vienna prior to Napoléon Bonaparte's invasion of Pavia. His younger brother, Francis Frank, who also was a medical graduate of Pavia, was appointed as one of his father's assistants at the General Hospital.

Working in overcrowded, unhygienic conditions, Francis Frank himself became ill a few days after treating a case of "nosocomial typhus." Despite treatment with Dover's powder, Malaga wine, quinine, opium, musk, camphor, blisters, and hot baths, he died on 19 March 1796. Of course, both Joseph Frank and his father were shattered by the catastrophe, and the anti-Brunonians charged that Brown's methods had caused his death.[58]

Joseph Frank gradually became disenchanted with Brown's ideas. He deviated from Brown's fundamental concept of the purely quantitative nature of excitability, proposing that the material composition of an organ would alter the manifestation of excitability, so that, for example, it would appear as an irritability in muscles in contrast to a sensibility in nerves.[59]

In 1797 Joseph Frank's observations at the medical clinic in Pavia in the year 1795 were published in Latin and German.[60] In the preface, Joseph's father expressed his reservations about certain aspects of Brunonian therapeutics: "Much of what this sagacious brain has produced, I approve of fully, but I am not pleased with all. I make use of the good and I throw the chaff away—but not ungratefully in the face of the praiseworthy man."[61]

Beethoven and Joseph Frank

In 1795 Beethoven paid tribute to the very fine amateur soprano Christine Gerhardi, who no doubt would have introduced him to her fiancé.[62] Joseph Frank loved to compose cantatas to celebrate the name days and birthdays of his illustrious father. Christine was often accompanied by Beethoven on the pianoforte at the fashionable soirees held at Johann Peter Frank's fine home at no. 20 Alserstrasse.[63]

No doubt Brunonianism would have been a frequent topic of conversation in the Frank household. According to Kalischer, Beethoven was also friendly with Dr. Bolderini, a physician who may have been the "disagreeable B" referred to in one of the composer's letters to Christine.[64] The "extremely stupid Joseph" referred to in that letter may have been a jocular reference to Joseph Frank.[65]

Although there is no record of it, it seems probable that Beethoven would have consulted Joseph Frank about his health. Perhaps Frank was the physician who treated his "terrible typhus" during the summer of 1796. Unfortunately, there is no record.

In 1800 Joseph Frank founded the Society of Physicians, a group of sympathetic Brunonians who held their meetings at the house of his assistant, Johann Malfatti. During Joseph's "scientific voyage" to Paris and London in 1802 and 1803, his breach with Brunonianism was completed and he was converted to the prevalent influence of rational empiricism.[66]

When Joseph Frank returned to Vienna in December 1803, Brunonianism had been replaced with Schelling's system of natural philosophy, which claimed that all natural phenomena could be deduced from reason alone.[67] Following the bitter anti-Brunonian attack mounted by the influential emperor's physician Dr. J. A. Stifft (1760–1836), Joseph Frank was forced for political reasons, together with his father, to take up an appointment at the University of Vilnius, where he continued to practice medicine for nearly twenty years.[68] He died in 1842.

THE PHRENOLOGICAL MOVEMENT OF
FRANZ JOSEPH GALL

In his book of recollections published in 1816, Dr. Aloys Weissenbach wrote,

Beethoven has greater bodily vigour and robustness than usually fall to the lot of men of high intellect. The whole man is visible in his countenance. If M. Gall, the phrenologist, is right in the position he has assigned to the faculties, musical genius may be grasped with the hand on Beethoven's head.[69]

Franz Joseph Gall was born on 9 March 1758 in Tifenbrunn, in the German state of Baden. Following his initial studies in Strasbourg, he moved to Vienna in 1781, where he graduated with an M.D. in 1785.[70] Even in his youth he had been fascinated with physiognomy, and he had, for example, observed a close correlation in his fellow students between prominence of eyes and excellence of memory.

Gall founded the science of craniology and cranioscopy after making a comparative study of the anatomy of hundreds of heads of musicians, actors, painters, and criminals. The bulk of his collection is preserved in the Rollett Museum at Baden.

From 1798 Gall turned to a comparative study of the anatomy and physiology of the brain, and from 1804 he was assisted by Carl Spurzheim, who coined the term phrenology.

Gall described the origins of the first eight cranial nerves, separated the divergent from the convergent fibers in the cerebellum, and confirmed the crossing of the pyramidal tract.[71] He was "the godfather of the principle of cortical localization of mental faculties."[72]

Gall concluded that humans and animals were subject to the same laws of organization, and that the brains of humans and animals shared in common nineteen centers of behavior in their cerebral cortex. He explained the superiority of man, in his possession of unique areas in the anterior-superior part of the human brain, which contained an additional eight centers for comparative sagacity, spirit of metaphysics, wit, poetic talent, goodness, imitative faculty, religious sentiment, and firmness.[73]

The human brain was unique because it controlled all the higher functions including instinctive urges and passions. Gall disassociated himself from the idealistic philosophies of Kant, Johann Gottlieb Fichte, Schelling, and G.W.F. Hegel.[74]

Following a bitter attack made by Dr. J. A. Stifft, the emperor decreed on 24 December 1801 that Gall's private lectures were forbidden, since his theory was materialistic and contrary to the basic principles of morals and religion.[75]

After leaving Vienna in 1805, Gall and Spurzheim set out on a lecture tour of Germany and adjacent countries, which met with sensational success. He arrived in Paris in 1807 and remained there till his death in 1828.

Although much of their phrenological doctrine is unacceptable today, the exuberance of their pioneering studies transcended science and psychology to affect philosophy, religion, education, and literature.

GALVANISM

In 1791 the electrophysiologist Aloysio Luigi Galvani (1737–1798), of Padua, published his paper "On Electrical Powers in the Movement of Muscles."[76] In his letter of 16 November 1801, Beethoven asked Wegeler for his opinion about the alleged spectacular cures of deafness by galvanism. Later Beethoven informed Herr Sandra that he was unable to endure such a treatment.

A renowned French neurologist, Guillaume Benjamin Amand Duchenne (1806–1875), of Boulogne, described his own personal experience of faradism, or the therapeutic application of a faradic current of electricity, of the external ear. The head was so placed that the external auditory meatus was perpendicular. After the ear was half filled with tepid water, an ear-rheophore was introduced into the ear canal, care being taken to avoid any contact with the walls of the canal or the tympanic membrane.[77] In order to avoid such contact during the procedure, it was essential to prevent any movement of the head.

A second moist electrode was placed over the mastoid process, and both electrodes were connected to an induction apparatus capable of very delicate graduation. Duchenne described his experience:

1. The rheophore having been placed in my own external auditory meatus (previously half-filled with water), and the apparatus being at its minimum, I perceived, on the instant that the intermission of the current took place, a little dry parchment-like sound, a crackling which I referred to the bottom of the external auditory meatus. When the intermissions were very rapid the sound resembled a crepitation, or the noise produced by the wings of a fly flying between a window-pane and the blind. The intensity of these sounds increased with the force of the current.
2. To the auditory phenomena was added a sense of tickling in the bottom of the ear, proportional to the strength of the current, and absolutely limited to the point at which the sound seemed to originate.
3. After a certain time, and with a certain degree of tension of the current, I felt very plainly a tickling in the right side of my tongue at the junction of the middle and posterior thirds. As the strength of the current increased, the tickling reached the point of the tongue, where I then felt a numbness and a disagreeable pricking which was not actually painful. This experiment is often followed by a numbness, and sometimes by an over-sensitiveness of the two front thirds of the edge of the tongue, which persists a considerable time.
4. It seemed also as if my tongue were dry and rapeuse [rough] on the side operated upon.[78]

Duchenne added three other effects: a peculiar metallic taste, a luminous sensation on the stimulated side, and sometimes increased salivation.

The gustatory sensations in the tongue were due to stimulation of the chorda tympani nerve in the tympanic membrane. Duchenne discovered that the crackling sound was not due to direct stimulation of the auditory nerve, but rather to the vibration of the middle ear ossicles through stimulation of their muscles.

Duchenne discovered that faradism of the external ear was very successful in curing cases of hysterical deafness, occasionally beneficial in quinine-induced hearing impairment, and rarely helpful in nervous deafness following obscure fevers.[79]

In Philipp Carl Hartmann's system of natural philosophy, the galvanic process was regarded as one of the general powers of nature. It was argued that the dynamic alternation of positive expansion and negative contraction was linked to a polarity of reproduction and disorganization.[80]

HOMEOPATHY

German physician Christian Friedrich Samuel Hahnemann (1755–1843) was born in Meissen on 10 April 1755, and he died in Paris on 2 July 1843. Hahnemann became disenchanted not only with the inadequate results of treating fevers with the traditional methods of bloodletting, purging, and emesis, but also with the dangers of the toxic effects of overdosage with mercury, digitalis, alcohol, opium, and other medicines.

While translating William Cullen's *Materia Medica* into German, he was struck by the observation that the effects of quinine given to a healthy person produced similar symptoms to the patient with intermittent fever, for whom it had been prescribed. In 1796 he formulated his healing law of similars, which stated that a disease could be cured by the administration of small doses of a refined medicine, which produced similar symptoms to the disease, when administered to a healthy person.

According to Hahnemann, a subtle infinitesimal amount of a properly dynamized medicament was able to release its spiritlike dynamic medicinal force in ways impossible to attain with even massive doses of the crude medicinal substance. His *Organon of Medicine* was published in 1810.[81]

Though Hahnemann was opposed to galvanic stimulation, he did permit such homeopathic adjuvants as bathing, massage, and even modified mesmerism. In 1821 the combined antagonistic efforts of orthodox physicians and apothecaries forced him to leave Leipzig.

The medical officer at the Prague Invalids' Home, Dr. Matthias Marenzeller (1765–1854), became an enthusiastic advocate of Hahnemann's methods, which despite the opposition of Stifft became popular in Vienna, especially in the court circles and among the Austrian military.

Indeed, in 1820, even though the homeopathic system was prohibited in Vienna, Prince Schwarzenberg, the famous field marshall of the Austrian army and commander in chief of the allied armies against Napoléon, went to Leipzig to consult and receive treatment from Hahnemann.

In 1831 the apparent successes of homeopathic treatments during an outbreak of cholera were praised from the pulpit of St. Stephan's Cathedral in Vienna by the physician-priest Johann Emanuel Veith (1787–1876).

A homeopathic hospital was established in 1834 at Gumpendorf, and the prohibition of homeopathic practice was lifted a year after Stifft's death in 1836. In 1841 lectures in homeopathy were permitted at the University of Vienna.[82]

JOHANN PETER FRANK

Born in the small town of Rodalben (Rotalben) in the Bavarian Palatinate, then in the possession of the Margraves of Baden-Baden, Johann Peter Frank (1745–1821) was one of the very great physicians of his time, an outstanding pioneer in clinical and social medicine, medical education, hospital administration, public health, hygiene, and medical police.[83]

Frank studied medicine at Heidelberg, transferred to Strasbourg after a dispute with his physiology lecturer, Dr. Harrer, and returned to Heidelberg in 1766 for his graduation.[84]

From 1772 until 1784, while serving as physician to the Prince-Bishop of Speyer at Bruchsal, on a salary of 400 florins, Frank wrote the first three volumes of his *System of Medical Police*.[85] This monumental treatise and his autobiography are important source materials for the social history of the period.

Three weeks after being offered a chair in Mainz in 1784, Frank received an invitation from Prince Kaunitz, following Stoll's recommendation, to succeed Simon André Tissot (1728–1797) at Pavia in Italy, as professor of medical practice, on a salary of 3,000 florins and a fine furnished house. In the wake of a delay in confirmation of this appointment, however, Frank accepted the post of professor of medical practice at the University of Göttingen, on a salary of 840 thaler.[86] On 25 May 1784 he gave his inaugural dissertation.[87]

During the ensuing harsh winter, however, when Frank became ill with loss of appetite and recurrent vomiting, he changed his mind and accepted the still vacant post at Pavia. At the emperor's command, during a stopover in Vienna in April 1785, Frank inspected the year-old Vienna General Hospital and gave his impressions to Joseph II during an audience. Frank arrived in Pavia on 18 May, just six weeks before the end of the academic year.

Much to his surprise, on 12 June, Emperor Joseph II and his brother, Grand Duke Leopold of Tuscany, arrived unexpectedly to undertake a detailed inspection of the university and the hospital. Shocked at the inadequate dimensions and squalor of an isolation ward for cases of infectious disease, the emperor was anxious to authorize any alterations or improvements that were advisable.[88]

Encouraged by the emperor's seal of approval, Frank extended the period of study for physicians to five years, and for surgeons to four. He doubled the number of lectures from 80 to 160, abolished free Thursdays, set up a pathology museum, founded new chairs, initiated new appointments, raised professional salaries (other than his own), and set aside twenty-two beds for clinical teaching.

He established a surgical clinic, a surgical ward, and an amphitheater. A model pharmacy was set up for the training of pharmacists, and the compilation of a new pharmacopoeia was encouraged. He held weekly meetings with his staff and improved the teaching of obstetrics and midwifery.

Little wonder that Pavia became a famous medical center which attracted students from near and far: by the turn of the century, he had trained 2,000 physicians. His appointment on 7 February 1786, as protomedicus and director-general of the medical services for Austrian Lombardy and the Duchy of Mantua, offered him further opportunities to develop his administrative skills and statesmanship.[89] In his academic address made on 5 May 1790, Frank elaborated on the evils of poverty as a cause of disease.[90]

Such were the skills of the physician whom Beethoven consulted in Vienna, although the relationship had begun on a social basis. In his letter of 29 June 1801 to Wegeler, Beethoven made reference to worsening deafness for three years, along with frequent diarrhea and debility since coming to Vienna. In that letter Beethoven stated, "Frank tried to tone up my constitution with strengthening medicines and my hearing with almond oil, but much good did it do me! His treatment had no effect, my deafness became even worse and my abdomen continued to be in the same state as before."[91]

It has been assumed that Beethoven was here probably referring to Dr. Johann Peter Frank, though as recently pointed out by Brandenburg, it could have been

Dr. Joseph Frank.[92] The toning up of his constitution with strengthening medicines was a Brunonian treatment for an asthenic disease, and at that time both
Johann Peter and especially Joseph Frank were advocates of such treatment.

Be that as it may, Beethoven then implied that he broke off relations with
Dr. Frank in the autumn of 1800, when in despair he consulted "a medical
asinus" who advised cold baths. Then he consulted another unnamed doctor
who prescribed tepid baths in the Danube, which resulted in a miraculous improvement of his diarrhea, although the deafness became worse. Following a
recurrence of colic and diarrhea during the winter, he consulted Dr. Vering four
weeks previously (i.e., 1 June 1801).

In a conversation-book entry in February 1820, Franz Oliva (1786–1848)
informed Beethoven that his physician was Dr. Frank, but it remains unclear
whether this was Johann Peter or Joseph Frank.[93]

After a year in Vilnius Johann Peter Frank moved to St. Petersburg, as physician in ordinary to the czar and as director of the first Medico-Chirurgical
Academy, on a salary of 42,000 rubles. Following a bout of dysentery, he decided to retire after three years in office, but before he departed, the Russian
government purchased his valuable library for 20,000 rubles, and Czar Alexander I granted him an annual pension of 3,000 rubles.

In 1809, during the war between France and Austria, Napoléon consulted
Frank twice, and invited him to Paris, though he refused tactfully. After a short
stay in Freiburg he returned to Vienna in 1811, where he completed his *System
of Medical Police*.[94]

GERHARD VON VERING

Born in Westphalia in northern Germany, Gerhard von Vering (1755–1823)
came to Vienna at the age of twenty, joined the army, and was soon promoted
to the post of regimental surgeon. Vering was one of a select band of doctors
whom Emperor Joseph II used to send on scientific scouting expeditions to
various European countries.[95]

Since the foundation of Joseph's Medical-Surgical Academy in 1785, Vering
was one of the three military surgeons on the staff. In 1804, when chief medical
officer (Feldstabsarzt) at Joseph's Academy, Vering founded the first institute
of surgeons and remained its director until 1813.[96]

When Beethoven first consulted Vering on 1 June 1801, Vering prescribed
tepid baths in the Danube, to which was added a bottle of strengthening ingredients. Though his diarrhea subsided with this treatment, his ears continued to
trouble him, and he began to feel weak. On 25 June, Vering, a Brunonian,
prescribed some pills for his stomach and an infusion for his ears.

Although he felt stronger after the pills, his ears continued to buzz day and
night. Vering then tried the painful blisters treatment, which resulted in an improvement of the tinnitus, but the deafness became worse.

A further exacerbation of abdominal symptoms improved for eight to ten days after tepid baths and one dose of stomach tonic, but Vering was opposed to shower baths. Beethoven, who felt Vering too casual for his liking, became dissatisfied with him and made enquiries about Dr. Schmidt.[97]

Beethoven later fell in love with Vering's daughter, Julie, who married Stephan von Breuning. Later Vering was appointed chief staff-surgeon of Lower Austria, while during the Napoleonic wars he was chief supervisor of the military hospitals.

Vering's son, Dr. Joseph Ritter Edler von Vering (1793–1862), was an otologist, dermatologist, psychiatrist, and writer. He was also Franz Schubert's physician. In 1821 his book *On the Treatment of Syphilis by the Effects of Mercury Application* was published in Vienna. In 1834 his book *Aphorismen über Ohrenkrankheiten* was published, but there was no mention in it of Beethoven's deafness, though he did state that diseases of the liver and gall bladder were often accompanied by hearing problems.[98]

LUDWIG VON TÜRKHEIM

Beethoven was also friendly with Baron Ludwig von Türkheim (1777–1846) who graduated in medicine in 1800, and who rose to become chancellor of the University of Vienna in 1816. Beethoven visited him in 1816 to ask a favor for his brother Johann.[99]

JOHANN NEPOMUK BIHLER

No doubt Beethoven would have discussed his health with his friend Bihler (or Biehler) for whom in 1817 he wrote letters of introduction to Xaver Schnyder von Wartensee and Hans Georg Nägeli. Though a trained physician, Bihler was employed as a tutor to the family of Archduke Karl.[100]

JOHANN ADAM SCHMIDT

An exceptional Swabian, born in Aub, near Würzburg, Johann Adam Schmidt (1759–1809) was the most talented of all of Beethoven's physicians and was his personal favorite. While initially Schmidt shared Brunonian principles in sympathy with the Franks and Vering, his wide reading and high intelligence enabled him to adapt his theories and practice of medicine to the newly evolving systems of Röschlaub's excitation theory, Schelling's natural philosophical speculations, and the vitalistic concepts of Romantic medicine.[101]

In 1788 Schmidt was appointed an associate professor of anatomy and surgery at Joseph's Academy, while from 1796 until his death Schmidt was a professor of general pathology, therapy, and *materia medica*. Indeed, his manuscript for a textbook of *materia medica* was published posthumously in 1811 in Vienna.[102]

However, Schmidt made his most important mark as the founder of ophthalmology, on which he gave from 1796 private lectures at Joseph's Academy. In

1789 he had been trained by Joseph Barth (1745–1818) in the art of cataract surgery, and he later wrote articles on the complications of such operations.[103] He also discovered new techniques for operating on the iris of the eye.[104] His pioneering studies into the pathology and treatment of diseases of the lachrymal gland culminated with the publication in 1803 of his authoritative textbook, which remained a standard reference for many years.[105]

The birth of medical specialization was witnessed in Vienna in 1812, when the first chair in ophthalmology was filled by Schmidt, who also established the first polyclinic for eye diseases.[106] He was also the first to clarify the nature of iritis.[107]

It is not surprising then that this talented, compassionate doctor, who had been personally recommended by his friend Wegeler, shared such a rewarding relationship with Beethoven, for there was also a musical affinity between them. It was presumably Schmidt who arranged for the faradism of his ears, but Beethoven could not tolerate it, and this treatment had to be abandoned.

Schmidt then wisely suggested the sparing of his hearing in a quiet country village for six months to give nature the opportunity to exert her own healing powers, which should never be underestimated. After despairing to the point of contemplating suicide, Beethoven resigned himself to his fate, as he expressed it in the *Heiligenstadt Testament*.

Although in that moving document Beethoven expressed his gratitude to Dr. Schmidt, he paid him the ultimate compliment in dedicating to his friend the Trio for Piano, Clarinet (or Violin), and Cello, Op. 38, a transcription of his very popular Opus 20 Septet. After remaining the exclusive property of Schmidt for a year, it was published in Vienna in January 1805.[108] Schmidt played the violin and his daughter the pianoforte, so what delightful music they could make when they shared with this gem.[109]

Schmidt treated Beethoven during the summer of 1807 for a dental abscess and headache, and probably also for the finger abscess and feverish attack he suffered in the spring of 1808. On 19 February 1809, Schmidt died unexpectedly in Vienna of a stroke.[110]

JOHANN MALFATTI VON MONTEREGGIO

Born in Lucca in Italy, Malfatti (1775–1859) studied medicine initially in Bologna with Aloysio Galvani and then with Johann Peter Frank in Pavia, following him to Vienna in 1795. After his graduation, Malfatti was appointed an assistant physician (*Sekundärarzt*) to Joseph Frank at the General Hospital.[111]

In 1800 Malfatti organized an ardent group of Brunonians into a Society of Physicians. The members at the hospital included the Franks, Johann Peter's assistant Thomas Cappellini, Carl Werner (the *Landschaftsprotomedicus*), and the recently appointed *primarius* Matthias von Sallaba. Several of the town physicians also joined this society. Members published an annual health guide and met in Malfatti's house. In 1802 Malfatti wrote an article, "On the Nursing Care of Disorders of the Organs of Hearing."[112] Stifft's ban on this society remained in force until after his death, when the society was reformed by Malfatti and Dr. Franz Wirer von Rettenbach.[113]

When the Franks quit Vienna in 1804, Malfatti resigned his post at the hospital and set up a private practice which soon became very successful. He was appointed physician to the Archduchess Beatrix von Este and the Archduke Carl, and during the Congress of Vienna he was in popular demand among various visiting diplomats.

Malfatti noted that certain diseases had a predilection for certain age groups; for example, rickets in childhood, tuberculosis (phthisis) in youth, and cancer in the elderly.[114]

He was also a friend of Ignaz Paul Vital Troxler (1780–1866), a follower of Schelling, and after the collapse of Brunonianism in Vienna, he changed over to the system of natural philosophy.[115] In his letter in September 1809 to Troxler, Beethoven sent his best wishes to Malfatti.[116]

In 1816 Malfatti treated patients suffering from paralysis and chronic hiccup with the mesmeric induction of magnetic sleep, modified to exclude a baquet.[117] His reputation was sullied when legal proceedings were taken against him for practicing magnetism.[118]

Following Dr. Schmidt's death in 1809, Dr. Malfatti remained Beethoven's physician until April 1817, when the composer changed his allegiance to Dr. Staudenheim. According to Thayer, Dr. Malfatti and Dr. Bertolini were too honorable to disclose the details of the breach.[119]

Even so, for many years, they had remained on cordial, friendly terms. Dr. Bertolini commissioned Beethoven to compose a small cantata to celebrate Malfatti's name day, on 24 June 1814, on the feast day of St. John. Beethoven set Clementi Bondi's text *Un lieto brindisi* for a soprano, two tenors, a bass, and a pianoforte, WoO 103.[120] During the party held at Malfatti's villa in Weinhaus, there was much feasting, drinking, and merriment, and the "thoroughly unbuttoned" Beethoven improvised brilliantly after the performance of the cantata.[121]

Malfatti made the following description of Beethoven: "He is a disorderly (*konfuser*) fellow—but all the same he may be the greatest genius."[122]

Beethoven retained some admiration for Malfatti's medical skills, for he asked his old friend to assist him during his final illness. Indeed Malfatti's cunning prescription of iced punch brought about a revival of the composer's spirits, albeit a temporary one.

In 1837 Malfatti was elevated to the nobility and took the title "von Montereggio."[123] In 1845 his book *Studies on the Anarchy and Hierarchy of Knowledge* was published in Leipzig.[124]

JOSEPH ANDREAS BERTOLINI

Malfatti's assistant Dr. Bertolini (1784–1861) was, during the years from 1806 to 1816, not only one of Beethoven's physicians, but also a close personal friend, in whom he was able to confide.

Convinced that his brother Caspar Carl had been poisoned, Beethoven persuaded Dr. Bertolini to perform an autopsy which affirmed death from tuberculosis.[125]

There was also a musical depth to their friendship, and during dinner with Bertolini at the Roman Emperor tavern in May 1814 Beethoven made sketches for the Overture to *Fidelio*. It was Dr. Bertolini who suggested the composition of a polonaise for pianoforte, Op. 89, and a small cantata, WoO 103.[126]

When Malfatti's patient, the music-loving Major-General Alexander Kyd heard Carl Czerny play, in several sessions, all the pianoforte works of Beethoven then in print, he was so impressed that he insisted Bertolini introduce him to the great composer. In September 1816 Kyd commissioned, through the person of Bertolini, a new symphony from Beethoven for 200 ducats, with the promise of additional lucrative profits from its performance by the London Philharmonic Society. However, when Kyd stipulated that the symphony was to be short and simple in the style of his earlier symphonies, Beethoven was insulted and withdrew. From that time he remained cool toward Bertolini, and later after a quarrel with Malfatti he broke with both of them.[127]

Beethoven also confided with Bertolini in writing. When in 1831 Bertolini contracted a severe bout of cholera, he burned all Beethoven's letters and notes, lest their highly confidential information should fall into careless hands.[128] Bertolini survived the cholera, and when he was interviewed by Otto Jahn in 1852 he passed on much valuable information, which was included in Thayer's biography.

JAKOB STAUDENHEIM

Born in Mainz, Staudenheim (1764–1830) studied chemistry in Paris with Antoine François Fourcroy, before continuing his studies at Augsburg and completing his medical degree with Maximilian Stoll in Vienna.[129] After curing Count Karl Harrach of a serious illness, he received the princely fee of 10,000 gulden, and he was appointed physician to Emperor Francis I. In 1826 he became personal physician to Napoléon's son, the duke of Reichstadt.[130]

In 1812 Dr. Staudenheim accompanied the imperial family to the Bohemian resorts, where he met Beethoven in Teplitz and advised him to take the waters at Carlsbad and Franzensbad. He was Beethoven's doctor from April 1817 until the spring of 1825, although the composer also consulted other physicians during these years.

Dr. Staudenheim remained an enthusiastic advocate of spa cures, and he sent Beethoven to take the baths at Heiligenstadt, Nussdorf, Mödling, Unterdöbling, Oberdöbling, and Baden. Though Beethoven liked the medicines and applications that he prescribed, he was loath to follow the doctor's advice regarding diet and restriction of alcohol. Staudenheim sternly reprimanded his patient whenever his instructions were not followed strictly.

In his letters of 15 February 1817 to Franz Brentano and Peter J. Simrock, Beethoven mentioned the lingering effects, since 15 October, of his feverish cold.[131] He was largely confined to his room and unable to attend one of Carl Czerny's Sunday musical soirees.[132]

In April he moved into new lodgings, near his nephew Carl's boarding school, on the second floor at no. 268 Glacis, in the Landstrasse district. Fed up with Dr. Malfatti and Dr. Bertolini, he again became a patient of Dr. Jakob Staudenheim (who he frequently miscalled Staudenheimer). The details were given in his letter of 19 June to the Countess Erdödy.

After feeling constantly unwell since 6 October 1816, I developed on 15 October a violent feverish cold, so that I had to stay in bed for a very long time; and only after several months was I allowed to go out even for a short while. Until now the after effects of this illness could not be dispelled. I changed my doctors, because my own doctor, a wily Italian, had powerful secondary motives where I was concerned and lacked both honesty and intelligence. That was in April, 1817. Well, from 15 April until 4 May I had to take six powders daily and six bowls of tea. That treatment lasted until 4 May. After that I had to take another kind of powder, also six times daily; and I had to rub myself three times a day with a volatile ointment. Then I had to come here [Heiligenstadt] where I am taking baths. Since yesterday I have been taking another medicine, namely, a tincture, of which I have to swallow 12 spoonfuls daily. . . . Although my health has improved a little, yet it will be a long time apparently before I am completely cured. . . . My hearing has become worse.[133]

Beethoven was a difficult patient who tended to modify the doctor's prescriptions according to his own inclinations and fancies. It would appear that he failed to follow strictly Dr. Staudenheim's advice, for he entered in his Tagebuch that on 2 May he took the powders and rubbed his chest.[134] Beethoven also consulted Christian Wilhelm Hufeland's medical treatise, which was in his library.[135] He decided that he should take the saltwater baths, like those at Wiesbaden, and then the warm sulphur baths like those at Aachen, and even the cold baths at Nenndorf.[136] However, Dr. Staudenheim directed him to the spas at Heiligenstadt and Nussdorf.

The advocates inclined to a diagnosis of syphilis have pounced on two documents relating to this period: first, the information that the volatile ointment contained a mercurial compound, and second, Beethoven's entry in his Tagebuch about sensual gratification.[137] It should be noted that Beethoven, in a letter of 7 July, informed Nanette Streicher: "I myself am inclined to distrust my present doctor who has finally pronounced my condition to be caused by a disease of the lungs."[138] It is therefore imperative that we carefully examine Dr. Staudenheim's treatments insofar as they might shed light on the diagnosis.

Powders, Tinctures, and a Volatile Ointment

Although Dr. Staudenheim's prescriptions are not extant, we do have access to the German pharmacopoeia of that period.[139] It is to be emphasized that the ingestion of powders and tinctures, as well as the application to the chest of a volatile ointment, was very much in vogue at that time for the treatment of chronic bronchial catarrh. The powders were made up from various species of datura mixed with nitrate of potash. The datura plants contained the alkaloid daturine, which consisted of varying quantities of atropine and hyoscyamine. Daturine was commonly prescribed not only in cases of bronchitis and asthma, but also for phthisis.[140]

Brunold Springer proposed that not only was Beethoven at this time treated with a mercury ointment for syphilis, but also that the treatment further damaged his hearing mechanism.[141] Yet the application of a lotion or volatile ointment, at that time, was invoked not only for the rheumatic complaints, but also for chronic afflictions of the chest. The volatile component of such applications consisted of ammonia, turpentine, camphor, eucalyptus, or some other volatile oils. Philipp Phoebus (1804–1880), a contemporary of Beethoven, noted that one such popular remedy consisted of the oil of poppy seeds in three parts to one part of *Liquor ammonii Caustici*.[142] It should also be mentioned that ammonia was introduced as an antisyphilitic remedy by Jacobus Vercellonus in 1722 and further, in 1774, Dr. B. Peyrilhe claimed that *Alkalis volatils* was of greater efficacy than mercury in the cure of luetic afflictions.[143] However such claims were invalid, and it was subsequently proved that ammonia was not an effective treatment for syphilis.

Since Dr. Staudenheim was aware that Beethoven's brother Carl Caspar had died of pulmonary tuberculosis in November 1815, no doubt he would have entertained the possibility of such a diagnosis in the composer during this illness. An old-fashioned remedy, popular in cases of phthisis, was the application of tartar emetic ointment, which was rubbed into the chest.[144]

Althaea Root

There is one other important clue. Beethoven made note of Althaea root in his Tagebuch.[145] The marshmallow root, *Radix althaea*, grows wild in temperate climates. Syrup of marshmallow was a popular cough suppressant in acute infections of the air passages, and it was often added to cough mixtures. *Radix althaea*, mixed with other emollient herbs, cumarin, and a volatile oil, was also applied to the skin as a volatile ointment.[146] Other powerful stimulants, used as counterirritants in chronic bronchitis, were *linimentum terebinthinae* and *linimentum camphorae compositum*.[147]

The Spa Logic

Why did Dr. Staudenheim direct Beethoven to take the baths at Heiligenstadt and Nussdorf? Even in the nineteenth century it was still erroneously believed that a primary gouty diathesis often gave rise to a diverse variety of secondary disorders, such as spasmodic asthma, bronchitis, hay fever, eczema, urticaria, and phlebitis. The patient was often therefore sent to a watering place for the alleviation of gout, in the hope that the secondary affliction (e.g., bronchitis) would clear up as a consequence.[148]

Tinctures

The tincture prescribed for Beethoven was most likely to have been *Tinctura lobeliae*, which was then a popular remedy for asthma and bronchitis. It may also have been a cough linctus such as a compound tincture of camphor, oxymel of squills, and syrup of tolu, or a bitter tonic containing an extract of quinine or *Aloës composita*, or even an opiate.[149] It was certainly not a tincture of iodine, since it was not until 1820 that a Swiss physician, Dr. Jean François Coindet, introduced iodine into medicine as a remedy for goiter. Iodine soon found widespread use as a treatment for syphilitic fevers, and especially for syphilitic, glandular, and rheumatic swellings. In about 1830, William Wallace of Dublin introduced potassium iodide into medicine.[150]

Nussdorf

Early in July, Beethoven moved from Heiligenstadt to Nussdorf, where he lodged in the still extant Greinerhaus at no. 26 Kahlenbergerstrasse. Apart from short visits to Vienna, he remained at Nussdorf until the middle of October. He was frustrated by his dependence on servants and the lack of nourishing food. He informed Nanette Streicher:

Much though I usually like solitude, yet at the moment it distresses me, the more so as with all the medicines and the baths I have to take it is hardly possible for me to occupy myself as I used to do. Furthermore, there is the distressing prospect that perhaps I may never be cured.[151]

Sassafrass

Beethoven again confided in Dr. Bihler, a physician, philologist, and musical enthusiast.[152] In his undated letter to Bihler he wrote, "Doctor Sassafrass, whom I told you of, is coming at noon today. So please turn up at my home too."[153] It is uncertain whether Beethoven is referring to a quack doctor, or alluding to Dr. Malfatti by way of one of his prescriptions. Sassafrass is the dried root of *Sassafrass officinale*, a plant of North America, which contains about 2 percent of ethereal oil, consisting of safrene and safrol, a liquid camphor. Sassafrass, with its strong aromatic, sweetish taste, had been used since 1560 as an antisyphilitic remedy.[154]

A Plaster on His Neck

In July Beethoven informed Nanette Streicher that "today I have had a fresh plaster put on the nape of my neck."[155] This might have been an application of

Emplastrum calefaciens, or a warm plaster, which induced a crop of pustules on the skin and was a popular remedy for the relief of chronic bronchitis or winter cough.[156] Or it may have been a vesicant such as a cantharides plaster. It was almost certainly not a mercurial plaster, which was then used to promote the cicatrization or absorption of syphilitic ulcers or tumors.[157]

In his letter of 25 August to Nanette Streicher he stated that he had become overheated and was ill again.[158] On 1 September he informed the Archduke Rudolph, "My ailing condition still persists; and although in some respects there is improvement, yet my complaint is still not absolutely cured. . . . Well, at last I must abandon the hope I so often cherished of making a complete recovery."[159]

Rheumatism

During the autumn of 1817 Beethoven suffered a frightful bout of rheumatism which confined him to his room for a day or two.[160] Dr. Staudenheim forbade him to be out of doors later than six in the evening.

On New Year's Day of 1818 he suffered pain so severe that he had to lie down on the couch.[161] Soon after he suffered another violent cold and cough.[162] Dr. Staudenheim sent him to take the baths at Mödling.

During the summer he was much better, apart from a short bout of indigestion, and he was able to complete the Opus 106 Sonata.

Beethoven retained a high regard for Dr. Staudenheim's abilities and requested a second opinion from him over Dr. Braunhofer's treatment. Staudenheim was recalled by Dr. Andreas Ignaz Wawruch for consultation prior to Beethoven's first abdominal paracentesis, and he also took part in the council of physicians, although he declined to take any fee for his services.[163]

CARL VON SMETANA

Although not a famous medical celebrity, Dr. Smetana (Smettana) (1774–1827) was a competent surgeon who had impressed Beethoven in 1816 when he performed a successful hernia operation on his nephew. In 1819 Beethoven's nephew Carl was attended at Mödling by Dr. Alois Hasenöhrl (1769–1846).[164]

Smetana had also gained a reputation in treating ailments of the ear. Following the embarrassment and shame of having publicly to quit the conducting of the revival of *Fidelio* in November 1822, Beethoven consulted Smetana about his deafness. Smetana prescribed a medicine to be taken by mouth. The prescription stated one teaspoon to be taken every hour, but Beethoven made a correction, as though it were a copyist's error on a musical score, and increased the dose to a tablespoon every hour. In the absence of dramatic benefit, Beethoven again consulted Father Weiss.[165]

Even so, when in April 1823 Beethoven was troubled with diarrhea and a burning irritation in his throat, he again consulted Dr. Smetana, who prescribed a strict diet, restriction of alcohol, and a spa cure, as recorded in a conversation-book.[166]

During the fourth week of April there were further entries by Dr. Smetana,[167] who inquired about Beethoven's digestion, appetite, and cough.[168] Dr. Smetana went on to recommend one of four bathing cures at Kalksburg,[169] Mödling, Baden, or Rodaun.[170]

A month later Beethoven again sought Dr. Smetana's assistance for his painful eye complaint. Finally, in July 1826, Beethoven requested his help following his nephew's attempted suicide, but the services of the surgeon Dr. Dögl, who had already been summoned, were retained.[171] Beethoven preferred Dr. Smetana to his brother Johann's physician, Dr. Joseph Saxinger, who married Therese van Beethoven's sister, Agnes.[172]

FATHER WEISS

Following the failure of Dr. Schmidt's treatment of faradism of the ear, it is stated in the *Fischhoff Manuscript* that Beethoven accompanied Nikolaus Paul Zmeskall on a visit to Father Weiss, who had gained an outstanding reputation for treating disorders of the ear at his rectory near St. Stephan's Cathedral. Father Weiss advised Beethoven to rest his ear as much as possible, and he instilled ear drops each day. In the absence of any dramatic benefit, Beethoven soon ceased attending and even refused Father Weiss's admission to his apartment.[173]

Even before Beethoven had completed Dr. Smetana's course of internal medicine in November 1822, the composer accompanied Schindler for a second course of treatment with Father Weiss. The priest hoped for some success in treating the deafness of the left ear by prescribing dietary precautions and ear drops, but Beethoven ceased attending after a few days.[174]

ANTON BRAUNHOFER

Beethoven's next physician, Dr. Braunhofer (1781–1846), was a professor of natural history and technology at the University of Vienna.[175] Despite his Viennese bluntness, there is no doubt that the patient-doctor relationship was warm and friendly because in 1820, after meeting Braunhofer, Beethoven dedicated a beautiful song to him. This setting of H. Goeble's text *Abendlied unterm gestirnten Himmel*, WoO 150, was published on 28 March 1820 in the *Wiener Zeitschrift für Kunst, Literatur, Theater und Mode*.[176]

It is fortunate that the conversation-book entries concerning Beethoven's serious illness during the spring of 1825 are extant. Beethoven sent his nephew several times to fetch Dr. Staudenheim, but he was not at home, and it would appear that he was not inclined to treat him. On 18 April Carl delivered the following note from his uncle to Dr. Anton Braunhofer at Bauernmarkt no. 588:

"My esteemed friend, I am not feeling well and I hope that you will not refuse to come to my help, for I am in great pain. If you can possibly visit me today, I do most earnestly beg you to come."[177]

Dr. Braunhofer came that day to visit Beethoven on the fourth floor at no. 969 Johannesgasse. The doctor took a medical history, examined Beethoven, and arrived at a diagnosis of intestinal inflammation. Dr. Braunhofer guaranteed him a complete recovery provided he would adhere to a strict diet without wine, coffee, or seasonings.

Beethoven could have chocolate for breakfast, cooked with milk or water, but without vanilla. He was to have soup for lunch, prepared with barley, but without any greens, especially not parsley, and without spices. If he had an appetite he could have soft boiled eggs, but nothing else.

Dr. Braunhofer insisted that Beethoven rest in bed, to be cared for by his brother Johann and his nephew Carl. Beethoven was also complaining of a thirst, and Dr. Braunhofer prescribed for this small doses of almond milk, made up by his brother, who was a pharmacist. Dr. Braunhofer stressed the importance of the strict diet and said that not much in the way of medicines would be needed. If tolerated, warm compresses were to be applied to the abdomen, and he was to continue using the *Goldene Ader* hemorrhoidal ointment.[178]

When his condition improved, the diet would be liberalized, a little alcohol would be permitted, and walks could be resumed as well as outings in Johann's carriage.

Beethoven, however, was unhappy about the lack of prescribed medicines, and he sent Carl to obtain Dr. Staudenheim's opinion. Dr. Braunhofer had promised to obtain a second medical opinion if his patient's progress proved unsatisfactory. Johann reassured his brother that the treatment was working, since there was an improvement in his stomach upset and diarrhea. Beethoven was encouraged to work and read during the day so that he would be more inclined to sleep at night. The warm abdominal compresses were not well tolerated.

At his next visit Dr. Braunhofer urged Beethoven to be more patient, and he again emphasized the superiority of a regular diet over taking medication. He also pointed out that it was not necessary to have a bowel movement every day.[179]

At his next visit, Beethoven, very much improved and no longer insistent on a second opinion, was reassured by Dr. Braunhofer.[180] A little later, Dr. Braunhofer lectured his patient about the scientific theory of his treatment:

Col tempo—no fever, no weakness—You can achieve complete strength only through an appropriate natural diet, and not through the so-called strengthening remedies. You feel weak because you are not quite well as yet. The ideas about strengthening exist only in the imagination of ignorant doctors who have no conception about life's energies. With their erroneous conceptions of treatment, e.g., blood letting, they weaken and completely ruin [the patient] with quinine, spirits and strengthening remedies. You need not drink warm water any more.[181]

When Beethoven, who was very keen to take strengthening and stimulating remedies, asked that Dr. Staudenheim's opinion be sought, he was reminded that he also had restricted his consumption of wine. Dr. Braunhofer advised Beethoven to work only during the day so that he could sleep better at night. He warned him that he was on the verge of an inflammation of his bowels, and that if he took alcohol, he would feel faint and weak within a few hours. Dr. Braunhofer wrote, "You would be Brown the Second if you had studied medicine [John Brown]. My studies have been based on his writings, and therefore I am a quasi-pupil of his."[182]

At his next visit Dr. Braunhofer permitted a little meat to be added to the soup, if he had an appetite for it. The almond milk seemed to be weakening him too much, and he should therefore drink only fresh water. There was no fever, but just a flutter in the head which causes heaviness, dizziness, and restless sleep.[183] Dr. Braunhofer prescribed a powder to be taken on a wafer to reduce the flutter. He also advised him to take a short walk the next day.[184]

During a subsequent visit Dr. Braunhofer advised Beethoven to restrict his baths to once or twice a week, until the tension in his belly had given way and his urine was no longer discolored.[185] It should be noted that the nephew Carl made mention of dark urine.[186]

Ludwig Rellstab, who visited Beethoven during the spring of 1825, described his complexion as "Brownish, yet not the strong, healthy tan which the huntsman acquires, but rather one transposed into a sickly, yellowish tone."[187]

His brother Johann wanted Beethoven to come to Gneixendorf for the summer, but the composer had again secured rooms in Baden at Schloss Gutenbrunn. On 6 May Johann wrote to Ferdinand Ries (living since 1824 in Godesberg, near Bonn), "He will write to you when he feels better. Unfortunately he suffered from an inflammation of the bowels, from which he is now saved, but his weakness is still very great, and he is unable to undertake anything."[188]

Dr. Braunhofer was in favor of Beethoven's going to the country, where he assured him he would be able to digest fresh milk.[189] Braunhofer also requested a small composition from his patient.[190]

On 7 May Beethoven went again to Baden, where each warm sulphur bath cost 1 fl.40 kr., so that the cost of the recommended course of thirty baths was twenty florins.[191] There is further information about his health in two letters written on 13 May. He informed Ferdinand Piringer, "The effects of the intestinal inflammation from which I have been suffering are very severe, for I feel so weak that as yet I can hardly walk properly, still less do any work."[192] The other letter, to Dr. Braunhofer, was written as an amusing dialogue between the doctor and his patient:

Esteemed Friend!
D[octor]: How are you, my patient?
Pat[ient]: We are rather poorly—we still feel very weak and are belching and so forth. I am inclined to think that I now require a stronger medicine, but it must not be consti-

pating—Surely I might be allowed to take white wine diluted with water, for that poisonous beer is bound to make me feel sick—my catarrhal condition is showing the following symptoms, that is to say, I spit a good deal of blood, but probably only from my windpipe. But I have frequent nose bleedings, which I often had last winter as well. And there is no doubt that my stomach has become dreadfully weak, and so has, generally speaking, my whole constitution. Judging by what I know of my own constitution, my strength will hardly be restored unaided.

On the third page of this letter, Beethoven wrote a four-part canon for Dr. Braunhofer: "Doktor, sperrt das Tor dem Tod," WoO 189[193] (Close the door 'gainst Death I plead, Doctor, notes will help in need).[194]

In this canon, Beethoven punned mischievously on the German words: *Noten* (notes) and *Nöten* (needs). It should also be noted that he concluded that he was spitting blood from his windpipe (haemoptysis) rather than his stomach (haematemesis), and it would appear most likely that this blood was emanating from his nose bleeds.

On 18 May he informed his nephew,

Tomorrow no doubt I shall have to drink coffee. Who knows, perhaps it may be better for me than chocolate. For the prescriptions of that B[raunhofer] have been a failure before now. And on the whole he strikes me as very narrow-minded and, therefore, a bit of a fool. He must have known about the asparagus—After the meal at the inn I am suffering a good deal today from diarrhoea.[195]

Beethoven was also losing weight: "I am getting thinner and thinner and feel more ailing than well and I have no doctor, not even a sympathetic soul at hand."[196]

He was soon feeling better and went on to compose the third movement of the String Quartet in A minor, Op. 132, which he called "Thanksgiving Offered to the Almighty by a Convalescent." In the letter of 9 June to his nephew, after referring to his weakness and faintness, he went on to write, "In any case Death with his scythe will not spare me very much longer."[197] At that point Beethoven had less than two years to live.

On 4 June he left another canon at Dr. Braunhofer's home when he found the doctor out: "Ich war hier, Doktor," WoO 190.[198]

On about 12 July Beethoven again consulted Dr. Braunhofer, who informed him that the sulphur baths were not agreeing with him because they excited him too much. The doctor again emphasized the importance of restricting spices in his food and drink. With regard to alcohol, Beethoven could consume only a small amount of wine diluted with water, but no spirits. Dr. Braunhofer advised him that he would send him to another doctor for his hearing at a later date.[199]

In Baden on fine days Beethoven usually took long walks, but one day in August he informed his new factotum, Carl Holz, "Since yesterday I have had a fresh and rather violent attack of my abdominal trouble."[200] Further details were written in his letter of 24 August to his nephew:

My stomach is in a very bad state and I have no doctor. . . . Since yesterday I have eaten nothing but soup and a couple of eggs and have drunk only water; my tongue is quite yellow; and without bowel motions and tonics my stomach will never, whatever the Cornö etc. Doktor[201] may say, never be cured.[202]

Two days later he asked Tobias Haslinger, "For more particulars about the *Mariabrunner* wine, for I must not drink red wine only, but white wine with water as well."[203]

In his letter from Baden on 4 October, Beethoven informed Carl,

I am hoping too to shake off my cold and catarrh while I am still here. But on the whole it is not very safe for me to be at Baden now with this catarrh. The winds, or rather, the hurricanes still persist. . . . Remember that I am stuck here and may easily fall ill.[204]

On the evening of Saturday 15 October, Beethoven moved into what was to be his last apartment in the Schwarzspanierhaus. Nearby, in the Rothes Haus, lived Stephan von Breuning and his family, who renewed their friendship with the composer. Madame von Breuning saw to the fitting out of his kitchen and supervised the engagement of his servants. She made mention of his distasteful habit of expectorating in the room, his shabby dress, his loud raucous voice, his ringing laugh, and his eccentric ways, which made her feel ashamed out on the street when people stopped, stared, and took him for a madman.[205]

ANDREAS IGNAZ WAWRUCH

Beethoven's last physician was born on 22 November 1773 in the Czech village of Niemczicz, a small town in the district of Prosnitz, about 35 kilometers south of Olmütz.[206] After matriculating he studied philosophy and theology at the University of Olmütz, before transferring to the University of Prague to study medicine.

In 1810 he became an assistant to Professor Johann Valentin Edler von Hildenbrand (1763–1818) in Vienna. The following year he gave lectures in Latin in the auditorium of the General Hospital on the history and literature of medicine.

After taking his doctorate of medicine in 1812, he was appointed full professor of pathology and pharmacology in Prague, a post he retained for seven years. His most famous pupil, Johann Evangelista Purkinje (1787–1869) after further studies in Berlin, became an eminent physiologist and histologist, rising to professor of physiology at Breslau and Prague.

In 1819 Wawruch was appointed director of the medical clinic in Vienna, while also serving as a professor of special pathology and therapy of internal medicine. In this post, which he retained till his death on 21 March 1842, Wawruch provided elementary training in internal medicine to rural surgeons and lower civilian surgeons in their second year of studies.[207]

Wawruch was a member of the Imperial & Royal Medical Society and a contributor to the journal *Medical Yearbooks of the I.R. Eastern Imperial State*.[208] During 1832 and 1833 he published five articles on East Indian cholera; in the same journal in 1841, he reviewed 206 cases of tapeworm infestation. These articles formed the basis of his monograph that was published in 1844.[209]

The unwarranted criticisms of Schindler and Gerhard von Breuning of Dr. Wawruch's treatment of Beethoven during his final illness will be discussed later. In the files of the Vienna State Archives, on 20 November 1827, it was stated that Dr. Wawruch received and acknowledged his fee of 250 florins, C.M., for his services to Beethoven during his last illness.[210]

On 20 May 1827 Wawruch wrote a manuscript, "Medical Review of L. van Beethoven's Last Days," which was unpublished at the time of his death. Wawruch was also an enthusiastic musician and very good cellist, so that when years later Aloys Fuchs called on his widow to search through his musical papers, Frau Wawruch offered him the manuscript for sale. Fuch's friend, Witthauer, paid the widow a considerable sum for its publication, on 30 April 1842, in the *Wiener Zeitschrift*. It was soon reprinted in other German and French papers.

JOHANN SEIBERT

The chief surgeon at the Vienna General Hospital, Dr. Johann Seibert (1782–1846), performed four abdominal paracentesis operations on 20 December 1826 and 8 January, 3 February, and 27 February 1827.

On 28 April 1827 Seibert submitted his bill for surgical services, home visits, and frequent medical consultations for the late Ludwig van Beethoven, during his last illness, between 20 December 1826 and 26 March 1827:

Four operations of paracentesis abdominis, including dressings and treatment
15 florins C.M. $\times$ 4 = 60 fl.C.M.
90 visits, frequently connected with medical consultations
1 fl. 30 kreuzer $\times$ 90 = 135 fl.C.M.
Total   195 fl.C.M.

The town council questioned the charges for ninety visits, and Schindler was asked for his opinion. He declared that the charge for the four operations was fair enough, but that several of the visits were very brief, involving only the exchange of a few words with the nurse or maid. Schindler suggested that only sixty visits, or at most sixty-five, were justifiably chargeable. The final outcome of the dispute was not recorded.[211]

JOHANN JOSEPH WAGNER

A native of Braunau in Bohemia, Dr. Wagner (1800–1834) became very proficient as a master of the art of dissection, following his appointment as assistant pathologist in Vienna. He passed on his skills to his now famous student-apprentice Carl Rokitansky.

In the wake of his declining health from 1825, Lorenz Biermayer delegated his duties to his young assistant, Wagner, who gained a wealth of experience in the performance of some 600 autopsies a year at the General Hospital, as well as forensic postmortem examinations. Wagner, a fast operator, could, for example, dissect the spinal canal from the second cervical vertebra in the neck to the sacrum in seven minutes.

Dr. Wagner wrote journal articles on rabies and intestinal ileus following internal perforation.[212] Yet, in his autobiography, Rokitansky wrote, "Not withstanding the daily contradictions between the results of dissection and the records on disease and diagnosis, [Wagner] was not able to grasp the lesson beyond casuistics or to form a clear idea of the reforming impact his subject was destined to make."[213]

No doubt Dr. Wagner's failure to issue a subsequent report on Beethoven's temporal bones was due not only to a lack of specialist knowledge in otology at that time, but also to his heavy workload and his own early demise with pulmonary tuberculosis.

On 29 April 1827 Dr. Wagner lodged his bill with the town council for the service of having performed Beethoven's postmortem examination. His claim of 20 florins C.M. plus 4 percent accrued interest is preserved in the files of the Vienna State Archives.[214]

NOTES

1. TDR, I, 502; L. Schiedermair, *Der junge Beethoven* (Leipzig: Quelle and Meyer, 1925), 233; T. Albrecht, ed., *Letters to Beethoven and Other Correspondence*, 3 vols. (Lincoln: University of Nebraska Press, 1996), no. 13.

2. Dr. Brenio Onetto-Bächler, "Letter to the editor," BN 7 (1992): 87–88. Dr. Johann Nikolaus Rovantini, a brother of Maria Magdalena Rovantini, was a medical practitioner in Würzburg. See B-Register, 7:249.

3. Hippocrates, 460–375 B.C.

4. Herman Boerhaave, 1668–1738.

5. Maximilian Stoll, 1742–1788.

6. In 1533 Pietro A. Mattioli (1500–1577) considered that mercury was a specific treatment for syphilis. In 1552 Thierry de Héry (1500?–1599) advocated mercury inunctions and internal guaic for luetic infection. See F. H. Garrison and L. T. Morton, *A Medical Bibliography*, ed. Leslie T. Morton (Aldershot, England: Gower, 1983), 4:2366, 2368.

7. Scurvy was described in 1250 by Jean de Joinville. In 1564 Spanish sailors cured themselves of scurvy by eating oranges and lemons. Garrison and Morton, *A Medical Bibliography*, 3710.

8. E. Lesky, *The Vienna Medical School of the Nineteenth Century* (Baltimore: Johns Hopkins University Press, 1976), 30, 80.

9. Michael G. Foster, *Baths and Medicinal Waters of Britain and Europe* (Bristol, England: John Wright, 1933), 87–88.

10. For a discussion of the waters and spas see also J. M. Gully, *The Water Cure in Chronic Disease* (London: John Churchill, 1851); T. Linn, *The Health Resorts of Europe, A Medical Guide to the Mineral Springs, Climatic, Mountain, and Seaside Health Resorts, Milk, Whey, Grape, Earth, Mud, Sand, and Air Cures of Europe* (New York: D. Appleton, 1893); C. E. Jones, "An Essay on the External Use of Water, by Tobias Smollett," *Bulletin of the History of Medicine* 3 (1935): 31–82; J. Wechsberg, *The Lost World of the Great Spas* (London: Weidenfeld and Nicolson, 1979); N. G. Coley, "Cures without Care: Chymical Physicians and Mineral Waters in Seventeenth-century English Medicine," *Medical History* 23 (1979): 191–214; R. Price, "Hydropathy in England, 1840–70," *Medical History* 25 (1981): 269–80; P. Hembry, *The English Spa 1560–1815: A Social History,* (London: Athlone Press, 1990); R. Porter, ed., *The Medical History of Waters and Spas* (London: Wellcome Institute for the History of Medicine, 1990); G. Weisz, "Water Cures and Science: The French Academy of Medicine and Mineral Waters in the Nineteenth Century," *Bulletin of the History of Medicine* 64 (1990): 393–416. In 1969 an exhibition of books on "Taking the Waters" was held at the Wellcome Institute of the History of Medicine in London, and I am grateful to Robin Price for the details.

11. Peter J. Davies, "Alexander Porfir'yevich Borodin (1833–1887): Composer, Chemist, Physician, and Social Reformer," *Journal of Medical Biography* 3 (1995): 207–17.

12. W. Winternitz, *Hydrotherapie auf physiologischer und klinischer Grundlage,* (Vienna: Urban und Schwarzenberg, 1877). For some years, Winternitz edited the periodical *Blätter für klinische Hydrotherapie.* See also R. F. Fox, *The Principles and Practice of Medical Hydrology* (London: University of London Press, 1913).

13. For a list of the arrivals see TF, 532.

14. Foster, *Baths and Medicinal Waters,* 130–131.

15. F. T. Frerichs, *A Clinical Treatise on Diseases of the Liver* (London: The New Sydenham Society, 1860) I:124–25; Foster, *Baths and Medicinal Waters,* 28–35, 183–84.

16. T. Lauder Brunton, *Lectures on the Action of Medicines* (London: Macmillan, 1897), 474.

17. Foster, *Baths and Medicinal Waters,* 184.

18. Ibid., 100–103, 184.

19. Ibid., 152.

20. Ibid., 103–4.

21. Gully, *Water Cure,* 220–24.

22. Lesky, *Vienna Medical School,* 1–2.

23. F. Wegeler and F. Ries, *Remembering Beethoven: The Biographical Notes of Franz Wegeler and Ferdinand Ries,* trans. F. Bauman and Tim Clark (London: A. Deutsch, 1987), 148. For a detailed study of the relation in Germany between philosophy and medicine, see Guenter B. Risse, "Kant, Schelling and the Early Search for a Philosophical Science of Medicine in Germany," *Journal of the History of Medicine* 27 (1972): 145–58; and "Philosophical Medicine in Nineteenth-Century Germany: An Episode in the Relation between Philosophy and Medicine," *Journal of Medicine and Philosophy* 1(1976): 72–91.

24. FRHB, I: 230; M. Zenger and O. E. Deutsch, *Mozart and His World in Contemporary Pictures* (Kassel: Bärenreiter, 1961), 354, no. 494; Gerhard von Breuning, *Memories of Beethoven,* ed. M. Solomon, trans. H. Mins and M. Solomon (Cambridge: Cambridge University Press, 1992), 34, 124, n. 31.

25. A-1371; B-1967.

26. Helmut Wyklicky, "Ergänzungen zur Kenntnis des Wiener Klinikers Maximilian Stoll," *Wiener klinische Wöchenschrift* 69 (1957): 507–9, which includes a survey of the literature on Stoll. The article was reprinted by Professor Doctor L. Schönbauer, director of the Institute of History of Medicine of the University of Vienna (University of Vienna, 1957), 1–6.

27. Prince Wenzel Kaunitz-Rietberg (1711–1794) was reich-chancellor in Vienna, having served as Austrian ambassador in Paris from 1750 to 1753.

28. Wyklicky, "Ergänzungen," 508, trans. Erna Schwerin.

29. A-227; B-391.

30. KHV, 608–10; M. Solomon, *Beethoven* (London: Cassell, 1978), 175; B. Cooper, ed., *The Beethoven Compendium* (London: Thames and Hudson, 1991), 266.

31. A-293; B-522 (Autumn 1811).

32. Wyklicky, "Ergänzungen," 508.

33. Ibid., 509, trans. Erna Schwerin.

34. Erich Ebstein, "Ein vergessenes Gedicht Blumauers an Stoll," *Janus* 75 (1907): 509–10. I am grateful to the Wellcome Institute for the History of Medicine in London for sending me the articles written by Wyklicky and Ebstein.

35. J. Pezzl, *Denkmal auf Maximilian Stoll* (Vienna: A. Blumauer, 1788).

36. M. Stoll, *Rationis medendi in Nosocomio practico Vindobonensi*, 7 parts (Vienna, 1777–1790). A German translation by G. L. Fabri was published in Breslau in 1791.

37. Even his son, William Cullen Brown, was uncertain of the precise date or place. For biographies of Brown, see John Brown, *The Elements of Medicine*, translated from the Latin with comments by the author, new ed. with biographical preface by Thomas Beddoes 2 vol. (London, J. Johnson, 1795), I: xxv–clxviii; W. C. Brown, *The Works of Dr John Brown*, 3 vols. (London: J. Johnson, 1804); Benjamin Ward Richardson, "John Brown, M.D., and the Brunonian System," in *Disciples of Aesculapius*, 2 vols. (London: Hutchinson, 1900), I: 245–61; Guenter Bernhard Risse, "The History of John Brown's Medical System in Germany during the Years 1790–1806" (Ph.D. diss., University of Chicago, 1971), 69–101. See also W. F. Bynum and Roy Porter, eds., *Brunonianism in Britain and Europe* (London: Wellcome Institute for the History of Medicine, 1988), 1–104.

38. Richardson, "John Brown," 246–49.

39. Risse, "History of John Brown's Medical System," 69–93. See also Christopher Lawrence, "Cullen, Brown and the Poverty of Essentialism," in *Brunonianism in Britain and Europe*, ed. W. F. Bynum and Roy Porter (London: Wellcome Institute for the History of Medicine, 1988), 1–21.

40. Richardson, "John Brown," 258–60.

41. Risse, "History of John Brown's Medical System," 101–11.

42. W. C. Brown, *Works of John Brown*, II: 136–38.

43. Richardson, "John Brown," 252–53.

44. W. C. Brown, *Works of John Brown*, II: 138–46.

45. Ibid., II: 153–55.

46. For an overview of Brunonian therapeutics, see G. B. Risse, "Brunonian Therapeutics: New Wine in Old Bottles?" in *Brunonianism in Britain and Europe*, ed. W. F. Bynum and Roy Porter (London: Wellcome Institute for the History of Medicine, 1988), 46–62; "The Brownian System of Medicine: Its Theoretical and Practical Implications," *Clio Medica* 5 (1970): 45–51.

47. W. C. Brown, *Works of John Brown*, II: 260–85.

48. Ibid., 286–310.

49. Ibid., III: 6–15.

50. For a discussion of Brunonianism in Vienna, see Lesky, *Vienna Medical School*, 8–12.

51. For a discussion of the rise and fall of Brunonianism in Germany, see Risse, "History of John Brown's Medical System," 136–350. See also Nelly Tsouyopoulos, "The Influence of John Brown's Ideas in Germany," in *Brunonianism in Britain and Europe*, W. F. Bynum and Roy Porter (London: Welcome Institute for the History of Medicine, 1988), 63–74. See also G. B. Risse, "Schelling, 'Naturphilosophie,' and John Brown's System of Medicine," *Bulletin of the History of Medicine* 50 (1976): 321–24.

52. George Rosen, "Biography of Dr. Johann Peter Frank: Written by Himself," in two parts, *Journal of the History of Medicine* 3 (1948): 11–46; 279–314; see p. 36. This is a translation of Frank's autobiography, which deals with his activities up to 24 December 1801, when he was fifty-seven years old. It was published in Vienna in 1802 by Karl Schaumburg & Co.

53. R. Jones, *An Inquiry into the State of Medicine on the Principles of Inductive Philosophy* (Edinburgh: Longman, Cadell and Elliot, 1781).

54. Ramunas Kondratas, "The Brunonian Influence on the Medical Thought and Practice of Joseph Frank," in *Brunonianism in Britain and Europe*, ed. W. F. Bynum and Roy Porter (London: Wellcome Institute for the History of Medicine, 1988), 75–88.

55. Risse, "Brunonian Therapeutics," 56.

56. Ibid., 57–59.

57. Rosen, "Biography of Dr. Johann Peter Frank," 304.

58. Kondratas, "Brunonian Influence," 81.

59. Ibid., 82.

60. J. Frank, *Ratio instituti clinici Ticinensis a mense Januario usque ad finem Junii 1795*, with a preface by J. P. Frank (Vienna: Camesina, 1797); *Heilart in der klischen Lehranstalt zu Pavia*, trans. by F. Schaeffer (Vienna: Camesina, 1797).

61. Gernot Rath, "Alexander von Humboldt and Brunonianism," *Journal of the History of Medicine and Allied Sciences* 15 (1960): 75–76.

62. FRHB, I: 163.

63. TF, 233.

64. A. C. Kalischer, *The Letters of Ludwig van Beethoven*, trans. J. S. Shedlock, 2 vols. (London: J. M. Dent, 1909), no. xxx.

65. A-24; B-34 (20 August 1798)

66. Kondratas, "Brunonian Influence," 82–85.

67. Tsouyopoulos, "Brunonianism," 67–73.

68. While Vilnius is now in Lithuania, it was then part of the Russian Empire. His experiences at the medical clinic in Vilnius were published in three volumes in Leipzig, 1808–1812. In 1814 Joseph Frank also wrote an interesting discourse on the effects of the French Revolution on medical practice. Frank's treatise, *Praxeos med.universae praecepta*," 1821, was published in two volumes. He considered otalgia and tinnitus to be independent disease entities, and he classified inflammations into "traumatic, catarrhal, metastatic, consensual, arthritic, scrofulous, and venereal, emphasizing that each type requires specialized treatment." See Adam Politzer, *History of Otology*, 2 vols. (Phoenix, Ariz.: Columella Press, 1981), I: 288.

69. Ludwig Nohl, ed., *Beethoven Depicted by His Contemporaries*, trans. E. Hill (London: W. Reeves, 1876), 144.

70. See Owsei Temkin, "Gall and the Phrenological Movement," *Bulletin of the History of Medicine* 21 (1947): 275–321; Lesky, *Vienna Medical School*, 4–8. See also E. Lesky, "Structure and Function in Gall," *Bulletin of the History of Medicine* 44 (1970): 293–314.

71. Lesky, *Vienna Medical School*, 5.

72. Temkin, "Gall," 275.

73. Ibid., 284.

74. Ibid., 281.

75. Lesky, *Vienna Medical School*, 7.

76. *Bonon. Sci. Art. Inst. Acad. Comment.* (Bologna) 7 (1791): 363–418. This appeared as a monograph in Modena in 1792. See Garrison and Morton, *Medical Bibliography*, no. 593, p. 77.

77. The ear-rheophore, designed by M. Charrière, consisted of a wire coated with ivory.

78. G. V. Poore, ed., *Selections from the Clinical Works of Dr. Duchenne (de Boulogne)* (London: The New Sydenham Society, 1883), 370.

79. Ibid., 371–77.

80. Lesky, *Vienna Medical School*, 80.

81. For an English translation of the sixth edition, the manuscript of which was completed the year before his death in 1842, see Samuel Hahnemann, *Organon of Medicine*, trans. J. Künzli, A. Naudé, and Peter Pendleton (London: Victor Gollancz 1986), 1–214. The work is subdivided into 291 suppositions.

82. Lesky, *Vienna Medical School*, 31–32.

83. Rosen, "Biography of Dr. Johann Peter Frank," 16. The most complete account of the lives of Johann Peter Frank and his son Joseph Frank is contained in their unpublished memoirs: *Mémoires biographiques de Jean Pierre Frank, et de Joseph Frank, son fils, redigés par ce dernier, MS*, University of Vilnius Library, Lithuania, 5 vols. (Leipzig, 1848).

84. Rosen, "Biography of Dr. Johann Peter Frank," 24–26.

85. Ibid., 36–44: I (1799), II (1780), III (1783). For a discussion, see Leona Baumgartner and Elizabeth Mapelsden Ramsey, "Johann Peter Frank and His *System einer vollständigen medicinischen Polizey*," in 2 parts, *Annals Med. Hist.* 5 (1933): 525–32; 6 (1934): 69–90.

86. Rosen, "Biography of Dr. Johann Peter Frank," 279–80. The University of Göttingen was founded in 1737 by George II of England.

87. J. P. Frank, "The Civil Administrator—Most Successful Physician," trans. from the Latin, with an introduction by Jean Captain Sabine, *Bull. Hist. Med.* 16 (1944): 289–318.

88. Rosen, "Biography of Dr. Johann Peter Frank," 280–84.

89. Ibid., 285–8. On 14 January 1786 Frank had been appointed director of the hospital at Pavia, where he received an annual increase in salary of 100 ducats.

90. J. P. Frank, "The People's Misery: Mother of Diseases," trans. from the Latin, with an introduction by Henry E. Sigerist, *Bull. Hist. Med.* 9 (1941): 81–100.

91. A-51; B-65.

92. A-51, 59, n. 2; B-65, n. 3; TF, 283, n. 14; Wegeler and Ries, *Remembering Beethoven*, 38, n. 7; W. Schweisheimer, "Beethoven's Physicians," *Musical Quarterly* 30 (1944): 289–98, cited from 291; P. Nettl, "Beethoven and the Medical Profession,"

Ciba Symposium 14 (1966): 96; H. Bankl and H. Jesserer, *Die Krankheiten Ludwig van Beethovens* (Vienna: W. Maudrich, 1987), 135–36.

93. LvBCB, I: 236, 17 v; 473, n. 540; D. W. MacArdle, *An Index to Beethoven's Conversation Books* (Detroit: Information Service, 1962), 12.

94. Rosen, "Biography of Dr. Johann Peter Frank, 12.

95. Nettl, "Beethoven and the Medical Profession," 97; A. Neumayr, "Notes on the Life, Works, and Medical History of Ludwig van Beethoven," trans. B. C. Clarke (Bloomington, Ind.: Medi-Ed Press, 1994), 338.

96. Lesky, *Vienna Medical School*, 44.

97. A-54; B-70.

98. FRHB, II: 366–67; Politzer, *History of Otology*, I: 288; O. E. Deutsch, *Schubert: A Documentary Biography* (London: J. M. Dent, 1946), 961.

99. A-700; B-816 (Summer 1815). See also FRHB, II: 341–43.

100. A-803, 804; B-1159, 1160; Albrecht, *Letters*, nos. 344, 395.

101. Lesky, *Vienna Medical School*, 62–3.

102. Ibid., 84.

103. Ibid., 62. Schmidt also wrote on purulent conjunctivitis of the newborn.

104. Ibid., 64. The operations of iridotomy, iridectomy, and iridodialysis.

105. *Über die Krankheiten des Thränenorgans*, Vienna, 1803.

106. Lesky, *Vienna Medical School*, 59.

107. Ibid., 65.

108. KHV, 94–95.

109. TF, 266.

110. Nettl, "Beethoven and the Medical Profession," 99; Lesky, *Vienna Medical School*, 59. The incorrect year of death in 1808 was given in FRHB, II: 135; Schweisheimer, "Beethoven's Physicians," 291; KHV, 95; and TF, 460.

111. For accounts of Dr. Malfatti, see FRBH, I: 384–86; Nettl, "Beethoven and the Medical Profession," 99–100; Bankl and Jesserer, *Die Krankheiten*, 136; Neumayr, "Notes," 340–41.

112. It was published in *Gesundheits-Taschenbuch für das Jahr 1802* (Vienna, 1802). See Politzer, *History of Otology*, I: 289.

113. Lesky, *Vienna Medical School*, 10–11, 33.

114. Ibid., 38–39.

115. Ibid., 79.

116. A-225; B-399.

117. Lesky, *Vienna Medical School*, 31.

118. For a brief account of Franz Anton Mesmer (1734–1815) and mesmerism, see P. J. Davies, *Mozart in Person: His Character and Health* (Westport, Conn.: Greenwood Press, 1989), 34–37.

119. TF, 648.

120. KHV, 565–66.

121. TF, 583.

122. TF, 460.

123. Nettl, "Beethoven and the Medical Profession," 99.

124. Lesky, *Vienna Medical School*, 85.

125. TDR, III: 519.

126. TDR, III: 428, 486.

127. TF, 648.

128. TDR, II: 554.

129. FRHB, II: 250–51.

130. P. Nettl, *Beethoven Encyclopedia* (London: P. Owens, 1957), 246; "Beethoven and the Medical Profession," 100.

131. A-758, 759; B-1083, 1084.

132. A-764; B-1093.

133. A-783; B-1132.

134. *Tagebuch*-130.

135. C. W. Hufeland, *Praktische Vebersicht der Vorzüglichsten Heilquellen Deutschlands* (Berlin, 1815).

136. *Tagebuch*-121.

137. *Tagebuch*-122.

138. A-785; B-1137.

139. The *Lectures on Pharmacology* by Dr C. Binz, the director of the Pharmacological Institute in the University of Bonn, is invaluable in this regard (London: New Sydenham Society, 1897). See also the books listed in the Bibliography by T. Lauder Brunton, Michael G. Foster, James M. Gully, and Edward John Waring.

140. C. Binz, *Lectures on Pharmacology for Practitioners and Students*, trans. from the second German ed. by Arthur C. Latham, 2 vols. (London: New Sydenham Society, 1895, 1897), I: 224–25; Brunton, *Lectures on the Action of Medicines*, 291–92.

141. Brunold Springer, *Die genialen Syphilitiker* (Berlin: Verlag der Neuen Generation, 1926), 21, 100, 105–6; W. Forster, *Beethovens Krankheiten und ihre Beurteilung* (Wiesbaden, Germany: Breitkopf and Härtel, 1956), 46.

142. Philipp Phoebus, *Spezielle ärztliche Rezeptierkunst* (Berlin, 1831), 239. Cited in Forster, *Beethovens Krankheiten*, 47, 67.

143. E. J. Waring, *Bibliotheca Therapeutica or Bibliography of Therapeutics, Chiefly in Reference to Articles of the Materia Medica* 2 vols. (London: New Sydenham Society, 1878), I: 222.

144. Brunton, *Lectures on the Action of Medicines*, 289.

145. *Tagebuch*-128.

146. Binz, *Lectures on Pharmacology*, II: 383–84.

147. Brunton, *Lectures on the Action of Medicines*, 288–89.

148. Ibid., 291; Foster, *Baths and Medicinal Waters*, 10–11.

149. Binz, *Lectures on Pharmacology*, II, 438; Brunton, *Lectures on the Action of Medicines*, 266.

150. Binz, *Lectures on Pharmacology*, I, 165, 182.

151. A-785; B-1137.

152. Dr. J. Bihler was tutor to the son of the wealthy banker, Baron Johann Baptist von Puthon. Bihler was later appointed tutor to the children of the Archduke Carl. See Kalischer, *Beethoven's Letters*, II: 95; E. Anderson, ed., *The Letters of Beethoven*, 3 vols. (London: Macmillan, 1961), 590, n. 3.

153. A-795; Kalischer, *Beethoven's Letters*, no. 715. This letter first appeared in the *Vienna Presse* of 21 December 1889, and it was published by T. von Frimmel, *Neue Beethoveniana* (Vienna: Carl Gerold's Sohn, 1890), 83. Anderson assigned it to July 1817. See also B-1115.

154. Binz, *Lectures on Pharmacology*, II, 173.

155. A-799.

156. Brunton, *Lectures on the Action of Medicines*, 289.

157. Binz, *Lectures on Pharmacology*, II, 138.

158. A-806; B-1164.

159. A-816; B-1166.

160. A-830; B-1179.

161. A-881; B-1203 (27 December 1817).

162. A-882; B-1226.

163. Albrecht, *Letters*, no. 472.

164. A-966; B-1322 (19 August 1819); TK, III: 14, n. 2.

165. FRHB, II: 185.

166. G. Schünemann, *Ludwig van Beethovens Konversationshefte*, 3 vols., trans. Erna Schwerin (Berlin: M. Hesses, 1941–1943), III: 127; LvBCB, III: 179–80.

167. The doctor in this entry was not named by either Schindler or Thayer. Schüne-mann entered Dr. Staudenheimer; Walther Nohl assumed it was Dr. Braunhofer. How-ever, Professor Köhler identified the writer as Dr. Smetana. See Schünemann, *Beethovens Konversationshefte*, III: 184; Walther Nohl, "Beethoven und sein Arzt Anton Braun-hofer," *Die Musik* 30 (1938): 823; LvBCB, III: 200.

168. Schünemann, *Beethovens Konversationshefte*, III: 184–5; LvBCB, III: 200.

169. Kalksburg was one of the most beautiful spas in the vicinity of Vienna. See Adolf Schmidl, *Wien's Umgebungen auf zwanzig Stunden im Umkreise*, 3 vols. (Vienna: 1835–1839), III: 174.

170. Rodaun was in the vicinity of Kalksburg, a two-hour journey from Vienna. See Schmidl, *Wien's Umgebungen*, III: 183.

171. TF, 997.

172. Albrecht, *Letters*, nos. 326, 327.

173. TF, 373–74.

174. Schindler-MacArdle, 238–39.

175. FRHB, I: 60; LvBCB, IX: 348–49, n. 99.

176. KHV, 621–22.

177. A-1359; B-1958. Dr. Braunhofer entered the date on the autograph, while Bee-thoven's address was entered in Carl's hand.

178. W. Nohl, "Beethoven und Braunhofer," 824; LvBCB, VII: 221–22. The conversation-book entries in Walther Nohl's article, translated by Erna Schwerin, have been rearranged in the chronological order deciphered by K-H. Köhler, G. Herre, and D. Beck, eds., *Ludwig van Beethovens Konversationshefte*, 9 vols. (Leipzig: VEB Deutsche Verlag für Musik, 1968–1988).

179. W. Nohl, "Beethoven und Braunhofer," 825. See also LvBCB, VII: 224.

180. Ibid. See also LvBCB, VII: 225.

181. Ibid. See also LvBCB, VII: 227–28.

182. Ibid. See also LvBCB, VII: 229.

183. Ibid. See also LvBCB, VII: 232.

184. Ibid. See also 826; LvBCB, VII: 233.

185. Ibid. See also LvBCB, VII: 234, 236.

186. LvBCB, VII: 246.

187. O. G. Sonneck, ed., *Beethoven: Impressions by His Contemporaries* (New York: Dover, 1967), 180.

188. TDR, V: 194, trans. Erna Schwerin.

189. LvBCB, VII: 243.

190. W. Nohl, "Beethoven und Braunhofer," 826; LvBCB, VII: 267.

191. LvBCB, VII: 308.

192. A-1370; B-1968.

193. A-1371; B-1967.

194. TF, 946.

195. A-1373; B-1973.

196. A-1375; B-1970.

197. A-1386; B-1988.

198. A-1385; B-1981.

199. W. Nohl, "Beethoven und Braunhofer," 826–27; LvBCB, VII: 319–20.

200. A-1422; B-2116 (February 1826).

201. This would appear to be a criticism of Dr. Braunhofer's treatment; however, Max Unger concluded that it referred to an oculist who treated his eye complaint in 1823. See M. Unger, *Beethovens Handschrift* (Leipzig: Quelle and Meyer, 1926), 21.

202. A-1416; B-2042.

203. A-1418; B-2045.

204. A-1438; B-2065.

205. TF, 967–68.

206. J. Klapetek, "Beethovens letzer Arzt," *Deutsche Medizinische Wöchenschrift* 93 (1963): 369. Frimmel's claim that he was born in 1782 is incorrect—see FRHB, II: 400.

207. Lesky, *Vienna Medical School*, 34.

208. *Medizinische Jahrbücher des des K.K.östlichen Kaiserstaates.*

209. Klapetek, "Beethovens letzer Arzt," 369–70.

210. Bankl and Jesserer, *Die Krankheiten*, 68. Dr. Wawruch had submitted his bill on 15 August 1827.

211. F. Kerst, *Die Erinnerungen an Beethoven*, 2 vols., (Stuttgart: Julius, 1925), II: 244; Bankl und Jesserer, *Die Krankheiten*, 67–68.

212. Lesky, *Vienna Medical School*, 77–78.

213. Ibid., 78.

214. Bankl and Jesserer, *Die Krankheiten*, 68.

2

The Accounts of Beethoven's Deafness

While Beethoven's recurrent respiratory catarrhs, dreadful gastrointestinal disorders, and depression were hard enough for him to bear, in some ways his deafness was the worst, the ultimate tragedy to afflict a musician. How fortunate it is that Beethoven himself wrote vivid accounts of his hearing impairment, accounts that must be quoted in full.

LETTER OF 29 JUNE 1801 TO FRANZ WEGELER

In this moving letter to his friend, physician Franz Wegeler,[1] Beethoven wrote,

But that jealous demon, my wretched health, has put a nasty spoke in my wheel; and it amounts to this, that for the last three years my hearing has become weaker and weaker. The trouble is supposed to have been caused by the condition of my abdomen which, as you know, was wretched even before I left Bonn, but has become worse in Vienna where I have been constantly afflicted with diarrhoea and have been suffering in consequence from an extraordinary debility. Frank[2] tried to tone up my constitution with strengthening medicines and my hearing with almond oil, but much good did it do me! His treatment had no effect, my deafness became even worse and my abdomen continued to be in the same state as before. Such was my condition until the autumn of last year; and sometimes I gave way to despair. Then a medical asinus advised me to take cold baths to improve my condition. A more sensible doctor, however, prescribed the usual tepid baths in the Danube. The result was miraculous; and my inside improved. But my deafness persisted or, I should say, became even worse. During this last winter I was truly wretched, for I had really dreadful attacks of colic and again relapsed completely into my former condition. And thus I remained until about four weeks ago when I went to see Vering.[3] For I began to think that my condition demanded the attention of a surgeon as well; and in any case I had confidence in him. Well, he succeeded in checking almost completely this violent diarrhoea. He prescribed tepid baths in the Danube, to which I had always to add a bottle of strengthening ingredients. He ordered no medicines until about four days ago when he prescribed pills for my stomach and an infusion for my ear. As a result I have been feeling, I may say, stronger and better; but my ears continue to hum and buzz day and night. I must confess that I lead a miserable life. For almost two years I have ceased to attend any social functions, just because I find it impossible to say to people: I am deaf. If I had any other profession I might be able to cope with my infirmity; but in my profession it is a terrible handicap. And if my enemies, of whom I have a fair number, were to hear about it, what would they say?—In order to give you some idea of this strange deafness, let me tell you that in the theatre I have to place myself quite close to the orchestra in order to understand what the actor is saying, and that at a distance I cannot hear the high notes of instruments or voices. As for the spoken voice it is surprising that some people have never noticed my deafness; but since I have always been liable to fits of absent-mindedness, they attribute my hardness of hearing to that. Sometimes too I can scarcely hear a person who speaks softly; I can hear sounds, it is true, but cannot make out the words. But if anyone shouts, I can't bear it. Heaven alone knows what is to become of me. Vering tells me that my hearing will certainly improve, although my deafness may not be completely cured—Already I have often cursed my Creator and my existence. Plutarch has shown me the path of resignation. If it is at all possible, I will bid defiance to my fate, though I feel that as long as I live there will be moments when I shall be God's most unhappy creature—I beg you not to say anything about my condition to any one, not even to Lorchen[4]; I am only telling you this as a secret; but I should like you to correspond with Vering about it. If my trouble persists, I will visit you next spring. You will rent a house for me in some beautiful part of the country and then for six months I will lead the life of a peasant. Perhaps that will make a difference. Resignation, what a wretched resource! Yet it is all that is left to me.[5]

LETTER OF 1 JULY 1801 TO CARL AMENDA

Two days later, Beethoven also confided in his very dear friend Carl Amenda,

You are no Viennese friend, no, you are one of those such as my native soil is wont to produce. How often would I like to have you here with me, for your B[eethoven] is leading a very unhappy life and is at variance with Nature and his Creator. Many times already I have cursed Him for exposing His creatures to the slightest hazard, so that the most beautiful blossom is thereby often crushed and destroyed. Let me tell you that my most prized possession, my hearing, has greatly deteriorated. When you were still with me, I already felt the symptoms; but I said nothing about them. Now they have become very much worse. We must wait and see whether my hearing can be restored. The symptoms are said to be caused by the condition of my abdomen. So far as the latter is concerned, I am almost quite cured. But that my hearing too will improve, I must hope, it is true, but I hardly think it possible, for diseases of that kind are the most difficult to cure. . . . But, in my present condition I must withdraw from everything; and my best years will rapidly pass away without my being able to achieve all that my talent and my strength have commanded me to do—Sad resignation, to which I am forced to have recourse. Needless to say, I am resolved to overcome all this, but how is it going to be done? Yes Amenda, if after six months my disease proves to be incurable, then I shall claim your sympathy, then you must give up everything and come to me. I shall then travel (when I am playing and composing, my affliction still hampers me least; it affects me most when I am in company) and you must be my companion.[6]

LETTER OF 16 NOVEMBER 1801 TO WEGELER

In his letter of response, which is not extant, Wegeler asked for further details about Beethoven's treatments. Beethoven responded,

You want to know how I am and what remedies I am trying. Despite my intense dislike to speak about this subject I am quite willing to do so to you—For the last few months Vering has made me apply to both arms vesicatories which, as you doubtless know, consist of a certain kind of bark.[7] Well, it is an extremely unpleasant treatment, inasmuch as for a few days (until the bark has drawn sufficiently) I am always deprived of the free use of my arms, not to mention the pain I have to suffer. True enough, I cannot deny it, the humming and buzzing is slightly less than it used to be, particularly in my left ear, where my deafness really began. But so far my hearing is certainly not a bit better; and I am inclined to think, although I do not dare to say so definitely, that it is a little weaker—The condition of my abdomen is improving, and especially when I have taken tepid baths for a few days I feel pretty well for eight or even ten days afterwards. I very rarely take a tonic for my stomach and, if so, only one dose. But following your advice I am now beginning to apply herbs to my belly—Vering won't hear of my taking shower baths. On the whole I am not at all satisfied with him. He takes far too little interest in and trouble with a complaint of this kind. I should never see him unless I went to his house, which is very inconvenient for me—What is your opinion of Schmidt?[8] It is true that I am not inclined to change doctors, but I think that V[ering] is too much of a practitioner to derive many new ideas from reading—In that respect S[chmidt], I consider, is a totally different fellow and, what is more, he might perhaps not be quite so casual—People talk about miraculous cures by *galvanism*; what is your opinion?—A medical man told me that in Berlin he saw a deaf and dumb child recover its hearing and a man who had also been deaf for seven years recover his—I have just heard that your Schmidt is making experiments with galvanism—I am now leading a slightly more pleasant life, for I am mixing more with my fellow creatures. You would find it hard to believe what an empty, sad life I have had for the last two years. My poor hearing haunted me everywhere like a ghost; and I avoided—all human society. I seemed to be a misanthrope and yet am far from being one.[9]

COTTON WOOL IN HIS EARS

During his first meeting with Beethoven in about 1800, Carl Czerny noted "that he had cotton which seemed to have been steeped in a yellowish liquid, in his ears."[10] This was probably a staining from Dr. Frank's almond oil ear drops, rather than a purulent discharge from the middle ear.

THE HEILIGENSTADT TESTAMENT

The subsequent course of Beethoven's deafness was vividly recounted in the *Heiligenstadt Testament*, one of the most profoundly moving documents ever written. It was discovered by Anton Schindler amongst Beethoven's personal papers during the summer of 1827. Schindler sent copies to Rochlitz in Leipzig, and to Moscheles in London.[11] Dr. Vering and Dr. Schmidt advised Beethoven to rest his hearing in the quiet solitude of the country for six months. He apparently went to Heiligenstädt in early April 1802, and the testament was written in response to a personal crisis that resulted in his contemplation of suicide.

The Heiligenstadt Testament
To Caspar Anton Carl and [Nikolaus Johann] van Beethoven
Heiligenstädt, October 6, 1802
For my Brothers Carl and [Johann] Beethoven
O my fellow men, who consider me, or describe me as, unfriendly, peevish or even misanthropic, how greatly do you wrong me. For you do not know the secret reason why I appear to you to be so. Ever since my childhood my heart and soul have been imbued with the tender feeling of goodwill; and I have always been ready to perform even great actions. But just think, for the last six years I have been afflicted with an incurable complaint which has been made worse by incompetent doctors. From year to year my hopes of being cured have gradually been shattered and finally I have been forced to accept the prospect of a permanent infirmity (the curing of which may perhaps take years or may even prove to be impossible). Though endowed with a passionate and lively temperament and even fond of the distractions offered by society I was soon obliged to seclude myself and live in solitude. If at times I decided just to ignore my infirmity, alas! how cruelly was I then driven back by the intensified sad experience of my poor hearing. Yet I could not bring myself to say to people: "Speak up, shout, for I am deaf." Alas! how could I possibly refer to the impairing of a sense which in me should be more perfectly developed than in other people, a sense which at one time I possessed in the greatest perfection, even to a degree of perfection such as assuredly few in my profession possess or have ever possessed—Oh, I cannot do it; so forgive me, if you ever see me withdrawing from your company which I used to enjoy. Moreover my misfortune pains me doubly, inasmuch as it leads to my being misjudged. For me there can be no relaxation in human society, no refined conversations, no mutual confidences. I must live quite alone and may creep into society only as often as sheer necessity demands; I must live like an outcast. If I appear in company I am overcome by a burning anxiety, a fear that I am running the risk of letting people notice my condition—And that has been my experience during the last six months which I have spent in the country. My sensible doctor by suggesting that I should spare my hearing as much as possible has more or less encouraged my present natural inclination, though indeed when carried away now and then by my instinctive desire for human society, I have let myself be tempted to seek it. But how humiliated I have felt if somebody standing beside me heard the sound of a flute in the distance and I heard nothing, or if somebody heard a shepherd sing and again I heard nothing—Such experiences almost made me despair, and I was on the point of putting an end to my life—The only thing that held me back was my art. For indeed, it seemed to me impossible to leave this world before I had produced

all the works that I felt the urge to compose; and thus I have dragged on this miserable existence—a truly miserable existence, seeing that I have such a sensitive body that any fairly sudden change can plunge me from the best spirits into the worst of humours— Patience—that is the virtue, I am told, which I must now choose for my guide; and I now possess it—I hope that I shall persist in my resolve to endure to the end, until it pleases the inexorable Parcae to cut the thread; perhaps my condition will improve, perhaps not; at any rate I am now resigned—At the early age of 28 I was obliged to become a philosopher, though this was not easy; for indeed this is more difficult for an artist than for anyone else—Almighty God, who look down into my innermost soul, you see into my heart and you know that it is filled with love for humanity and a desire to do good. Oh my fellow men, when some day you read this statement, remember that you have done me wrong; and let some unfortunate man derive comfort from the thought that he has found another equally unfortunate who, notwithstanding all the obstacles imposed by nature, yet did everything in his power to be raised to the rank of noble artists and human beings.—And you, my brothers Carl and [Johann], when I am dead, request on my behalf Professor Schmidt, if he is still living, to describe my disease, and attach this written document to his record, so that after my death at any rate the world and I may be reconciled as far as possible—At the same time I herewith nominate you both heirs to my small property (if I may so describe it)—Divide it honestly, live in harmony and help one another. You know that you have long ago been forgiven for the harm you did me. I again thank you, my brother Carl, in particular, for the affection you have shown me of late years. My wish is that you should have a better and more carefree existence than I have had. Urge your children to be virtuous, for virtue alone can make a man happy. Money cannot do this. I speak from experience. It was virtue that sustained me in my misery. It was thanks to virtue and also to my art that I did not put an end to my life by suicide—Farewell and love one another—I thank all my friends, and especially Prince Lichnowsky, and Professor Schmidt. I would like Prince L[ichnowsky]'s instruments to be preserved by one of you, provided this does not lead to a quarrel between you.[12] But as soon as they can serve a more useful purpose, just sell them; and how glad I shall be if in my grave I can still be of some use to you both—Well, that is all—Joyfully I go to meet Death—should it come before I have had an opportunity of developing all my artistic gifts, then in spite of my hard fate it would still come too soon, and no doubt I would like it to postpone its coming—Yet even so I should be content, for would it not free me from a condition of continual suffering? Come then, Death, whenever you like, and with courage I will go to meet you—Farewell; and when I am dead, do not wholly forget me. I deserve to be remembered by you, since during my lifetime I have often thought of you and tried to make you happy—Be happy

Ludwig van Beethoven

For my brothers Carl and [Johann]
To be read and executed after my death—
Heiligenstadt, October 10, 1802—Thus I take leave of you—and, what is more, rather sadly—yes, the hope I cherished—the hope I brought with me here of being cured to a certain extent at any rate—that hope I must now abandon completely. As the autumn leaves fall and wither, likewise—that hope has faded for me. I am leaving here—almost in the same condition as I arrived—Even that high courage—which has often inspired

me on fine summer days—has vanished—Oh Providence—do but grant me one day of pure joy—For so long now the inner echo of real joy has been unknown to me—Oh when—oh when, Almighty God—shall I be able to hear and feel this echo again in the temple of Nature and in contact with humanity—Never?—No!—Oh, that would be too hard.[13]

In the original autograph, Beethoven misspelled the place "Heiglnstadt." The name of his younger brother, Johann van Beethoven, was omitted twice in the letter and also in the postscript.

THE ACCOUNT OF FERDINAND RIES

Ferdinand Ries wrote a moving account of Beethoven's deafness, pertaining to the year 1801:

The beginning deafness was for him such a sensitive subject that one had to be very careful not to let him feel this deficiency by speaking in a loud voice. If he had not understood something, he usually related it to his absent-mindedness, which was characteristic of him anyway. He stayed in the country much of the time, where I went for a lesson. Occasionally he said at 8 o'clock in the morning, after breakfast: "Let's first go for a little walk." We did, but did not return until between 3 and 4, after we had eaten something in the village. On one of these walks Beethoven offered (to me) the first, striking proof of his decreased hearing, about which I had already heard from Stephan von Breuning. I called his attention to a shepherd playing a flute in the woods. For half an hour Beethoven could not hear any such sound, and although I repeatedly assured him that I no longer heard anything either (which was not the case), he became quiet and gloomy.—Whenever he occasionally appeared to be merry, it was always to a point of exuberance, but this occurred only rarely.[14]

LUDWIG RELLSTAB'S ACCOUNT

Ries' account was embellished in the memoirs of Ludwig Rellstab:

After we had walked for about one hour, we sat down in the meadow. Suddenly the tunes of a shawm [in German, *Schalmei*, an ancient instrument, made of elderwood, resembling the flute] were heard from the distant mountains of the valley. This unexpected sound beneath the light-blue sky of spring, in the deepest quiet of the woods, had a startling effect on me. I could not refrain from calling Beethoven's attention to it; he sat next to me deep in thought, apparently unaware of it [the sounds]. He listened attentively, but I recognized from his expression that he did not hear the continuing sounds. Then for the first time I became convinced of his severe hearing impairment. I had already suspected it earlier on, but since at the start the affliction was periodic, I thought I was mistaken. But this time I was thoroughly convinced, for the sounds were so loud and clear, that not even one was lost, and Beethoven did not hear anything! In order not to upset him, I pretended not to hear anything either. After a while we were off again, and the sounds accompanied us on the lonely wood path for a long while, but escaped Beethoven's notice completely.[15]

CHARLES NEATE'S ANECDOTE

We should now consider the puzzling anecdote of the English pianist Charles Neate who, in 1815, when encouraging Beethoven to visit England, offered further inducement by suggesting that he consult a London physician about his deafness. Beethoven replied,

No, I have already received all kinds of advice from doctors. I will never be cured. I will tell you, how it all started. I was once at work to write an opera. Neate: *Fidelio?* Beethoven: No. It was not *Fidelio*. I was in contact with a very moody and unpleasant first tenor. I had already composed two great arias on identical text, with which he was not satisfied, and still a third, which he seemed to approve of at the first try, and which he took with him. I thanked the Heavens that I had finally finished with him, and immediately sat down to work at a composition which I was very keen to finish, and which I had set aside on account of these arias. I was not at work for half an hour, when I heard a knock at my door, which I immediately recognized as that of my first tenor. I jumped up from my chair in such excitement and rage that, when he entered the room, I threw myself upon the floor, as they do on the stage (here Beethoven opened his arms wide, making an explanatory gesture), and I fell on my hands. When I got up again, I was deaf and have remained that way ever since. The doctors say that the nerve was injured.[16]

Alexander Thayer concluded that the aria in question was the insertion arietta for Ignaz Umlauf's *Die schöne Schusterin*, composed during 1796 or 1797 (*O welch' ein Leben*, WoO 91). However, Theodor von Frimmel and Romain Rolland proposed that the work in question was the oratorio "Christ on the Mount of Olives" (*Christus am Ölberg*, Op. 85).[17]

RECONCILED TO HIS DEAFNESS

J. E. Dolezalek informed Otto Jahn that, during the rehearsals of the Eroica Symphony in 1804, Beethoven had much difficulty in hearing the wind instruments.[18] Two years later, Beethoven was becoming reconciled to his deafness. On a page of sketches for the finale of the Third Razumovsky Quartet (Op. 59, no 3), he wrote, "Just as you are now plunging into the whirlpool of society— just so possible is it to compose works in spite of social obstacles. Let your deafness no longer be a secret—even in art."[19]

CORRECTION OF ERRORS BY WILHELM CARL RUST

In 1808 Beethoven's hearing was still sufficiently keen for him to detect two subtle errors in the playing of the former child prodigy Wilhelm Carl Rust

(1787–1855) of Dessau: "In a scherzo I had not played the notes crisply enough and at another time I had struck one note twice instead of binding it."[20]

PANDEMONIUM AT HIS AKADEMIE IN DECEMBER 1808

During the second half of a long program, Beethoven cut the lengthy da capo in the scherzo of the Fifth Symphony, and he improvised the introduction to the choral *Fantasia*, Op. 80, prior to the development of utter chaos and a breakdown of the orchestra.

At the somewhat hurried rehearsal, Beethoven had arranged with Ignaz Seyfried that the second variation was to be played without the repeat. However, at the performance in the evening, Beethoven forgot his proposal of change, and he played the repeat at variance with the orchestra until a halt was called, after which it was played through without any error.[21]

Johann Friedrich Reichardt, who listened to the concert on a bitter cold evening from 6:30 until 10:30, in Prince Lobkowitz's box, described the final number:

A long Fantasia, in which Beethoven displayed all his masterly power; and, last of all, another Fantasia, in which the orchestra and chorus took part (the so-called Choral *Fantasia*). The rendering of the original ideas contained in this piece was spoilt by such a complete confusion among the band, that Beethoven, carried away by his feelings, and quite unmindful of the place and the audience, called out to the performers to leave off and go back to the beginning. You can imagine our sensations. For the moment I wished I had had the courage to leave sooner.[22]

Beethoven's own account of the mistake was expressed in his letter of 7 January 1809 to Breitkopf and Härtel:

In spite of the fact that various mistakes were made, which I could not prevent, the public nevertheless applauded the whole performance with enthusiasm. . . . The musicians, in particular, were enraged that, when from sheer carelessness a mistake had been made in the simplest and most straightforward passage in the world, I suddenly made them stop playing and called out in a loud voice: "Once more."—Such a thing had never happened to them before. The public, however, expressed its pleasure at this.[23]

BEETHOVEN TAKES REFUGE IN A CELLAR

During the third French occupation of Vienna, at 9:00 P.M., on 11 May 1809, a battery of twenty howitzers opened fire and continued to shell the city from a battery on the Spittelberg, until the white flag was raised at 2:30 P.M., on the next day. Beethoven took refuge in the cellar of his brother Caspar Carl's house in the Rauhensteingasse: "Beethoven was excessively alarmed; he passed most of the time in a cellar at his brother Caspar's, where, besides, he covered his head with pillows that he might not hear the cannon."[24] During our discussion of the mechanism of Beethoven's deafness, we will see that this incident provides an important clue for the diagnosis.

BEETHOVEN CHOOSES A STREICHER PIANO

Baron Georg Schall von Falkenhorst (1761–1831), a major general in the Imperial Army, who gave musical soirees at his residence in the Weihburggasse, asked Beethoven to choose one of Johann Streicher's pianos for him. In his letter to Streicher (shortly before 27 July 1810), Beethoven made light of his tinnitus: "I can't help it, the pianoforte beside the door near your entrance is constantly ringing in my ears—I feel sure that I shall be thanked for having chosen this one."[25]

ENTRY IN THE "PETTER SKETCHBOOK"

During the late summer of 1811, Beethoven made the following entry on the first page of the "Petter Sketchbook":

> Baumwolle in den
> Ohren am Klavier
> benimmt meinen Gehör
> das unangenehm
> Rauschende.—
> (Cotton in my ears at the piano
> takes away the disagreeable
> ringing in my ears.)[26]

LOUIS SPOHR'S ACCOUNT

During the fall of 1812 composer Louis Spohr met Beethoven at a restaurant in Vienna. In his autobiography, he wrote, "Beethoven was very talkative, which greatly surprised the company, as he generally sat silent and gloomy; but conversing with him was hard work, for one had to shout loud enough to be heard three rooms off."[27]

Soon after, Spohr was overcome with sadness when he heard Beethoven at the clavier while rehearsing his Trio in D major (Op. 70, no. 1):

This was no pleasure, for in the first place, the piano was very much out of tune, which was of very little consequence to Beethoven for he could not hear it; and secondly, the artist's deafness had left little trace of his once famous powers as a virtuoso. The poor deaf-man played the forti so loudly that the strings clattered, and the piani so softly that whole groups of notes were inaudible, thus rendering an understanding of the work impossible unless one could look over the piano part. The contemplation of so hard a fate, made me profoundly melancholy. If deafness be a heavy misfortune to an ordinary man, how is a musician to bear it without despairing? Beethoven's constant gloom no longer seemed a mystery to me.[28]

THE EAR TRUMPETS

Carl Czerny informed Otto Jahn that between 1812 and 1816 it gradually became more difficult, even with shouting, to converse with Beethoven.[29] In desperation Beethoven sought the assistance of hearing aids; at that time, only mechanical devices were available. Beethoven became friendly with a musical acoustic mechanic and entrepreneur, Johann Nepomuk Mälzel, who had recently invented the panharmonicon, a mechanical orchestra for trumpet, clarinet, viola, and cello.[30] In 1812 Mälzel promised Beethoven that he would manufacture for him a set of ear trumpets to assist his conversation and hearing of music. Beethoven received four ear trumpets from Mälzel, as recounted by Schindler: "By degrees four acoustic machines were produced, but only one of which Beethoven found serviceable, and used for a considerable time, especially in his interviews with the Archduke Rudolph and others, when it would have been too tedious to keep up a conversation in writing."[31]

The four ear trumpets, made by Mälzel in 1814, are now in the Beethoven House in Bonn. One of them, with stars near the opening, was referred to by Beethoven in his Tagebuch: "An ear trumpet could be such that the stars of the opening [amplify] the entrance of the sound and the sound would be transmitted around the ear and in this way could be heard towards all openings."[32] Beethoven also wrote comments about the construction of ear trumpets in the desk sketchbooks of 1814 and 1815.[33]

Two of these ear trumpets were used for conversation; the smaller one was taken by the composer on his walks and outings. When composing at the keyboard, Beethoven would attach the larger ear trumpets by a headband, so that his hands remained free to play the piano. In 1815 he wrote in his Tagebuch, "If possible, bring the ear-trumpets to perfection and then travel. This you owe to yourself, to Mankind and to Him, the Almighty. Only thus can you once again develop everything that has to remain locked within you."[34]

Beethoven used other ear trumpets too. In 1815 he wrote in his Tagebuch, "Next to the—, the Mälzel ear-trumpet is the strongest. One should have different ones in the room for music, speech, and also for halls of various sizes."[35]

Another of his ear trumpets is preserved at the Gesellschaft der Musikfreunde in Vienna.[36] A silver trumpet was reserved for him at Steiner's music shop.[37] On one occasion he loaned one of his ear trumpets to Nanette Streicher for a day.[38] In January 1820 Beethoven was invited to inspect three hearing aids belonging to a neighbor, who had presented them to Baron Andreas Joseph von Stifft.[39] According to Dr. Rattel, Beethoven, while at the piano, used a wooden rod with one end grasped between his teeth, while the other end rested on the sound box of the instrument.[40] The dubious authenticity of this anecdote is not substantiated in other sources.

In 1977 Beethoven's hearing aids were featured on a postage stamp issued by the Republic of Maldives.[41]

THE REHEARSAL OF THE SEVENTH SYMPHONY

During the rehearsals of the Seventh Symphony in December 1813, Louis Spohr, a violinist in the orchestra, observed that Beethoven did not hear the soft passages of the music, and while conducting the allegretto he overlooked a hold in pianissimo.[42]

After playing the *Archduke Trio* with Ignaz Schuppanzigh at a morning concert in the Prater, in the middle of 1814, Beethoven played in public only as an accompanist. At his last public appearance as a pianist, on 25 January 1815, at the Rittersaal, on the occasion of a special concert to honor the Russian empress's birthday, Beethoven accompanied the singer Franz Wild in a revised version of his song "An die Hoffnung," Op. 32.[43]

1816: THE ACCOUNTS OF CARL VON BURSY AND PETER JOSEPH SIMROCK

During his visit to Beethoven in June 1816, Dr. Carl von Bursy made a record in his diary[44]: "He asked me to speak loudly as his hearing was very bad just then. . . . He often misunderstood me, and had to pay the greatest attention to catch what I said. This of course much disconcerted me, and sharing my embarrassment he spoke the more himself and very loudly."[45]

During his visit to Vienna in 1816, Peter Joseph Simrock, the son of the Bonn publisher Nikolaus Simrock, often dined with Beethoven at Baden in his lodging in the Sailerstätte, or in the inn Zur goldenen Birn. He told Thayer "that he had no difficulty in making Beethoven understand him if he spoke into his left ear; but anything private or confidential must be communicated in writing."[46]

POTTER'S IMPRESSION IN 1817

The director of the Royal Music Academy in London, Cipriani Potter, came to Vienna in 1817 for instruction in composition. Potter brought letters to Beethoven from Charles Neate, Ferdinand Ries, Pierre Rode, Domenico Dragonetti, and others. Beethoven recommended him to Aloys Förster. Noting that Beethoven spoke Italian, Potter communicated in that language.[47] Potter made himself heard "by using his hands as a speaking-trumpet; Beethoven did not always hear everything, but was content when he caught the meaning."[48]

A year later, regular communication in writing became necessary.

THE CONVERSATION-BOOKS

Beethoven's conversation-books (*Konversationshefte*) are among the most unique documents in the history of music. Some 400 of them, spanning the years from 1818 to three weeks before his death in 1827, were inherited by Stephan von Breuning, whose widow handed them over to Anton Schindler. When, in 1846, Schindler sold the collection to the Royal Prussian Library in Berlin (formerly the Deutsche Staatsbibliothek in East Berlin), two thirds of the books were missing. After carefully sifting through this treasury of literature, Schindler destroyed 264 of this collection, which he tried to justify by telling S. W. Dehn that the missing books contained only minor trivialities of no importance, as well as distasteful, "licentious assaults" against members of the imperial family. No doubt Schindler also destroyed any material that could have tainted his own idealized portrait of Beethoven, or any derogatory references to himself.[49]

Furthermore, expert handwriting analyses, conducted by Grita Herre and Dagmar Beck, have established that Schindler forged some 240 entries in the extant conversation-books.[50]

The earlier editions published by Walther Nohl, Georg Schünemann, and Jacques-Gabriel Prod'homme were incomplete. For example, Schünemann included thirty-seven of the books, spanning the period from February 1818 to July 1823. Donald MacArdle's invaluable index was published in 1962.[51] The complete edition is published by Deutscher Verlag für Musik in Leipzig. Between 1968 and 1993, 127 of the books were published in ten volumes. Unfortunately, during Beethoven's move back to Vienna from Baden in 1823, quantities of his personal papers, including some of the conversation-books, were lost.[52] There is a hiatus in the periods: September 1820 to June 1822, June to November 1822, and November 1822 to January 1823.

Beethoven himself less often wrote entries in the conversation-books, since he usually responded viva voce. However, he sometimes copied passages from a newspaper or journal, as in January 1820 when he copied a notice from the *Austrian Observer* that Thaddäus Hänke had died: "Hänke, the naturalist from Bohemia, died in South America."[53]

Unfortunately for posterity, on some occasions, as for example during Beethoven's final illness, the visitor's conversation entries, recorded with a slate pencil on a slate, were later erased.

It is emphasized that, in 1855, the Royal Library in Berlin loaned Alexander Wheelock Thayer the 138 conversation-books then in its possession. Thayer made practically a complete transcript of them and laboriously deciphered the many hieroglyphic scrawls in his effort to establish the chronological order of the conversations.[54] Unfortunately, Thayer's complete transcriptions have been lost, though many extracts were quoted in his monumental biography.

JULY 1817: BEETHOVEN REQUESTS A LOUDER PIANO FROM STREICHER

We should now resume the poignant story of Beethoven's deafness. In his letter of 7 July 1817 to Nanette Streicher Beethoven wrote, "Now I have a great favour to ask of Streicher. Request him on my behalf to be so kind as to adjust one of your pianos for me to suit my impaired hearing. It should be as loud as possible. That is absolutely necessary."[55]

Streicher obliged by producing a new model with a compass of six and a half octaves. Streicher also connected ear trumpets to the upright sound board. It should be remembered that the more elegant, lighter, wooden-framed instruments used by Beethoven (Stein, Streicher, Walter, Schanz, Erard, Broadwood, and Graf) yielded clearer, softer tones, over a restricted compass, when compared to the modern, heavy, iron-framed pianos.[56]

AUGUST VON KLÖBER'S DESCRIPTION

On 19 May 1818, Beethoven, in the company of his nephew Carl, a housekeeper, and a maid, went to Mödling, where they lodged at the Hafner House at what is now no. 79 Hauptstrasse.[57] Beethoven also took along his superb six-octave Broadwood grand pianoforte (now in the National Museum at Budapest), which had arrived from London in February but which was damaged in transit.

August von Klöber, an artist, made mention of Beethoven's deafness in his reminiscences and stated that it was necessary for him to converse in writing in Carl's presence, or alternatively by shouting into his ear trumpet. A large metal dome, to amplify the sound, was attached to the piano:

Beethoven then sat down, and the boy had to begin practising the piano, a gift from England and equipped with a large metal dome. The instrument stood roughly four to five paces behind him, and Beethoven, despite his deafness, corrected every mistake the boy made, had him repeat single passages, etc.[58]

INTEREST IN ACOUSTICS

Beethoven developed a keen interest in the science of speech and acoustics. In May 1819 he jotted down in his conversation-book the titles of two books which were available at Gerold's on the Stephansplatz: (1) Franz König's *The Easiest Way to Teach Children Arithmetic in a Pleasant Manner*, 2d ed., Prague, 1819, costing 4 fl. 30 kr. (w.w.); and (2) Heinrich August Kerndörffer's *Material for First Instruction in Declamation*, Leipzig, 1815, costing 1 fl. 18 kr.[59]

Beethoven also copied a notice from the *Allgemeine Musikalische Zeitung* of a lecture to be given by Dr. Ernst Florens Friedrich Chladni (1756–1827) on "Acoustics and Meteor Masses."[60] Dr. Chladni, born in Wittenberg, was the famous discoverer of two unusual musical instruments: the euphon ("sound figures") and the clavicylinder (glass staff clavier).[61] On 15 May 1819, Chladni's book on acoustics was advertised in the *Wiener Zeitung*.[62] Beethoven noted in his Tagebuch that he had consulted Dr. Chladni's book *Die Akustic*,[63] and in his letter of 10 March 1815 to Breitkopf and Härtel he stated, "One of my acquaintances would like to have Chladni's address."[64]

SIEGMUND WOLFSSOHN'S HEAD MACHINE FOR
THE DEAF

An article about a new device for the deaf, discovered by Dr. Siegmund Wolfssohn, was published on 29 February 1820 in the scientific journal *Wiener Conversationsblatt*: "The head machine for the deaf. It is an ingenious contraption shaped like a flat compressed tiara which, covered by a wig, can be worn unnoticed. Wolfssohn assures me that our immortal Beethoven uses it to decided advantage."[65] Incensed by this article, Beethoven wrote in a conversation book, "He[rr] Wolfssohn lies about me."[66]

It would appear that Beethoven asked Carl Bernard to lodge an objection to the journal, with the following correction, which appeared in the journal on 9 March 1820: "That Beethoven did look at the machine but never used it."[67]

Dr. Wolfssohn, a physician, mechanical instrument maker, and manufacturer of medical supplies for the court, consulted in his premises at no. 629 Bauermarkt.

CARL JOSEPH MEYER'S ELECTRO-VIBRATION MACHINE

On 17 April 1819, a notice appeared in the *Wiener Zeitung*.[68] It was an advertisement for a new method of treatment conducted by Dr. Carl Joseph Meyer, a physician and surgeon, who was practicing in the Elisabethiner House at no. 317 Landstrasse. Dr. Meyer's electro-vibration machine was claimed to be of benefit in the treatment of such difficult conditions as rheumatism, gout, ringing in the ears, hearing difficulties, and deafness.[69] Beethoven jotted down details in his conversation-book, but there is no record that he ever consulted Dr. Meyer.[70]

Dr. Jakob Staudenheim sent Beethoven to take the baths at Mödling, where he arrived on 12 May and took the same lodgings as he had in the previous year at the Hafner House. Early in June, he informed the Archduke Rudolph from his sickbed that "[he had] caught a violent cold."[71] In July he was again very unwell, and he went into town several times to consult Dr. Staudenheim. On 31 August, while working on the *Missa solemnis*, he was again unwell and taking medicines.[72]

There are also undated references to "another attack"[73] and "catarrh."[74]

On 10 October he enclosed a note for Dr. Staudenheim in his letter to Anton Steiner, but unfortunately it is not extant.[75]

HORSERADISH EAR DROPS

Heinrich Seelig owned an expensive delicatessen and wine store on the Neuen Markt, no. 1124. Beethoven often shopped there, and many of his conversation-book entries were made in Seelig's store. Seelig, also an art collector, owned a Leonardo da Vinci masterpiece, then valued at 20,000 florins.[76]

In November 1819 Seelig told Beethoven and Franz Oliva about a new treatment for deafness, recommended by a Dr. Graff. A piece of cotton, saturated with the juice of freshly plucked horseradish, was to be inserted into the ears as often as possible. The wife of a nearby count had allegedly been cured of deafness within four weeks by this treatment.[77] No doubt Beethoven would have tried such a simple remedy.

WINTER EARACHE IN 1822

While there is no documented history of earache during the early evolution of his deafness, in his letter to the cellist Bernhard Romberg, dated 12 February 1822, Beethoven wrote, "Last night I again succumbed to the earache which I usually suffer from during this season. Even your playing would only cause me pain today."[78]

CLOCK CHIMES OF CHERUBINI'S OVERTURE TO *MEDEA*

There was retention of some hearing in his left ear, and on 3 October 1822, the emperor's name day, he conducted from the piano the *Consecration of the House* Overture, Op. 124, to a packed house in the Josephstadt Theater, with his left ear turned toward the stage. There was, in the restaurant adjacent to this theater, a musical clock that chimed Cherubini's overture to *Medea*. Beethoven was fond of this piece and strained with his left ear to hear it.[79] Though a regular concertgoer until 1820, he attended only sporadically after that year.

In contrast to the early loss of high-tone frequencies, the lower tones were retained, so that Beethoven could hear the clatter of wagon wheels, claps of thunder, and gunshots.[80] On one occasion, according to Schuppanzigh, after having struck the wall violently with a bootjack, Beethoven held it to his ear in a desperate bid to hear the after vibrations.[81]

REVIVAL OF *FIDELIO* IN 1822

The fourth revival of *Fidelio* on 3 November 1822 was a benefit performance for a seventeen-year-old soprano, Wilhelmine Schröder (later Madame Schröder-Devrient, reputedly the greatest ever Fidelio). Her pathetic tale of Beethoven's attempt to conduct the dress rehearsal describes one of the most painful, embarrassing events in his life.

At that time the Master's physical ear already was deaf to all tone. With confusion written on his face, with a more than earthly enthusiasm in his eye, swinging his baton to and fro with violent motions, he stood in the midst of the playing musicians and did not hear a single note! When he thought they should play *piano*, he almost crept under the conductor's desk, and when he wanted a *forte*, he leaped high into the air with the strangest gestures, uttering the weirdest sounds. With each succeeding number we grew more intimidated, and I felt as though I were gazing at one of [Ernst Theodore] Hoffmann's fantastic figures which had popped up before me. It was unavoidable that the deaf Master should throw singers and orchestra into the greatest confusion and put them entirely off beat until none knew where they were at. Of all this, however, Beethoven was entirely unconscious, and thus with the utmost difficulty we concluded a rehearsal with which he seemed altogether content, for he laid down his baton with a happy smile. Yet it was impossible to entrust the performance itself to him, and Conductor Umlauf had to charge himself with the heart-rending business of calling his attention to the fact that the opera could not be given under his direction. He is said to have resigned himself with a sorrowful heavenward glance; and I found him sitting behind Umlauf in the orchestra the following evening, lost in profound meditation. You probably know with what enthusiasm the Vienna public greeted *Fidelio* on that occasion, and also that since that performance this immortal work has found a permanent place in the repertoire of the German operatic stage. Every artist taking part in the performance accomplished his task that evening with enthusiastic devotion; for who would not gladly have given his last breath for the wretched Master who heard nothing of all the beauty and glory he had created! Beethoven followed the entire performance with strained attention, and it seemed as though he were trying to gather from each of our movements whether we had at least half understood his meaning.[82]

The next day, Beethoven consulted Dr. Carl von Smetana, who prescribed internal medicines without benefit. In desperation he then returned to Father Weiss, whose instillation of ear drops had resulted in an apparent, transient improvement in the hearing in his left ear. When Beethoven realized that there was no cure, he abandoned the treatment and resigned himself to his fate.[83]

CONVERSATIONS WITH HERR SANDRA

During April 1823 Beethoven met a deaf man named Herr Sandra, who made several entries in the conversation-books.[84] These conversations are reproduced in Appendix 1. Sandra asked him in writing, not only about the efficacy of the various general treatments, but also specifically about the value of mechanical aids and faradic stimulation. Beethoven replied that deafness was indeed a very sad malady, about which the doctors knew very little. He recommended the various bathing cures and walks in the country air but advised him to spare the hearing mechanism by the use of writing for conversations and the avoidance of using hearing machines. He told Sandra that he had sustained a little hearing in his left ear because he had refrained from using the ear trumpets. As to the faradic treatment, he said that he had tried it earlier on but was unable to tolerate it.[85]

THE PREMIERE OF THE NINTH SYMPHONY

A moving account of the wild, enthusiastic applause given after the first performance of the Ninth Symphony in the Kärntnerthor theater on 7 May 1824 was related to Sir George Grove by Madame Caroline Sabatier-Unger, during her visit to London in 1869.

At the close of the performance an incident occurred which must have brought the tears to many an eye in the room. The master, though placed in the midst of this confluence of music, heard nothing of it at all and was not even sensible of the applause of the audience at the end of his great work, but continued standing with his back to the audience, and beating the time, till Fräulein Ungher, who had sung the contralto part, turned him, or induced him to turn round and face the people, who were still clapping their hands, and giving way to the greatest demonstrations of pleasure. His turning round, and the sudden conviction thereby forced on everybody that he had not done so before because he could not hear what was going on, acted like an electric shock on all present, and a volcanic explosion of sympathy and admiration followed, which was repeated again and again, and seemed as if it would never end.[86]

BEETHOVEN'S REHEARSALS OF OP. 127

The first performance, in Beethoven's absence, of the String Quartet in E-flat, Op. 127, by Schuppanzigh's Quartet, on 6 March 1825, went badly. However, the second rendering, led by Joseph Böhm, after several rehearsals supervised by Beethoven, received a storm of applause. Böhm recalled,

The unhappy man was so deaf that he could no longer hear the heavenly sound of his compositions. And yet rehearsing in his presence was not easy. With close attention his eyes followed the bows and therefore he was able to judge the smallest fluctuations in tempo or rhythm and correct them immediately.[87]

BEETHOVEN DIRECTS OP. 132

Sir George Smart attended the premiere of the String Quartet in A minor, Op. 132, on Friday 9 September 1825, at the tavern Zum wilden Mann. This quartet was played twice by Ignaz Schuppanzigh on first violin, Carl Holz on second violin, Franz Weiss on viola, and Joseph Linke on cello: "He [Beethoven] directed the performers, and took off his coat, the room being warm and crowded. A staccato passage not being expressed to the satisfaction of his eye, for alas, he could not hear, he seized Holz's violin and played the passage a quarter of a tone too flat."[88]

THE VISIT OF AN ENGLISH LADY

An English lady who visited Beethoven at Baden during the autumn of 1825 recounted the following anecdote: "I conversed with him in writing, for I found it impossible to render myself audible; and, though this was a very clumsy mode of communicating, it did not signify, as he talked on, freely and willingly, and did not wait for questions, or seem to expect long replies."[89]

GRAF'S PIANO AND CONTRAPTION

Following his severance of relations with Mälzel, Beethoven sought help from the imperial pianoforte maker Conrad Graf, who was also a drinking companion. Graf made a gift to Beethoven of one of his new models, with quadruple strings, in lieu of the usual three to each key. Although it was a stronger instrument, this model was not a success. The thinner wire produced a softer sound, especially in the higher octaves and had a poor tone in the treble.[90] Beethoven moved from Baden into the Schwarzspanierhaus on Saturday, 15 October 1825. In the center of his large bedroom, in this apartment at no. 200 Alsergrund Glacis, the Broadwood and Graf pianos stood head to tail. Graf attached an ingenious device to amplify the sound.[91] According to Schindler,

The imperial court pianoforte-maker, Conrad Graf, made for Beethoven a sound-conductor, which, being placed on the pianoforte, helped to convey the tone more distinctly to his ear; but though this contrivance was ingenious, it afforded no assistance in Beethoven's case of extreme deafness. The most painful thing of all was to hear him improvise on stringed instruments, owing to his incapability of tuning them. The music which he thus produced was frightful, though in his mind it was pure and harmonious.[92]

THE VISIT OF CLARA SCHUMANN'S FATHER

Beethoven improvised on his favorite Broadwood pianoforte for Clara Schumann's father, Friedrich Wieck, during his visit with Andreas Stein.

Then he improvised for me during an hour, after he had mounted his ear-trumpet and placed it on the resonance-plate on which already stood the pretty well battered, large grand piano, with its very powerful, rough tone. . . . He played in a flowing, genial manner, for the most part orchestrally, and was still quite adept in the passing over of the right and left hands (a few times he missed the mark), weaving in the clearest and most charming melodies, which seemed to stream to him unsought, most of the time keeping his eyes turned upward, and with close-gathered fingers.[93]

THE RESONANCE HOLDER

Dr. Samuel Spiker, after his visit to Beethoven in September 1826, wrote in his reminiscences,

Unfortunately his deafness—which also explained a peculiar mechanism fastened to his grand piano, a kind of resonance-holder, beneath which he sat when he played, and which was meant to catch up and concentrate the sound about him—made conversation with him a very wearisome matter which, however, in view of his uncommon liveliness, one seemed to feel but little. Paper and pencil were immediately at hand when we entered, and a page was soon covered with writing, answers to his queries and new questions asked him.[94]

Johann Andreas Stumpff described Graf's contraption as follows:

This top constructed for Beethoven to aid his hearing impairment, consisted of a semi-circle of thin resonating wood (*Resonanzholz*), closed at both ends, and raised above the keys of the piano from bass to treble, enveloping the head of the player at the height of the semicircle—viz., resembling a dome shaped hollow roof—; thus, the sound waves remained concentrated inside it, exerting a beneficial effect on deaf ears, as was the case with Beethoven.[95]

Neither the resonance holder nor an illustration of it have survived.[96]

STONE DEAF IN 1826

With the gradual decline of the faint traces of hearing in his left ear, Beethoven used to pound his Broadwood piano mercilessly in a desperate bid to hear it. Little wonder that many of its strings were broken. The deaf composer would also on occasion thump on the wall with a boot last in desperation to capture the tones.

On one occasion, while visiting the Breunings' Rothes Haus, which must have been subsequent to October 1825, Beethoven showed delight when he heard the high piercing shriek of one of Gerhard's sisters.[97]

Gerhard von Breuning established beyond any doubt that Beethoven was stone deaf during his last year. On one occasion, when Beethoven was late for dinner at the Rothes Haus, Gerhard von Breuning was sent to fetch him. Upon entering Beethoven's apartment in the Schwarzspanierhaus, the boy found him at work on one of the Galitzin Quartets. Beethoven beckoned him to wait for a while until he had written down the inspiration of that moment. Gerhard went to the Graf piano, with its attached resonance holder, and began to strum softly on the keys. When the boy observed that Beethoven showed no reaction, he deliberately began pounding the keys very loudly. However Beethoven did not hear him, and kept on writing until he had finished, when he told the boy to go. In the street Beethoven asked the boy a question. Gerhard screamed the answer directly into his ear, but Beethoven understood his gestures rather than his words.[98]

At the end of August 1826, however, there was further optimistic mention of a possible cure for his deafness in the conversation-books. A friend of the cellist Joseph Linke had experienced an improvement in hearing by the instillation of ear drops made from cooking green nut shells in milk.[99]

Gerhard von Breuning also stated that many people in Vienna maintained that Beethoven's ears were impaired only to the perception of speech and general noise, but not to music.[100]

IGNATIUS VON SEYFRIED'S ACCOUNT

The progress of Beethoven's deafness was well summarized by his friend, Ignatius von Seyfried: "The disease of the ear which caused his deafness developed itself, indeed, very gradually, but refused, from the very first, to yield to any means adopted against it, and at length ended in a total deprivation of hearing, which rendered oral communication with him impossible."[101]

ADOLF BERNARD MARX'S DESCRIPTION

The early biographer Adolf Bernard Marx gave the following description:

As early as 1816 it is found that he is incapable of conducting his own works; in 1824 he could not hear the storm of applause from a great audience; but in 1822 he still improvises marvellously in social circles; in 1824 he studies their parts in the Ninth Symphony and Solemn Mass with Sontag and Ungher, and in 1825 he listens carefully to a performance of the Quartet in A-minor, Op. 132.[102]

LABLACHE: DO YOU HEAR THE BELL?

The most famous Italian bass of his generation, Luigi Lablache (1794–1858), with an incredible deep compass and control of voice power, is given favorable mention in the conversation-books during the summer of 1823 at Hetzendorf.[103]

Franz Grillparzer noted that "Lablache, and in a degree Fodor, are better actors than the Germans ever had."[104]

Lablache sang with the Italian Opera Company at the Kärnthnerthor theater during the seasons 1823 to 1825 and 1827 and 1828.[105] In the Vienna theaters at that time it was customary for a bell to be rung to signal a change of scene. Lablache claimed that Beethoven, when dying, made the extraordinary remark to him: "Do you hear the bell? They are changing the scene!"[106]

NOTES

1. Beethoven's failure to insert the year led to a controversy over the date of this important letter. Wegeler, Schindler, Nohl, and Kalischer concluded that it was written in 1800, but Thayer argued persuasively in favor of 1801, and he was supported by MacArdle, Anderson, and Elliot Forbes. See Wegeler and Ries, *Remembering Beethoven*, 27–32, 174, n. 18; Schindler-Moscheles, II: 205; Schindler-MacArdle, 61; Ludwig Nohl, *Beethoven's Letters (1790–1826)*, trans. Lady Wallace, 2 vols. (London: Longmans, Green, 1866), no. 14, p. 20; Kalischer, *Beethoven's Letters*, no. 36, I: 29, 33; TDR, II: 271–74; TK, I: 299–301; TF, 283–85. For a lucid discussion of the controversy, see Alan Tyson, "Ferdinand Ries (1784–1838): The History of His Contribution to Beethoven Biography," *Nineteenth Century Music* vol. 7 (1984): 217.

2. Dr. Johann Peter Frank.

3. Dr. Gerhard von Vering.

4. Eleonore von Breuning.

5. A-51; B-65.

6. A-53; B-67.

7. Wegeler quoted this letter in the *Biographische Notizen*, and in the note he

identified the bark of *Daphne mezereum.* See Wegeler and Ries, *Remembering Beethoven*, 42.

8. Dr. Johann Adam Schmidt.

9. A-54; B-70. Beethoven also omitted the year of this letter, but Wegeler noted 16 November 1801 at the side of the autograph.

10. Sonneck, *Beethoven: Impressions*, 26.

11. Rochlitz published it in the AMZ, Leipzig, of 17 October 1827. Moscheles published a translation in the first English edition of Schindler's biography—Schindler-Moscheles, I: 80–87. The autograph is now in the State Library at Hamburg. For a facsimile, see *Beethovens Heiligenstädter Testament*, ed. W. Tiemann, (Offenbach, Germany: Wilhelm Kumm Verlag, 1984). See also TDR, II: 333–35.

12. The four string instruments given to Beethoven by Prince Carl Lichnowsky were a violin and a cello by Guarneri, a violin by Amati, and a viola dated 1690.

13. Anderson, *Letters*, Appendix A, pp. 1351–54; B-106.

14. F. G. Wegeler and F. Ries, *Biographische Notizen über Ludwig van Beethoven*, trans. Erna Schwerin (Koblenz, Germany: K. Bädeker, 1838), 98–99.

15. F. Kerst, *Die Erinnerungen an Beethoven*, 2 vols., trans. Erna Schwerin (Stuttgart: Julius Hoffmann, 1925), I: 105–6.

16. TDR, II: 168, trans. Erna Schwerin.

17. FRHB, II: 303; R. Rolland, *Beethoven the Creator; The Great Creative Epochs*, vol. I *From the Eroica to the Appassionata* (London: Victor Gollancz, 1929), 275.

18. TF, 373.

19. TF, 400; Rolland, *Beethoven the Creator*, 273.

20. TF, 439.

21. TF, 448–449.

22. L. Nohl, *Beethoven Depicted by His Contemporaries*, 68.

23. A-192; B-350.

24. Wegeler and Ries, *Remembering Beethoven*, 108. The validity of this anecdote was contested by Josef Bergauer who argued that, in view of Ludwig's recent quarrel with Caspar Carl, he would have been more likely to have taken refuge in the house of the poet Ignaz Franz Castelli at no. 4 Ballgasse. See George R. Marek, *Beethoven: Biography of a Genius* (London: William Kimber, 1974), 397.

25. A-267; B-459.

26. Trans. Erna Schwerin. I am most grateful to Dr. Sieghard Brandenburg, who personally checked this entry. The "Petter Sketchbook," containing seventy-four leaves, now in the H. C. Bodmer collection at the Beethoven-Archiv in Bonn (Mh 59), was written between September 1811 and December 1812. See JTW, 207–19. Thayer and Max Unger concluded erroneously that the first nine leaves belonged to the year 1809. See TDR, III: 152; TF, 473–74.

27. L. Nohl, *Beethoven Depicted by His Contemporaries*, 116.

28. Ibid., 122.

29. TF, 690.

30. Nettl, *Beethoven Encyclopedia*, 129.

31. Schindler-Moscheles, I: 149.

32. *Tagebuch*-27.

33. *Tours*, Conservatoire de Musique, SV 383, fols. 3 r, 2 v; *Paris Ms* 90, fol. 3 r. See JTW, 240.

34. *Tagebuch*-41.

35. *Tagebuch*-52. See also A-459; B-691.

36. It is illustrated in J. Schmidt-Görg and H. Schmidt, *Beethoven* (Bonn: Beethoven Archiv, 1972), 24.

37. TF, 690–91; George Thomas Ealy, "Of Ear Trumpets and a Resonance Plate: Early Hearing Aids and Beethoven's Hearing Perception," *Nineteenth Century Music* 17 (1994): 262–73.

38. A-844; B-1177.

39. Schünemann, *Beethovens Konversationshefte*, I: 186; LvBCB, I: 190, 463, n. 444. Baron A. J. von Stifft (1760–1836) was Imperial & Royal state and conference councillor, protomedicus, and president of the medical faculty. He lived at Ballplatz no. 29.

40. Dr. Gelineau, *Hygiène de l'oreille et des sourds*, 162, cited by Klotz-Forest, "La surdité de Beethoven," *La Chronique Médicale* 12 (1905): 331.

41. Robert Brilliant, "Beethoven on stamps," BN 3 (1988): 12–13.

42. TF, 565–66.

43. TF, 610–11.

44. TDR, III: 556–59. Bursy's diary was first published in the St. Petersburg Zeitung in 1854. Certain passages were censored.

45. L. Nohl, *Beethoven Depicted by His Contemporaries*, 153–54.

46. TDR, III: 566; TF, 647.

47. TDR, IV: 55–58. Potter also noted that Beethoven was less fluent in French.

48. TF, 683.

49. For a further discussion of the conversation-books, see TF, 730–32; Karl-Heinz Köhler, "The Conversation-Books: Aspects of a New Picture of Beethoven," in *Beethoven, Performers, and Critics*, ed. Robert Winter and Bruce Carr (Detroit: Wayne State University Press, 1980), 147–61; Marek, *Beethoven*, 642–46.

50. D. Beck and G. Herre, "Anton Schindlers fingierte Eintragungen in den Konversationsheften," in *Zu Beethoven*, vol. 1 *Aufsätze und Annotationen*, ed. Harry Goldschmidt, (Berlin: Verlag Neue Musik, 1979), 11–89; Peter Stadlen, "Schindler's Beethoven Forgeries," MT 118 (1977): 549–52; Peter Stadlen, "Schindler and the Conversation-Books," *Soundings* 7 (1978): 2–18; William S. Newman, "Yet Another Major Beethoven Forgery by Schindler?" JM 3 (1984): 397–422; D. Beck and G. Herre, "Anton Schindlers 'Nutzannendung' der Cramer-Etüden," in *Zu Beethoven*, vol. 3 (Berlin: Verlag Neue Musik, 1988), 177–208.

51. MacArdle, *An Index to Beethoven's Conversation-Books*.

52. See *Wiener Allgemeine Theater Zeitung*, no. 137, 15 November 1823; LvBCB, IV: 369, n. 447; Stadlen, "Schindler's Beethoven Forgeries," 551–52.

53. Schünemann, *Beethovens Konversationshefte*, I: 197; LvBCB, I: 200, trans. Erna Schwerin. The notice, that Hänke had died in 1817 in Bolivia, appeared on p. 82 of the *Austrian Observer* of 17 January 1820.

54. TK, I:xi; TF, 730–31.

55. A-785; B-1137.

56. For a discussion of Beethoven's pianos, see Derek Melville, "Beethoven's Pianos," in *The Beethoven Reader*, ed. D. Arnold and N. Fortune (New York: W. W. Norton, 1971), 41–67; William S. Newman, "Beethoven and the Piano: His Options, Preferences, Pianism, and Playing," in *Beethoven on Beethoven: Playing His Piano Music His Way*, ed. W. S. Newman (New York: W. W. Norton, 1988), 45–82.

57. For details of Beethoven in Mödling, see Frimmel, *Neue Beethoveniana*, 173–88.

58. AMZ, no. 18, 4 May 1864, trans. H.C.R. Landon, in *Beethoven: A Documentary Study*, 296. Emily Hill translated the device as a "leaden sounding-board." See L. Nohl, *Beethoven Depicted by His Contemporaries*, 164.

59. Schünemann, *Beethovens Konversationshefte*, I: 34; LvBCB, I: 42, 417 n. 48, and 49.

60. Ibid., I: 34; LvBCB, I: 42, 417 n. 50. The announcement of Dr. Chladni's lectures in Vienna, to commence on 14 April, appeared in the AMZ, Vienna, no. 28, 7 April 1819, p. 227.

61. LvBCB, I: 417, n. 51.

62. Breitkopf and Härtel published two of Dr. Chladni's books: *Die Akustic* (Leipzig, 1802); and *Neue Beiträge zur Akustic* (Leipzig, 1817).

63. *Tagebuch-54*.

64. A-533; B-789. Dr. Chladni had earlier written *Entdeckungen über die Theorie des Klanges* (Leipzig, 1787).

65. *Weiner Conversationsblatt*, no. 25, 225, in Schünemann, *Beethovens Konversationsheft*, I: 286, n. 1, trans. Erna Schwerin.

66. Schünemann, *Beethovens Konversationsheft*, I: 286; LvBCB, I: 291.

67. *Wiener Conversationsblatt*, no. 29, 273, in Schünemann, *Beethovens Konversationsheft*, I: 287, n. 2, trans. Erna Schwerin. See also LvBCB, I: 484, n. 673.

68. No. 87, p. 347.

69. LvBCB, I: 423, n. 101.

70. Schünemann, *Beethovens Konversationsheft*, I: 41–42, 49; LvBCB, I: 50, 57.

71. A-948; B-1292 (3 March 1819).

72. A-952, 963; B-1312, 1327.

73. A-995; B-1047 (1816/17).

74. A-997; B-1904 (November–December 1824).

75. A-977; B-1343.

76. FRHB, II: 176; Nettl, *Beethoven Encyclopedia*, 230.

77. Schünemann, *Beethovens Konversationsheft*, I: 91; LvBCB, I: 100.

78. A-1072; B-1457.

79. TF, 808.

80. L. Nohl, *Beethoven, Liszt, Wagner* (Vienna: Braumüller, 1874), 112; Solomon, *Beethoven*, 123.

81. FRHB, II: 163.

82. Sonneck, *Beethoven: Impressions*, 130–31.

83. TF, 812–13.

84. See LvBCB, III: 146, 157, 165, 166, 169, 170, 172–74, 449 n. 400.

85. See LvBCB, III: 169, 170; Jesserer and Bankl, *Die Krankheiten*, 38–39; Frida Knight, *Beethoven and the Age of Revolution* (London: Lawrence and Wishart, 1973), 111–12.

86. George Grove, *Beethoven and His Nine Symphonies*, 2nd ed. (London: Novello, Ewer, 1896), 334–35.

87. TF, 940–41.

88. Sonneck, *Beethoven: Impressions*, 192.

89. From *The Harmonicum*, December 1825, in Schindler-Moscheles, I: 296. The author was probably Mrs. Sarah Burney Payne, the daughter of a famous music historian, Dr. Charles Burney. During her visit on 27 September 1825, Beethoven inscribed a piano piece of thirteen measures to her, WoO 61a. See KHV, 507–8; TF, 956–57.

90. Melville, "Beethoven's Pianos," 45–46. For further information about Conrad Graf, see TDR, V: 252, 498; FRHB, I: 179.

91. Breuning, *Memories of Beethoven*, 72.

92. Schindler-Moscheles, II: 175–76.

93. Sonneck, *Beethoven: Impressions*, 208. Writing from memory to his second wife, Wieck placed his visit in May 1826. However, Riemann argued that it was probably at Hietzing in May 1824, since Beethoven's Broadwood piano was undergoing repairs by Graf in May 1826.

94. Ibid., 211.

95. TDR, V: 128, n. 4, trans. Erna Schwerin.

96. Ealy, "Of Ear Trumpets and a Resonance Plate," 271.

97. Breuning, *Memories of Beethoven*, 72.

98. Sonneck, *Beethoven: Impressions*, 202.

99. LvBCB, X: 148, 2 r, trans. Erna Schwerin.

100. Breuning, *Memories of Beethoven*, 72.

101. I. Von Seyfried, BS, trans. Henry Hugh Pierson (Hamburgh and New York: Schuberth, Leipzig, 1853), Appendix, 8.

102. Henry Krehbiel and Friedrich Kerst, *Beethoven: The Man and the Artist As Revealed in His Own Words* (New York: Dover, 1964), 109–10.

103. LvBCB, III: 374. For a discussion of Lablache, see Philip Robinson, "Luigi Lablache," in *New Grove* 10: 341–42.

104. LvBCB, III: 403; TF, 862.

105. LvBCB, III: 491, n. 881.

106. Wilhelm von Lenz, *Beethoven: Eine Kunststudie* (Hamburg: Hoffmann and Campe, 1885), I: 78; Rolland, *Beethoven: The Creator*, 405, n. 301.

3

Beethoven's Appearance

Beethoven was short and stocky with a height of 168.5 centimeters or 5 feet, 6 inches.[1] His sturdy, compact, muscular figure emanated great strength. Above the broad shoulders his large head was attached to a short neck.

His massive, high, wide forehead featured central vaulting between the frontal eminences so that it appeared like a shell. There were well-marked furrows above the root of the nose.

Beneath the attractive, thick, low brows were small, deep-set, expressive brown eyes. The nose was short, broad, and square, with finely shaped nostrils.

There was a prominent central philtrum in the upper lip, together with a slight protruding of the lower lip. The mouth was strong and sensitive, while under the oral fissure there was a deep transverse furrow.

The lower jaws were prominent, and the asymmetrical broad chin, unequally divided by a deep cleft, was especially irregular on the right side. His ruddy cheeks contrasted with a swarthy, dark-brown complexion, and his face was disfigured with numerous pockmarks and scars, especially in the forehead, glabella, nose, cheeks, and chin.[2]

Beethoven's abundant, bushy, long black hair fell in admirable, unruly disarray over his forehead, almost completely covering his ears, and he liked to toss it back when he extended his neck. By 1816 his hair had turned grey, and when he neglected shaving to allow his beard to grow, as he did frequently, there was accentuation of a wildness in his appearance which could on occasion incite fear. His fingers were short and stubby, and he always leaned forward a little when walking on his short legs.

It has been emphasized that every mood of Beethoven's being found instant powerful expression in his features, which were subject to sudden striking changes in appearance. When he laughed his eyes appeared to recede into their sockets, while when he was excited during musical inspirations, his eyes distended and gained prominence. During his melancholy spells his gaze was either devoid of any trace of pleasure of living, or piercing with an indefinable sadness. At the other extreme of exhilarated high mood, his arresting gaze and fiery expressive eyes would sparkle, or roll wildly, full of rude energy, in a radiant, vivid, animated countenance.[3]

Beethoven remained slim until his early thirties. Among his contemporaries there is disagreement about the color of his eyes. Anton Schindler stated they were brown,[4] as recently did Anne-Louise Coldicott.[5] Beethoven's eyes were painted brown in the portraits executed by C. Hornemann (1803), W. J. Mähler (1815), F. Schimon (1818–1819), J. Stieler (1819–1820), and F. Waldmüller (1823); however, they are green in B. Höfel's copper engraving after Louis Letronne (1814). A. Klöber, who painted his portrait over several sittings during the summer at Mödling in 1817, stated that his eyes were bluish-grey.[6] The unreliable K. J. Braun von Braunthal asserted they were grey.[7]

BEETHOVEN'S DRESS

At Mödling in 1817, Klöber noted that Beethoven was dressed in a light-blue coat with yellow buttons and white waistcoat and neckcloth, as was then the fashion, but his dress was "negligé."[8] Perhaps that outfit was purchased the previous year, which would account for Dr. Carl von Bursy's description of his "gala costume."[9]

Johann A. Schlosser's claim that "Beethoven's dress was always immaculate" is untrue.[10] Even in the late 1790s Frau von Bernhard found his very ordinary attire below standard,[11] and Franz Grillparzer noted that his dress was less elegant after 1805.[12] His preference for clean linen was often offset by his irregular domestic disorder.

In 1821 Sir John Russell stated that Beethoven's neglect of his person contributed to a wild appearance.[13] In 1822 Gioacchino Rossini was saddened at his apparent destitution and shabbiness,[14] and Johann Rochlitz noted a neglected, almost uncivilized outward appearance.[15] The following year, Carl Maria von Weber described a rough, repellent man who was dressed in a shabby house robe with torn sleeves.[16] While Dr. W. C. Müller found him in unconventional dress without a collar,[17] Samuel Spiker considered that his plain grey morning suit blended well with his cheerful, jovial face and disordered hair.[18]

Admittedly it should be emphasized that Beethoven held no court appointment in Vienna, which would have obliged him to dress appropriately for official ceremonies. No doubt his depression, thriftiness, and withdrawal from society all contributed to his negligent dress. In 1821 this great genius was actually arrested as a tramp.[19]

Gerhard von Breuning stated that Beethoven dressed like a plain townsman, and he gave an excellent description of the composer in his later years.[20] Beethoven's dress is well captured in the pencil drawings made by J. D. Böhm,

J.P.T. Lyser, M. Tejcek, and J. Weidner. It is not difficult to imagine his pockets bulging with a thick carpenter's pencil, an ear trumpet, a sketchbook, and a pad to use for conversation.

In his estate Beethoven's clothing and personal linen were valued at 37 fl. C.M. His wardrobe included two cloth coats, two spencers, two Prince Alberts, one blue cloth overcoat, sixteen knee stockings, eight pairs of trousers, two hats, six pairs of boots, fourteen shirts, eighteen pairs of socks, night attire, and underwear. His silver watch was valued at 8 fl., and an oval ring with precious stones was estimated at 90 fl.[21]

BEETHOVEN'S VOICE

In Bonn Beethoven acquired a strong provincial Rhenish accent, which he retained in Vienna where it was blended in an odd mixture with the colloquial Viennese dialect. Following the onset of deafness he tended to shout, especially when upset. His singing voice was a deep bass which lost its sonority after his hearing impairment developed. His laugh was loud, exaggerated, and unpleasant.[22]

SMALLPOX

There is no documentation of illness during his childhood, but of course he no doubt would have suffered the usual coughs and colds that afflict us all, despite the absence of a record.

Most authors, including Alexander Wheelock Thayer and Theodor von Frimmel, have nevertheless concluded that Beethoven suffered smallpox in his childhood, which would account for his pockmarked face.[23] In 1829 Johann Andreas and Nanette Streicher, intimately acquainted with Beethoven, were interviewed in Vienna by Vincent and Mary Novello. The Streichers placed an 1812 Franz Klein bust of Beethoven before the Novellos, and they asserted that the facial pockmarks and the scarred chin, especially on the right side, were the result of smallpox.[24] In his letter to publisher Franz Anton Hoffmeister of Leipzig, dated 8 April 1802, Beethoven made passing mention of several errors in the new edition of his Opus 18 Quartets (published by Mollo and Co.) and went on to pun on the word *Stich* (which translates as prick, stitch, sting, bite, stab, cut, engraving): "My skin is quite full of pricks and scratches."[25]

I also support the substantial medical view that Beethoven's facial pockmarks were presumably the sequela of smallpox contracted during his childhood.[26] Johann van Beethoven's face was also pockmarked, suggesting the possibility that father and son contracted smallpox together, although that was not necessarily so. Furthermore, physician Dr. Gerhard von Breuning affirmed that Beethoven's face was spotted with "brown smallpox depressions," which were evident in Klein's life mask.[27]

Edward Larkin, while conceding that the smaller, discrete, and confluent scars on Beethoven's face were compatible with previous smallpox, argued, however, that the larger lesions and indurations were not typical of it, but rather suggestive of systemic lupus erythematosus. Larkin drew particular attention to the 5 cm × 2 cm area of deep scarring in the middle of the forehead, extending down the nose, and especially the elongated 1.5 cm × 0.5 cm atrophic scar on the right side of the nose, as being typical of systemic lupus erythematosus. He proposed an onset at the age of sixteen.[28] While the precise date of onset of Beethoven's facial scars is unknown, it was probably before 1783, since the pockmarks are evident in the anonymous portrait made at the age of thirteen that Beethoven gave to Zmeskall.[29] It is highly improbable, however, that Beethoven would have survived over forty-three years from such a serious disorder as systemic lupus erythematosus without effective treatment.

Dr. T. G. Palferman advocated that the existing scars from smallpox in childhood were later affected by sarcoidosis, causing "lupus pernio" or "nodular granulomatous infiltration."[30] However, that is unlikely not only because there is no mention in the literature of any alteration of the scars, but also because there is no significant change in the appearance of the scars in Carl Danhauser's death mask, when compared with Klein's life mask.

Voltaire estimated that sixty out of every hundred people would contract smallpox during their life. Wolfgang Amadeus Mozart came down with a serious attack of smallpox in 1767 during an epidemic in Vienna.[31] Even though Edward Jenner had published his pioneering studies into the discovery of vaccination in 1798, in 1806 there were 2,330 deaths in Vienna from smallpox.[32]

NOTES

1. According to Schindler, he was 5 Fuss 4 Zoll Wiener Mass: Schindler-Moscheles, II: 191; Bankl and Jesserer, *Die Krankheiten*, 70. 1 Wiener Fuss = 31.6 cm; 1 Wiener Zoll = 2.63 cm.

2. The pockmarks are well reproduced in the life mask and the death mask.

3. For accounts of Beethoven's appearance, see L. Nohl, *Beethoven Depicted by His Contemporaries*, 1–374; T. von Frimmel, "Beethovens Äussere Erscheinung," in BS (Munich: Georg Müller, 1905), I: 1–170; T. von Frimmel, *Beethoven im zeitgenössischen Bildnis* (Vienna: Karl König, 1923), 1–114; Sonneck, *Beethoven: Impressions*, 1–231; W. Barclay Squire, "Beethoven's Appearance," Music and Letters, 8 (1927): 122–5; Nettl, *Beethoven Encyclopedia*, 5–7.

4. Schindler-Moscheles, II: 192.

5. B. Cooper, *Beethoven Compendium*, 102.

6. L. Nohl, *Beethoven Depicted by His Contemporaries*, 166.

7. Ibid., 301; O. E. Deutsch, *Schubert: Memoirs by His Friends* (New York: Macmillan 1958), 249.

8. L. Nohl, *Beethoven Depicted by His Contemporaries*, 166.

9. Ibid., 157.

10. J. A. Schlosser, *Beethoven: The First Biography*, ed. B. Cooper, trans. R. G. Pauly (Portland, Oreg.: Amadeus Press, 1996), 105.

11. Sonneck, *Beethoven: Impressions*, 20.

12. Ibid., 154.

13. Ibid., 114.

14. Ibid., 117.

15. Ibid., 122.

16. Ibid., 161.

17. L. Nohl, *Beethoven Depicted by His Contemporaries*, 189–90.

18. Sonneck, *Beethoven: Impressions*, 210.

19. TF, 777–78.

20. Breuning, *Memories of Beethoven*, 70–2.

21. TF, 1074.

22. Nettl, *Beethoven Encyclopedia*, 239–40.

23. TF, 253; Frimmel, *Neue Beethoveniana*, 216; P. Bekker, *Beethoven* (London: J. M. Dent, 1925), 41; A. de Hevesy, *Beethoven: The Man* (London: Faber and Gwyer, 1927), 52; J. Schmidt-Görg and H. Schmidt, eds., *Ludwig van Beethoven*, 246.

24. N. Medici di Marignano and R. Hughes, *A Mozart Pilgrimage: Being the Travel Diaries of Vincent and Mary Novello in the Year 1824* (London: Novello, 1955), 194.

25. A-57; B-84.

26. Klotz-Forest, "La dernière maladie et la mort de Beethoven," *La Chronique Médicale* 13 (1906): 246; Forster, *Beethovens Krankheiten*, 8; M. Piroth, "Beethovens letzte Krankheit auf Grund der zeitgenössischen medizinischen Quellen," *Beethoven-Jahrbuch* (1959–1960): 11; S. J. London, "Beethoven: Case Report of a Titan's Last Crisis," *Archives of Internal Medicine* 113 (1964): 444; Bankl and Jesserer, *Die Krankheiten*, 10.

27. Breuning, *Memories of Beethoven*, 44.

28. Edward Larkin, "Beethoven's Illness—A Likely Diagnosis," *Proceedings of the Royal Society of Medicine* 64 (1971): 496; Edward Larkin, "Beethoven's Medical History," in *Beethoven: The Last Decade 1817–1827*, ed. Martin Cooper (Oxford: Oxford University Press, 449.

29. H. C. Landon, *Beethoven: A Documentary Study* (London: Thames and Hudson, 1970, abr., 1974), no. 4, p. 6 (abridged ed.); Samuel Geiser and Rita Steblin, "The Unknown Portrait of Beethoven As a Thirteen-year old," BN 6 (1991): 57, 64–67.

30. T. G. Palferman, "Classical Notes: Beethoven's Medical History: Variations on a Rheumatological Theme," *Journal of the Royal Society of Medicine* 83 (1990): 644.

31. For an account of Mozart's smallpox, see Davies, *Mozart in Person*, 25–30.

32. A. M. Hanson, *Musical Life in Biedermeier Vienna* (Cambridge: Cambridge University Press, 1985), 12.

4

Final Illness, Death, and Burial

The details of Beethoven's last illness have been documented by Alexander Wheelock Thayer,[1] Anton Schindler,[2] Gerhard von Breuning,[3] Ludwig Nohl,[4] Stephan Ley,[5] and other scholars.[6] Previous accounts by other physicians should also be consulted.[7]

It must be emphasized that Schindler's spiteful, vengeful attacks on Johann van Beethoven, the nephew Carl, Dr. Andreas Ignaz Wawruch, and Dr. Johann Malfatti, endorsed in good faith by Gerhard von Breuning, were completely unfounded.[8]

THE HASTY RETURN TO VIENNA FROM GNEIXENDORF

Schindler's scandalous assertion that Beethoven's precipitate return to the Austrian capital was related to maltreatment by his brother Johann, who refused him the use of his carriage, was untrue. The conversation-book entries, extracted by Thayer, show that in the latter part of November 1826, Beethoven became restless to return to Vienna.

There is also a reflection of perennial quarrels with Johann and his wife, together with the frequent reproaches of Carl. However, it is submitted that Beethoven's major concern at that time was the deterioration of his health, and he felt an urgent need to consult with his doctors. We have seen that he was troubled with weight loss, abdominal distention, swollen feet, excessive thirst, loss of appetite, diarrhea, and abdominal discomfort.

Following an argument with Johann, Beethoven decided hastily to return to Vienna. At such short notice it would appear that the only available transport was an open milkwagon (*Leiterwagen*). In his retrospective report Dr. Wawruch wrote,

He was anxious about the possibility to become helpless in the event of acute illness and isolation in the country, and therefore longed to return to Vienna. According to his own, jokingly made report, he used the most wretched transportation of the devil for his return home.

December was rough, wet, and cold. Beethoven's clothing was not fit for this unfriendly season, yet he was driven by an inner unrest, a gloomy premonition for disaster. It was necessary for him to stay overnight in a country inn, where he could only obtain an unheated room which was without window insulation. Toward midnight he felt the first chill and fever, accompanied by strong thirst and pain in his sides. He drank ice cold water in large quantities, looking forward hopefully to the first beam of light. Tired and ill he had himself placed on the carriage, finally arriving in Vienna ill and exhausted.[9]

HIS LAST ABODE IN THE HOUSE OF THE BLACK-ROBED SPANIARDS

It was on Saturday, 2 December 1826, that Beethoven returned for the last time to his lodgings in the Schwarzspanierhaus, which originally had been a Jesuit seminary. He sent Carl to fetch Dr. Anton Braunhofer, who refused to come because the distance was too far. Then Dr. Jakob Staudenheim was sent for, but though he agreed to come, he failed to attend immediately.

Beethoven then implored Carl Holz to find him a physician. Holz initially tried to secure the services of the medical consultant Dr. Dominik Vivenot, but he was unable to come because he himself was sick.[10] Holz therefore turned next to Carl Bogner's physician, Dr. Wawruch, who was a professor at the hospital. Wawruch agreed to come after dinner.[11]

Schindler's charge that Dr. Wawruch was summoned by a billiards marker in a coffeehouse frequented by Carl is yet a further example of his bitter scandalmongering.[12] Nanette Streicher's criticism of Dr. Wawruch to Vincent and Mary Novello was also unwarranted:

Beethoven's life might probably have been prolonged for some time had he continued to employ the King's Physician whom he had consulted at the commencement of his illness—but he was fearful that his means would be inadequate to meet the fees that might be thus incurred and he had too high a spirit to accept any attendance as a favour conferred upon him.[13]

It will become apparent that effective medical treatment for Beethoven's final illness was not then available and that Dr. Wawruch's treatment at that time was exemplary.

DR. WAWRUCH'S INITIAL VISIT

After dinner on 5 December, Dr. Wawruch visited his deaf, bedridden patient for the first time. He obtained the medical history by having Beethoven's nephew Carl write down a series of direct questions in the conversation-book.

Dr. Wawruch asked Beethoven whether he suffered from hemorrhoids or headache and when his bowels last moved. The doctor studied Beethoven's chest and abdomen as he took a deep breath. He inquired how long had his abdomen been so distended, how frequently was he passing urine and was there any difficulty with the passage, how long had his feet been swollen, had he ever passed blood from the rectum, and had he ever before this suffered with a chill or feverish attack. After the examination, Dr. Wawruch reassured him that he would make every effort to make him well.[14]

Unfortunately, several of Dr. Wawruch's entries were removed, presumably by Schindler.[15] Nor have his visitors' entries on slate survived.[16] Fortunately, the entries concerning Dr. Wawruch's initial treatment are extant. He prescribed weak tea to promote perspiration. Towels soaked in juniper were to be applied to the abdomen every one and a half to two hours. A laxative was also prescribed, and if he had not moved his bowels by 7 P.M., the maid Thekla was to fetch the barber to administer an enema. Two tablespoons of lukewarm medicine were to be taken every hour, while prunes and sugar were encouraged.

On 11 December Dr. Wawruch found Beethoven's abdomen to be less distended. He prescribed raspberry juice and permitted a little white wine diluted with water. He also encouraged liberal amounts of parsley and celery soup.[17]

In his retrospective report Dr. Wawruch wrote:

I was called only on the third day. I found Beethoven with ominous symptoms of pneumonia [*Lungenentzündung*]: his face hot, he had bloody sputum, he was in danger of choking, and the pain in his side permitted only an uncomfortable position on his back. Anti-inflammatory treatment soon brought about the desired relief: his nature was victorious, and freed him from the apparent mortal danger by the passing of the crisis. On the fifth day he was able to sit up and to describe to me his plight with great emotion. On the seventh day he was sufficiently recovered to be able to get up, walk around, and read and write.

But on the eighth day I was shocked to observe on my morning visit to find him very upset, and jaundiced all over his body; terrible diarrhoea with emesis [*Brechdurchfall*] had become life-threatening the previous night. A powerful rage over his undeserved illness resulted in a strong emotional explosion. He trembled, writhing in pain in his liver and bowels, and his feet, heretofore only moderately swollen, were now severely oedematous. From that point on, dropsy developed: he urinated less, his liver showed clear signs of hardened nodes, the jaundice increased. The loving support of his friends appeased his excitement, and he soon forgot his ordeal. But the illness progressed rapidly. Already during the third week attacks of nocturnal choking appeared: the enormous volume of the accumulated water required immediate intervention, and I felt compelled to suggest an abdominal puncture to prevent the possibility of a sudden rupture. After a few moments of serious thought, Beethoven agreed to the operation, supported by the opinion of Ritter von Staudenheim who had been called in for consultation, and who recommended the same procedure as indispensable and urgent. The Chief Surgeon of the General Hospital, Dr. Seibert, made the incision with the skill usually attributed to him, so that Beethoven happily exclaimed at the appearance of a stream of water that the surgeon impresses him like Moses who struck the rock with his staff, drawing water in this way.

Relief was soon obtained. The liquid amounted to 25 lbs. [7.7 liters],[18] and the secondary flow was certainly five times this amount.

A carelessness resulting in the loosening of the dressing during the night, presumably for the purpose of removal of the water as quickly as possible, almost spoiled the pleasure of the improvement. A severe erysipeloid inflammation, exhibiting signs of incipient gangrene, appeared, but careful drying of the edges of the wound soon arrested this unhealthy development. Happily, the three subsequent operations were without the least sequelae.

During his final illness Beethoven at last found a faithful, devoted house-keeper and cook, Sali, who had been recommended by the von Breunings. His maid, Thekla, who served him in Gneixendorf, had to be dismissed when she was found to be dishonest. Carl was always close at hand to attend to his every need, and the apothecary, Johann, was in regular attendance, from about 10 December, with advice about diet and medications. A warning bell was placed close by on the bedside table.

The main ingredients of Dr. Wawruch's anti-inflammatory treatment were bed rest, warmth, the promotion of sweating by the administration of sudorific drugs or diaphoretic herbs, and especially regular evacuations of the bowel. If aperients and purgatives failed to stimulate a bowel action, then a barber was to be called at 7:00 P.M. to administer an enema. On such occasions Carl encouraged Beethoven to take a deep breath to assist in retaining the enema for as long as possible. Carl also obtained a chamber pot and a urine bottle for his uncle. All urine was to be kept until examined by Dr. Wawruch.

Rice soup, fruit, or soup containing barley, parsley, and celery were encouraged. The von Breuning kitchen assisted with his meals. Alcohol was restricted to a little diluted white wine. Only one cup of coffee was permitted, though herbal tea and raspberry juice were encouraged.

Dr. Wawruch prescribed liberal quantities of almond milk and two table-spoons of lukewarm medicine every hour. Hot towels, dipped in juniper, were to be applied repeatedly to his swollen abdomen during the day and also at night, if he awakened with discomfort. His maid was to remain close at hand for the necessary changing of the towels.[19]

WAS THE DIAGNOSIS OF PNEUMONIA CORRECT?

Dr. Wawruch was most attentive to Beethoven. Following the initial consultation on 5 December, he made two visits the next day, and then called every day until 14 December.[20]

In his first edition, Schindler criticized Dr. Wawruch's delay in the diagnosis of dropsy:

The malady which brought him back to Vienna, on the occasion just mentioned, was an inflammation of the lungs, soon followed by symptoms of dropsy. These at first Professor

Wawruch refused to recognise, but they increased so rapidly that it was no longer possible to doubt the nature of the disease.[21]

In his third edition, Schindler changed his wording.

The illness from which Beethoven was suffering was an inflammation of the lungs, a complication that developed from his intestinal chill. This condition was diagnosed much too late by Dr. Wawruch and, by the time the correct diagnosis was made, the phase of dropsy was already far advanced.[22]

Schindler's criticisms of Dr. Wawruch were unwarranted since we have already seen that Beethoven showed evidence of fluid retention in Gneixendorf, well before his departure to Vienna.

However there is more substance to Dr. Gerhard von Breuning's criticism of Professor Wawruch's diagnosis of pneumonia. Dr. von Breuning postulated three reasons to support his contention that Beethoven's "pain in his side" emanated from a peritonitis, an inflammatory disorder within his abdomen, rather than pneumonia:

Firstly, only peritonitis, and not pneumonia, can produce dropsy; secondly, although there was a catarrhal irritation of the respiratory organs at the beginning of the illness, he did not cough throughout his illness, his voice remained strong and he had no pain in breathing except to the extent that later the excessive accumulations of liquid in the abdomen exerted an alarmingly constricting pressure upwards; and finally, during the three days of his struggle for life his lungs were so completely healthy and strong that there could be no question of a previous pneumonia.[23]

Breuning's first objection was invalid, for it is now known that in patients with hepatic cirrhosis and portal hypertension, a severe infection anywhere in the body may precipitate hepatic decompensation, as manifested by fluid retention and other symptoms. His second point, that Beethoven's attacks of breathlessness were apparently due to the accumulation of intra-abdominal ascitic fluid, rather than a primary respiratory disorder, seems to be true. Breuning's third objection was incorrect. The absence of respiratory symptoms during the last three days of Beethoven's life does not exclude the possibility of pneumonia at the onset of his final illness nearly four months earlier.

In the early stages, ascites is easily overlooked, but the abdomen becomes gradually distended, assuming a barrel shape, giving way to breathlessness caused by the impaired action of the diaphragm. Unfortunately, Dr. Wawruch made no mention of his findings from a physical examination of Beethoven's chest. Admittedly, a history of coughing pink or "rusty" sputum, as opposed to "blood-streaked" sputum, would have supported a diagnosis of pneumonia, but such a history is not certain.

The specific German words for hemorrhage from the lungs, or pulmonary hemorrhage are *Lungenbluten, Hämoptoe, Lungenblutung*, or *Blutsturz*.[24] Dr.

Wawruch's description, "*Er spuckte Blut*," lacks specificity in translation. The literal translation is "He spat blood." Perhaps Dr. Wawruch was uncertain as to the origin of the hemorrhage. Although, as indicated above, it implies that "he had bloody sputum," it could also mean that "he expectorated blood." We have seen that Beethoven was subject to nose bleeds. Perhaps the blood in his spit emanated from the back of his nose?

A less likely possibility is that the blood regurgitated from the stomach from gastro-oesophageal varices, which may occur in patients with cirrhosis and portal hypertension.

Though Beethoven's clinical improvement between the fifth and seventh day of his illness is in keeping with resolution of pneumonia by crisis, his relapse and second rigor on the eighth day is not typical of pneumonia. Prior to the antibiotic era, the resolution of pneumococcal pneumonia by crisis occurred between the seventh and tenth day. The crisis was manifested by diaphoresis, abrupt defervescence, and a dramatic improvement in well-being. Recurrent rigors in a patient with pneumonia suggest either a microorganism other than the pneumococcus, or the development of a septic complication such as empyema, lung abscess, meningitis, or endocarditis.[25]

There is therefore significant doubt about the validity of Dr. Wawruch's diagnosis of pneumonia. Furthermore, while at the autopsy Beethoven's lungs were normal, there was evidence of renal papillary necrosis.[26] The composer's symptoms and the course of his final illness are in keeping with this diagnosis.

However there is no doubt that the initial affliction, whatever it was, precipitated further hepatic decompensation, made evident by jaundice and worsening fluid retention, by way of ascites and edema.

In the middle of December, the arrival of George Frideric Handel's works provided a pleasant distraction from his sufferings.[27] Around 19 December he received a visit from Johann Baptist Jenger, who noted that he had not shaved in three weeks and that "he himself lay in bed suffering terribly." Jenger was informed that Beethoven was suffering from "dropsy in the chest."[28]

WAS AN OPERATION APPROPRIATE?

Dr. Wawruch's decision, in consultation with Dr. Staudenheim, to recommend an operation to relieve the abdominal distention and difficulty in breathing caused by a tense ascites was correct because effective diuretic agents were then not available. Today, a therapeutic abdominal paracentesis would not be performed for the relief of ascites complicating hepatic cirrhosis because it is now known that such a procedure aggravates the already existing electrolyte disturbances and protein depletion. Today, after the aspiration of a little fluid for diagnostic purposes, the ascites would be treated with restricted intake of salt and effective modern diuretic drugs.

At the first operation on 20 December 1826, in Beethoven's apartment, Seibert was assisted by Wawruch; nephew Carl, brother Johann, and Schindler were also present. Dr. Wawruch reassured Beethoven that he would obtain relief in half an hour. Five and one-half Mass (equivalent to 7.7 liters) was measured off. After the operation he was to remain lying on his side.[29]

Beethoven's grim humor did not desert him for, after the puncture, he exclaimed, "Better water from the body, than water from the pen."[30]

Dr. Seibert made daily visits at 1:00 P.M. from 20–23 December. Johann van Beethoven prepared a Salep decoction.[31] Further enemas were administered. Only one cup of coffee was permitted in the morning, but herbal tea and almond milk were encouraged. Thekla carried barley soup from the von Breuning's kitchen.

JANUARY 1827

It was not a happy new year for the seriously ill composer. On 2 January Carl departed to join Lieutenant Field Marshall Baron Josef von Stutterheim's regiment at Iglau. The following day, Beethoven drafted a copy of his will nominating Carl as his sole heir.[32]

Within a few days of the first abdominal paracentesis, there was a recurrent buildup of fluid. As is evident in the conversation-book entries, 5–8 January, Dr. Seibert was trying to delay a second operation, and Beethoven was disgruntled about Dr. Wawruch's treatment.

THE SECOND OPERATION

On 8 January, Dr. Seibert performed a second abdominal paracentesis. He noted that the ascitic fluid was clearer, and he drew off 10 Mass (14 liters).[33]

Beethoven was increasingly concerned at his lack of progress, and on being informed of Dr. Wawruch's impending arrival he would turn to the wall saying, "Oh, that ass!" Gerhard von Breuning later criticized Wawruch's excessive prescription of drugs, recalling two occasions when the housekeeper, Sali, returned 80 six-ounce bottles to the dispensary to collect the refund. Dr. Wawruch also prescribed two teaspoons of cream of tartar and sugar to be added to his drinking water.[34]

Schindler also later criticized Dr. Wawruch's prescribing habits: "He ruined him with too many medications; during this period he had counted 75 bottles, not including the different powders, of consumption, and generally, he had no confidence in this doctor."[35]

Johann also clashed with Dr. Wawruch over the medication prescribed. For example, aware that digitalis was beneficial in cases of cardiac dropsy, he advocated that it should be prescribed for his brother. Aware of the potentially fatal toxic effects of digitalis in this situation, Dr. Wawruch refused. It is now known that the toxic effects of digitalis on the heart are enhanced by the presence of potassium depletion (hypokalemia), which is commonly present in patients with ascites due to cirrhosis.

THE COUNCIL OF PHYSICIANS

According to Schindler, Beethoven expressed a preference to be treated by Dr. Malfatti, with whom he had parted company in 1817. Over his concern with his responsibility to comply with medical ethics, Dr. Malfatti initially refused to become involved: "Tell Beethoven that he, the Master of harmony, must know that I have to live with my colleagues also in harmony." However, after several requests from Schindler, Dr. Malfatti agreed to come, albeit to attend initially in consultation with other physicians who had been involved in Beethoven's care.[36] The council of physicians, involving a consultation among Wawruch, Staudenheim, Braunhofer, and Malfatti, took place on 11 January. No doubt Dr. Wawruch, who would have been aware of the serious prognosis, would have been relieved to share the responsibility for the medical care of so famous a patient.

The deaf composer agreed to this consultation which had been urged by Schindler and Beethoven's brother Johann.[37] According to Schindler, after a reconciliation between Beethoven and Malfatti at a private meeting on 19 January, the wily Italian physician made frequent visits, although Dr. Wawruch remained in charge and continued to call daily.[38]

In his letter of 12 January 1827 to Frau Marie Pachler Koschak, Jenger commented on the council:

A consultation about Beethoven took place yesterday, the outcome of which I wanted to await in order to give you as much detailed information as possible about the illness of the great Master.

Until now, Professor Wawruch, reputed to be quite intelligent as a doctor, has treated B. However, at the consultation the highly respected Dr. Malfatti declared that B. (whose former doctor Malfatti had been, and who asserted to be thoroughly familiar with B's nature) was not treated correctly. He prescribed nothing: fruit ices and stomach rubs with ice cold water—nothing else—with which Malfatti has supposed to have completely cured a patient with similar complaints.

But will B. be able to tolerate this remedy? This is a question which only time can answer. After the second puncture 5–6 days ago, B. seems to feel somewhat better; but for his complete recovery there is little, but perhaps still some hope.[39]

The revival of Beethoven's spirits engendered by the initial small doses of alcohol was spectacular, as noted by the composer in a note to Schindler: "Miracle, miracle, miracle! Both most learned men [Wawruch and Seibert] have been beaten. I will be saved only by Malfatti's knowledge. It is necessary for you to come to me this morning for a moment. Yours Beethoven."[40]

Let us now resume Dr. Wawruch's report:

Beethoven was fully aware that the paracentesis was only palliative, and expected the renewed increase in fluid, the more so as the rainy and cold winter season favours the recurrence of the malady, thus exacerbating the basic medical problems of chronic liver disease and organic illness of the lower digestive system. It is strange that Beethoven was unable to tolerate almost none of the medications, even after his successful operations, except those that were easily soluble. His appetite decreased from day to day, and his strength was bound to diminish significantly from the frequent loss of fluids. Now Dr. Malfatti who supported me with his advice from that time on, and understood Beethoven's inclination towards alcoholic beverages (he had been a long-time friend of his), hit upon the idea to suggest frozen punch. I must confess that this remedy worked extremely well at least for a few days. Beethoven felt so restored by this ice, laced with wine, that he slept right through the first night quietly, sweating profusely. He was lively and often full of humorous ideas, and even dreamed that he would be able to finish his oratorio *Saul and David* which he had begun. As can be expected, his joy was short-lived. He misused the prescription and heartily imbibed in punch. The alcohol soon caused a strong congestion of blood in the head; he became soporous, he gurgled like someone deeply under the influence of alcohol, began to talk incoherently, and a few times he suffered from an inflammatory sore throat with hoarseness, even voicelessness. He became more active, and as soon as he had caught a chill in his bowels, causing colic and diarrhea, it was time to withdraw this delicious treat.

A HAYSEED VAPOR BATH

On 25 January Schindler brought word from the mother of the singer Fräulein Schechner about a remedy that had cured her seventy-year-old husband: juniper berry tea and a hayseed vapor bath (*Heublumenbad*). Dr. Malfatti, aware that these remedies had been prescribed by Dr. Harz for the late king of Bavaria, also recommended them for Beethoven.[41]

After jugs of hot water had been poured over dried birch leaves, Beethoven sat immersed in the water while the bath and his body up to his neck were covered with a sheet. The excessive sweating induced by this "sauna" was supposed to be beneficial, but Beethoven was unable to tolerate the treatment because of increasing abdominal distention.[42] To make matters worse, the herbal tea caused diarrhea.

If Dr. Malfatti himself could not come, his assistant, Dr. Röhrich, came in his place. On 27 January the proof corrections of the E-flat Major Quartet, Op. 127, were sent to B. Schott's Sons at Mainz.

THE THIRD OPERATION

Following the third abdominal paracentesis on 3 February, Beethoven was to remain on his back during the morning, but was to turn onto his right side in the afternoon. Dr. Malfatti wondered whether a tube might be inserted into the wound so as to allow free drainage of the fluid, but Dr. Seibert said that this was not possible.

Dr. Malfatti also advised that Beethoven should remain out of bed for half an hour twice a day, so as to prevent bed sores. Oil cloth was purchased to prevent the bed sheets becoming wet from fluid dripping from the wound.[43]

Juniper berries heated in herbal tea were prescribed to promote the flow of urine. A little veal was permitted, together with ice for sucking. During Dr. Wawruch's visit on 11 February, Beethoven asked him if he could drink wine. Dr. Wawruch and Dr. Malfatti both recommended a fine Mosel wine. Stephan von Breuning supplied a fine bottle while Dr. Malfatti sent a very old Gumpoldskirchner.[44]

Subsequently, on two occasions, Beethoven placed an order with Bernard Schott's Sons for a few bottles of unadulterated old white Rhine or Moselle wines.[45] It would appear that Malfatti and Wawruch, aware of the hopeless prognosis, did not want to deny him the pleasure of imbibing old German wines of excellence, though Beethoven himself believed that these wines would bring him refreshment, strength, and health. In his letter of 17 February to Franz Gerhard Wegeler, he stated, "My recovery, if I may call it so, is still very slow. Presumably I must expect a fourth operation, although the doctors have not yet said anything about this. I cultivate patience and think: well, sometimes some good comes from all this evil."[46]

MELANCHOLY

During his final illness, Beethoven remained subject to recurrent spells of melancholy.[47] He missed Carl and was concerned not only about his survival but especially about his lack of income. The latter worry prompted his importunate letters to Stumpff, Moscheles, and Smart in London.[48] Admittedly he was also troubled by the failure of Prince Galitzin to honor his debt for the string quartets. The exaggeration of this problem in his mind by his depression is well accounted for by the development of a delusion of poverty.

In mid-February Antonio Diabelli gave him a recently published lithograph of Joseph Haydn's birthplace at Rohrau in Lower Austria. Gerhard von Breuning's piano teacher, Anton Heller, hurriedly made a frame of black polished wood and added the caption, "Jos. Hayden's Birthplace in Rohrau." When the misspelling of Haydn's name was pointed out to Beethoven, he became angry and upset and remained irritable about it till the error was erased.[49]

GERHARD VON BREUNING'S VISITS

During the early months of 1827, Stephan von Breuning was also ill with liver disease. How Beethoven would have looked forward to the frequent visits of fourteen-year-old Gerhard von Breuning.

In his letter of 22 February to Moscheles, Schindler wrote, "As it is already apparent, the dropsy will cause emaciation [*Abzehrung*]; for he is only skin and bone now; but his constitution will still resist this horrendous end for a long time."[50]

THE OTHER VISITORS

Apart from the regular visits made by his family, Schindler, and the Breunings, Carl Holz also came frequently. His friend Ignaz von Gleichenstein made several visits, including one with his wife and son. Of course, Schuppanzigh, Dolezálek, and Linke came to see him, and Count Moritz Lichnowsky entertained him with gossip from the theaters. Although he was confined to his room with gout, Nikolaus Zmeskall kept in touch through Schindler, and on 18 February Beethoven wrote him a note of condolence.

Beethoven's other visitors included Tobias Haslinger and his son Carl, Diabelli, the banker Heribert Rau, J. Schikh, Johann Andreas Streicher, violinist Franz Clement, soprano Nanette Schechner and her fiancé tenor Ludwig Cramolini, Schindler's sister, and wealthy merchant Johann Nepomuk Wolfmayer.[51] Wolfmayer, who had earlier commissioned a Requiem Mass, was rewarded with the dedication of the String Quartet in F, Op. 135.

Beethoven read Sir Walter Scott's *Kenilworth* and some of his old favorites by Plutarch, Homer, Plato, Aristotle, and Friedrich von Schiller. Gerhard von Breuning also offered him a world history written by Schröckh and some descriptions of summer travel.[52]

Johann Streicher, Stephan Breuning, and Dr. Malfatti gave Beethoven gifts of fine wine.

THE FOURTH OPERATION

On 27 February Dr. Seibert performed a fourth abdominal paracentesis. Some of the fluid leaked onto the floor forming a big puddle which extended to the center of the large bedroom with two windows.[53]

On this occasion 7 Mass, 1 Seitl (10.25 liters) of fluid was removed. A bandage was applied to the wound for a day. Gerhard von Breuning noted that Beethoven passed more urine after the operation.

Dr. Seibert ordered the skin over pressure points to be rubbed, to prevent bed sores. A doeskin was also obtained for Beethoven to lie on. The maid placed a wooden bowl under the bed to catch any fluid escaping the wound. Stephan von Breuning sent extra linen sheets to absorb the fluid. Dr. Malfatti's locum tenens, Dr. Rohrich, visited Beethoven on some mornings.

THE LEAKING WOUND AND THE BEDSORES

The conversation-book entries highlight two of the major problems faced by Beethoven's physicians: the leaking wound and bedsores.

Following each abdominal paracentesis, the ascitic fluid would continue to ooze through the wound for eleven days or more. This problem was addressed by frequent changes of bed linen, or the application of oilcloth to the sheets, or the positioning of a bowl under the bed to catch the drip, or regular changes of hay under the bed to absorb the moisture.

Furthermore, a large "grandfather's chair" was purchased for 50 florins, W.W., so that while his bed was being made up, Beethoven could rest in the chair for at least half an hour a day.

The real extent of his bedsores was not fully appreciated until his corpse was removed from his bed for the autopsy.[54] Modern nursing methods try to prevent the development of bedsores by making two hourly changes of position of the patient confined to bed, as well as early mobilization. Lying on a sheepskin is beneficial, and the rubbing of pressure points with spirit or a soothing lotion is still appropriate.

MARCH 1827: HIS LAST MONTH

In his report Dr. Wawruch continued,

Under these described circumstances, attended by a rapidly increasing emaciation and ebbing of his life's strength, the months of January, February, and March went by. Beethoven himself prognosticated his approaching death during his many sad hours, at the time of his fourth operation, and he was not wrong. He was unable to accept any comfort, and when I expressed hope for improvement with the coming of a revitalizing spring temperature, he responded with a smile: "My work is done; if any doctor could still help, his name shall be called wonderful!" This sad reference to Handel's *Messiah* moved me so greatly that I had to confirm to myself the truth of this statement.

Physical, Mental, and Spiritual Consolation

During this last month of his life, the devoted Baron Pasqualati excelled himself in providing permissible dishes of delicious food to satisfy Beethoven's palate, such as stewed peaches, stewed cherries cooked simply without added lemon, and delicacies of field fare and game. This kind friend not only provided him with vintage champagne, but also with a fine glass to drink it.[55] On 10 March four bottles of 1806 Rüdesheimer Berg arrived from Schott's, with the promise of a further case to follow.[56]

On several occasions Beethoven took much pleasure in reading through the music of his beloved Handel. Leaning the scores against the wall, while turning the pages, he would often pause with emotion to express his utmost joy in superlatives.[57]

He obtained spiritual consolation through prayer and submission to God's will.[58] He was very grateful for the 1,000 gulden sent by the Royal Philharmonic Society.[59]

Beethoven and Schubert

Of course there is no need to doubt that Beethoven perceived a divine spark in Franz Schubert.[60] However there is controversy in the literature with regard to the number of their personal meetings, or indeed if they ever met at all.[61] Although Anselm Hüttenbrenner (1794–1868) made no mention of it in his recollections of Schubert in 1854, he informed Ferdinand Luib in writing in 1858 that Schubert had visited Beethoven on his deathbed about a week before he died.[62] Two years later, he informed Thayer that this historic visit had taken place on the very day of Beethoven's death.

Against the backdrop of Schindler's unreliability as a witness, why should we doubt Hüttenbrenner's credibility as a witness, thirty-one years after the event, even though we sympathize with his difficulty or inability to recall the precise date of this auspicious event in history?

The Visits of Hummel and Hiller

On 8 March Hummel made the first of three visits to Beethoven, accompanied by his fifteen-year-old pupil Ferdinand Hiller, whose account of the meeting did not appear in print until 1871.[63] Hiller initially recounted the news that had reached Weimar:

He was suffering from dropsy. In Vienna, the artists who had visited Hummel reported the worst with regard to his condition. On the one hand it was hopeless; on the other unspeakably sad. Absolute deafness, a continually increasing distrust of everyone on earth, and now, added to this, bodily sufferings—unsuccessful operations—discontent and loneliness—and an appearance which almost excited horror.[64]

At the first visit they were surprised to find Beethoven sitting out of bed at the window:

He wore a long, gray dressing-gown, completely open at the moment, and high boots which reached to his knees. Emaciated by his evil malady he seemed to me, as he rose, to be tall in stature. He was unshaven, his heavy, partly gray hair hung in disorder over his temples, the expression of his features grew very mild and gentle when he caught sight of Hummel, and he seemed to be extraordinarily glad to see him. The two men embraced with the utmost heartiness.[65]

At the second visit on 13 March they found that his condition had deteriorated: "He lay in bed, seemed to be suffering violent pain and occasionally gave a deep groan, although he talked a good deal and with animation."[66]

At the third visit, on 23 March, Hummel brought his wife, Elizabeth Hummel née Röckel, as Beethoven had requested:

He lay there faint and wretched, at times sighing gently. No further word passed his lips; the perspiration stood out on his brow. Seeing that by some chance he did not have his handkerchief at hand, Hummel's wife took her dainty wisp of battiste and at different times dried his face. Never shall I forget the grateful glance which his broken eyes sent up to her when she did this.[67]

Holz's Last Visit

The precise date of Carl Holz's last visit is not recorded, but according to Fanny Linzbauer, he was accompanied by Tobias Haslinger and Ignaz Castelli. It was a moving scene, and after the dying Beethoven had with great effort blessed the three kneeling friends, they kissed his hands and wept.[68]

A CODICIL OF HIS WILL

Beethoven's state of mental alertness had deteriorated into a stupor. Stephan von Breuning, anxious that Beethoven add a codicil to his will, could delay no longer. While Johann and Schindler propped up the sick composer on pillows, Breuning kept the pen moistened with ink and supervised Beethoven to copy out the prepared text.[69] The tremulous script, errors, repetitions, and omissions reflect the author's state of stupor:

Mein Neffffe Karle Soll alleini Erbe sejn, dass Kapital meines
Nachlalasses soll jedoch Seinen natürlichen oder testament arischschen
Erben zufallen.
Wien am 23.März 1827
     Lwig van Beethen.

My nephew Karl shall be the sole heir. The capital of my estate shall,
however, go to his natural heirs, or those he names in his own Will.
Vienna, 23 March 1827
     Ludwig van Beethoven.[70]

These were his last written words.[71]

A further description of Beethoven's condition at this time is given in Schindler's letter of 24 March to Moscheles. It should be noted that there was no mention in this letter of Beethoven's reception of the Last Sacrament. More about this later.

His dissolution approaches with rapid steps, and indeed it is the unanimous wish of us all to see him released from his dreadful sufferings. Nothing else remains to be hoped for. One may indeed say that, for the last eight days, he has been more like a dead than living man, being able only now and then to muster sufficient strength to ask a question, or to inquire for what he wanted. . . . He is in an almost constant state of insensibility, or rather of stupor; his head hanging down on his chest, and his eyes staringly fixed for hours upon the same spot. He seldom recognises his most intimate acquaintances, and requires to be told who stands before him. This is dreadful to behold, but only for a few days longer can such a state of things last: since yesterday all the natural functions of the body have ceased. . . . The exaltation of his mind is indeed so great, that he at times borders upon the childish. We were also obliged to procure for him a great arm-chair, which cost fifty florins, on which he rests daily at least for half an hour, whilst his room and bed are arranged. . . . Everything he eats or drinks I must taste first, to ascertain whether it might not be injurious for him. . . . [After some hours] I have just left Beethoven. He is certainly dying; before this letter is beyond the walls of the city, the great light will have become extinct for ever. He is still in full possession of his senses. The enclosed lock I have just cut from his head.[72]

HIS RECEPTION OF THE LAST RITES OF THE CATHOLIC CHURCH

At that time Austrian law decreed that the physician attending a dying Christian patient was obliged to offer to arrange a visit from a priest to confer the consolation of reception of the Last Sacrament and Holy Viaticum. The religious Dr. Wawruch did not neglect his responsibility.

The portentous day approached more rapidly. My frequently so difficult duty and responsibility as a physician made it necessary to point out the coming end to him, so that he may be able to fulfil his duties as a citizen and those prescribed by his religion. With the greatest discretion I wrote the necessary message on a sheet of paper, our customary medium of communication. Beethoven read it slowly with exemplary composure, his face resembling that of someone transfigured. He shook my hand heartily and seriously saying: "Have the priest come!" Then he was quiet and thoughtful, nodding in a friendly manner: "I will see you soon again." Soon thereafter Beethoven made his devotions with devout resignation which looks confidently to eternity, and, turning to the friends surrounding him, said: *"Plaudite amici! Finita est comoedia."*

The truth of this account was affirmed by Schindler in his letter of 12 April 1827 to Schott's Sons, later published in the journal *Cäcilia*[73]:

When I went to him on the morning of 24 March, I found him very much changed, and so weak that it was with the utmost effort that he uttered two or three words intelligently. Dr. Wawruch, the medical man in attendance, soon arrived, and after looking at him for some moments, he said to me: "Beethoven is dying rapidly!" As we had some days previously concluded as well as we could all arrangements about his will, all we desired was that he should make his peace with heaven, and thus show the world that he died a true Christian. The doctor wrote, requesting him in the name of all his friends to receive the Last Sacrament. He answered calmly and composedly: "I will." Dr. Wawruch then went away, leaving me to arrange this. . . . The priest came about 12, and his ministrations were very edifying. Beethoven seemed then himself to realise his approaching end, for scarcely had the minister left the room when he said to young Herr von Breuning (son of the Hofrath) and myself: "Plaudite amici, comoedia est finita. Did I not always

say that it would be so?" . . . At that moment, Herr Hofrath von Breuning's office servant
came into the room with the case of wine which you sent. It was now about a quarter
to 1 o'clock. I placed the two bottles of *Rudesheim* and the two other bottles with the
potion on the table by his bed. He looked at them and said: "What a pity! what a pity!—
too late." These were his last words. He immediately afterwards fell into an agony which
prevented him from uttering a syllable.
Towards evening he lost consciousness, and his mind began to wander. This lasted till
the evening of the 25th, when signs of death were unmistakably visible. But he did not
cease to breathe till a quarter to six in the evening of the 26th. The death struggle was
fearful to behold, for the strength of his constitution, especially his chest, was enormous.
He partook of your *Rudesheim* by teaspoonfuls until the end.[74]

The later assertion, by Schindler in his third edition, and by Gerhard von
Breuning, that Beethoven had said, "Applaud, friends, the comedy is over," on
an earlier occasion after a consultation with one of the doctors, seems therefore
to be incorrect.[75]

In his letter of 20 August 1860 to Thayer, Anselm Hüttenbrenner stated,

Owing to a request from the wife of the late music publisher, Tobias Haslinger, I may
have been the cause of Beethoven having been asked, in the gentlest manner, by Jenger
and Mdme. van Beethoven, to receive the Holy Communion; but I never entreated him
to partake of the Last Sacrament, neither was I present at its dispensation in the forenoon
of 24 March 1827. It is also a pure invention that Beethoven ever said to me: "Plaudite
amici, finita est comoedia." . . . Mdme. van Beethoven told me that after the administration of the sacrament on the day of his death, her brother-in-law said to the priest:
"Reverend sir, I thank you. You have given me consolation."[76]

During Thayer's visit to Graz in June 1860, Hüttenbrenner confused the identity of Mdme. van Beethoven with the nephew Carl's mother, who later complained that she did not learn of Beethoven's death until after the event. Stephan
Ley proposed that the woman in question was the maid, Sali, but that seems
less likely.[77] On the other hand, Beethoven's alleged last words, spoken after
the arrival of the wine, seem appropriate.[78]

According to Ludwig Nohl, Beethoven received Holy Viaticum in the presence of Johann and Therese van Beethoven, Jenger, Breuning, and Schindler.
Johann, in his brief report of his brother's last illness, stated that when the priest
was leaving, Beethoven said, "I thank you for this last service."[79]

In his letter of 26 March to Moscheles, the banker Rau wrote,

I found poor Beethoven [on 15 March] in the most wretched condition, more like a
skeleton than a living being. He was in the last stage of dropsy, and it had been necessary
to tap him four or five times. His medical attendant is Doctor Malfatti, so he is in
excellent hands, but Malfatti gives him little hope. It is impossible to say for certain how
long his present state will continue, or if recovery may yet be possible; but the recent
news of the help afforded him [the gift of 1,000 florins from the Philharmonic Society]
has worked a remarkable change. The emotion of joy was so excessive as to rupture, in

the course of the night, one of the punctured wounds that had cicatrized over; the water which had accumulated for fourteen days flowed away in streams. I found him on my visit next day [16 March] remarkably cheerful, and feeling a wonderful sense of relief. I hurried off to Malfatti's to tell him of this occurrence, which he considers a very favourable one. They intend to apply a hollow probe for some time, so as to keep his wound open and allow the water to escape freely. May God bless these means![80]

Earlier Dr. Malfatti had favored the introduction of a hollow tube through the wound to allow free drainage of the ascitic fluid, but Dr. Seibert must have been opposed to such a treatment. Effective antiseptics such as carbolic acid were not then available, and the vital importance of an aseptic technique in surgery was not appreciated.[81] The introduction of a hollow tube into the wound then would have been associated with a serious of risk of septic complications such as peritonitis.

THE TERMINAL COMA

On the evening of 24 March, Beethoven lapsed into a coma and he remained unconscious till his death forty-eight hours later. Schindler described it as a state of almost constant delirium. Dr. Wawruch concluded his report:

After a few hours he lost consciousness, became comatose, and the death rattle began. The next morning all signs of approaching death were present. The 26 March was stormy, gloomy; a snowstorm with thunder and lightning started around 6 P.M.—Beethoven died.—Would a Roman augury not have concluded that the chance uproar of the elements was related to his apotheosis?[82]

Gerhard von Breuning described Beethoven's sad plight during his last two days:

On the next day and the day after that the powerful man lay there unconscious, breathing with a very audible rattling noise. His strong body and unimpaired lungs struggled titanically with approaching death. It was a terrible sight. And yet we knew that the poor man was no longer suffering; all the same, it was hideous to see this noble being so irrevocably disintegrating that all communication with him was impossible. On 25 March it was not expected that he would survive the night; but on the twenty-sixth we found him still alive, breathing even louder than before.[83]

BEETHOVEN'S LAST MOMENTS

In his letter of 20 August 1860 to Thayer, Hüttenbrenner wrote an account of Beethoven's last moments:

Your valuable letter from Vienna, of 17 July, greatly pleased me. Although correspondence is not so easy as it was thirty years ago, and I do not willingly recall melancholy circumstances in which I once took part, I will comply with your wish, and write down what, after an interval of thirty-three years, I, who was an eye-witness, can remember of Beethoven's last moments. I often thought of writing an account in some newspaper, but never carried out my intentions, for I keep in the background as much as possible, and am very loath to draw attention to myself and my affairs. When I entered Beethoven's bed-room on 26 March 1827, about three o'clock in the afternoon, I found there Herr Hofrath Breuning and his son, Frau van Beethoven (wife of Johann van Beethoven), landowner and apothecary at Linz, and my friend Joseph Teltscher, a portrait painter. Professor Schindler was, I believe, also present. After a while these gentlemen left, with little hope of finding the composer alive when they returned. During Beethoven's last moments, no one was in the room except Frau van Johann Beethoven and myself. He had been lying unconscious, and struggling with death from 3 till 5 o'clock, when there came a loud peal of thunder, accompanied by a flash of lightning, which vividly illuminated the room. (Snow was on the ground.) After this unexpected phenomenon, which made a deep impression upon me, Beethoven opened his eyes, raised his right hand, and gazed fixedly upwards for some seconds, with clenched fist, and a solemn threatening expression, as if he would say: "I defy you, ye adverse powers. Depart! God is with me." Or his appearance may be described as that of a brave general, exclaiming to his fainting troops: "Courage, soldiers! Forward! Trust in me! Victory is ours!"

His hand dropped, and his eyes were half closed. My right hand supported his head, my left lay on his breast. He gave no sign of life. The spirit of the great master had passed from this false world to the kingdom of truth. I closed his half-shut eyes, and kissed his brow, mouth, hands, and eyes. At my request Frau van Beethoven cut a lock of his hair, and gave it to me as a sacred memorial of Beethoven's dying hour.

Deeply agitated, I hastened immediately to the city to communicate the news to Herr Tobias Haslinger, and a few hours after returned to my home at Styria.

Beethoven's personal appearance was repellent rather than attractive; but the lofty spirit which pervaded his creations made a strong, irresistible, and magical impression on the mind of every highly cultivated lover of music. It was impossible not to esteem, love, and admire Beethoven.[84]

Of course Johann van Beethoven and Sali were also present in Beethoven's bedroom, that last day, and a nurse from Dr. Wawruch's clinic also assisted the unconscious patient. Teltscher began to make some preliminary sketches of the dying composer until, at Breuning's displeasure, he left the room, though he returned later.[85]

Stephan von Breuning and Schindler left the death chamber to find a suitable site for a grave in the Währing Cemetery. Gerhard von Breuning was called home at 5:15 P.M. for a lesson with his teacher.[86] In his letter of 28 March to J. A. Stumpff, Johann Baptist Streicher stated, "At 5:45 P.M., Beethoven suddenly and violently sat up in bed, and passed away in the arms of his brother, in the presence of Herr Hüttenbrenner and a painter who still attempted to draw the great artist in his last moments."[87]

THE DEATH CERTIFICATE

The page in the Municipal Register of Deaths with the original entry was removed as a souvenir, and in its place there is a typewritten copy from the appropriate listing in the *Wiener Zeitung*:

Register of Death, tom. 160, fol.B 29:
Beethoven, Ludwig van, Composer, 57 years old, am Alsergrund no 200, of dropsy (Wassersucht).
On Monday, 26 March 1827, at "a quarter to six" in the evening.[88]

In fact, at the time of his death, Beethoven's age was 56 years, 3 months, and 10 days. The still extant official records at the Vienna meteorological bureau support the contentions of Wawruch, Schindler, Hüttenbrenner, and Streicher that Beethoven died during a storm. On 26 March 1827, stormy weather developed at 3:00 P.M., giving way to lightning, thunder, and strong winds an hour later.[89]

Two men kept the death watch that first night, the next morning Dr. Johann Joseph Wagner performed an autopsy. On the afternoon of 27 March, Holz discovered in a secret drawer in a cupboard seven bank shares, valued at 7,441 florins, along with the letter to the Immortal Beloved, and two ivory miniature portraits, recently identified as Giulietta Guicciardi and Antonie Brentano.[90] The inventory of Beethoven's estate is extant.[91]

THE DEATH MASK

According to the anecdotal account in F. Kerst, written at Währing by the eighty-year-old Carl Danhauser, early on the morning after Beethoven's death, he and his brother Joseph were awakened to hear the sad news from noted animal painter Ranftl. They all hastened off, together with a stucco worker, Hofmann, to the Schwarzspanierhaus, with a view to obtain an impression for a death mask.

Upon their arrival, however, they found that Beethoven's beard was so thick that they had to call a barber to shave him. Finding themselves short of cash, when the barber wanted to charge them a ducat, they decided to do it themselves. After Danhauser had soaped it, Ranftl shaved his face clean. Only then did Joseph Danhauser and Hofmann obtain a good casting, and they also cut two locks of hair from his temple for a souvenir.[92]

However, since in Danhauser's death mask there is an accurate reproduction of distortion of the right jaw, secondary to the autopsy, the casting must have been taken after Dr. Wagner's postmortem, almost certainly on 28 March. Furthermore, in his letter of 27 March to Schindler, Stephan Breuning stated expressly that Danhauser had applied for permission to take the impression the next morning, estimating that it would take only from five to eight minutes.[93]

Several death masks and busts were molded by Joseph Danhauser from the
original casting. The more faithful of the two extant death masks is the one
located at the Historischen Museen der Stadt in Vienna. The fine details are less
distinct in the copy at the Beethoven-Haus in Bonn, which also displays a more
accentuated deformity beneath the right cheek.[94] The mask in Vienna was given
by Danhauser to Franz Liszt in 1840, and it was later acquired by the museum
from Princess Marie von Hohenlohe.

Danhauser sent a plaster bust to Moscheles in London, with a view to the
execution from it of a marble copy, but it shattered in transit. The fine bust by
Danhauser in the Beethoven-Haus in Bonn also shows the influence of Franz
Klein's life mask.[95] Danhauser also produced oil sketches of Beethoven's head
and hands.[96] His lithograph of Beethoven's face was widely distributed.

Following his visit on 28 March, Schubert's friend Franz von Hartmann noted
in his diary that he was awestruck by the celestial dignity in the death chamber,
despite the disfiguration of the head, the bluish postmortem discoloration of the
chest, the swollen abdomen, and the cadaverous stench. The attendant exchanged
a lock of Beethoven's hair for a tip.[97] During their visit on 29 March the Breunings observed that his hair had been cut off.[98]

THE FUNERAL

Invitations to the funeral were issued by Haslinger's Music Store:

INVITATION
to
LUDWIG van BEETHOVEN'S
FUNERAL

which will take place on 29 March at 3 o'clock in the afternoon. Participants will meet
in the apartment of the deceased in the Schwarzspanier Haus no. 200, at the Glacis before
the Schottenthor. The procession will go to the Trinity Church of the Minorites in the
Alsergasse.
The musical world sustained the irreplaceable loss of the famous composer on 26 March
1827, at about 6 o'clock in the evening. Beethoven died as a result of dropsy in the 56th
year of his age, after receiving the Holy Sacraments.
The day of the Exequies will be announced later by L. van Beethoven's Admirers and
Friends.
(This card is distributed in Haslinger's Music Store.)[99]

An official account of Beethoven's funeral is kept in the archives of the
Vienna Supreme Court.[100] The clothed corpse was laid in a polished oak coffin;
the hands clasped a wax cross and a lily. The head, adorned with a wreath of
white roses, rested on a white silk pillow, while large lilies were placed on the
left and right sides of the body. On each side of the coffin there were eight
candles burning, while on a table at the foot was a crucifix, a bowl of holy

water for blessing, and ears of corn. The maid, Sali, tirelessly received the many visitors wishing to pay their last respects to Beethoven.

Toward noon Andreas Zeller distributed rose bouquets to the invited mourners.[101] Near three o'clock valedictory poems written by Johann Gabriel Seidl and Ignaz Franz Castelli were distributed.[102] As anticipated by Stephan von Breuning, the surge of the huge crowd into the courtyard in front of the Schwarzspanierhaus was so great that the entrance gate had to be locked and help sought from the soldiers at the Alser barracks. Even the schools were closed. The crowd was further swelled by the curious on a mild, pleasant spring afternoon.

At 3:00 P.M., the lid of the coffin was sealed, and the casket was carried out into the court. After the solemn blessing of the dead man by nine priests from the Schottenstifte, a funeral chorale from Bernhard Anselm Weber's opera *Wilhelm Tell* was chanted.[103] The eight singers from Domenico Barbaia's Italian Opera Company at the Kärntnertor theater and the Theater an der Wien were Borschitzky, L. Cramolini, Eichenberger, Hofmann, Müller, Rupprecht, Schuster, and Anton Wranitzky. They also carried the coffin into the church.

The solemn procession to the Holy Trinity Church on the Alserstrasse was led by the crossbearer followed by members of the Grundspital and the students of the Musik Verein.[104] Then came the four trombone players: the Blöch brothers, Tuschka, and Weidle; followed by M. Assmayer's choir with the singers Frühwald, Geissler, Gros, Kokrement, Leidl, Nejebse, Perschl, Pfeifer, Rathmayer, Schnitzer, Seipelt, Sykora, Tiebe, Weinkopf, and Ziegler. The trombonists and choir alternated the verses of the psalm *Miserere mei Deus*.[105] The *Amplius lava me ab iniquitate* was also sung.[106]

Following the choir came the parish crucifer, the nine priests from the Schottenstifte, and the director of ceremonies. Then followed the coffin, carried on the shoulders of the eight opera singers. The coffin was covered by a fine embroidered pall, ordered by Schindler from the 2d Civil Regiment. The edges of the pall were held by eight Kapellmeisters: on the right, J. Eybler, J. Hummel, R. Kreutzer, and I. Seyfried; on the left, Gänsbacher, A. Gyrowetz, J. Weigl, and W. Würfel. They were dressed in black with white ribbons suspended from their scarfs, and they carried candles wrapped in crepe.

On either side of the coffin there marched the torchbearers, each of whom carried a lighted wax torch adorned with flowers: Heinrich Anschütz, J. K. Bernard, J. L. Blahetka, Joseph Böhm, I. L. Castelli, Carl Czerny, David, F. Grillparzer, Conrad Graf, J. C. Grünbaum, Haslinger, Hildebrandt, C. Holz, Kaller, Krall, E. Lannoy, J. Linke, J. Mayseder, Meric, Merk, P. Mechetti, Meier, Paccini, F. Piringer, Rodicci, Raimund, P. J. Riotte, F. Schoberlechner, Franz Schubert, J. Schickh, Schmiedl, Streicher, I. Schuppanzigh, S. A. Steiner, Weidmann, J. N. Wolfmayer, and others.

Behind the coffin marched Johann and Therese van Beethoven, Stephan and Gerhard von Breuning, Schindler, Hofrat von Mosel, and Count Moritz Dietrichstein. Then followed the pupils of the Kapellmeister of St. Anna, Joseph Drechsler, the students of the conservatory, and numerous friends and admirers. The splendid ceremonial hearse, drawn by four horses, hired from St. Stephan's Cathedral, brought up the rear.

Estimates of the crowd at Beethoven's funeral vary from 10,000 to 20,000.[107] Though it was only some 500 paces from the house to the church, it took an hour and a half for the procession to make this journey. As the coffin rounded the corner of the Breunings' Rothes Haus, a brass band played the Funeral March from the Opus 26 Sonata.

The Holy Trinity Church was also crammed to overflowing, and it was only with much difficulty that the official party gained admittance. The many that fainted were taken across to the nearby General Hospital.

The three main altars of the church were illuminated brightly with six and a half pounds of wax candles. But that was not all, for Johann Wolfmayer lit, at his own expense, all the candles at the side altars, wall brackets, and chandeliers.

While the nine priests from the Schottenstifte performed the sacred blessing of Beethoven's remains, in front of the main altar, the choir chanted the solemn *Libera me, Domine*, composed for the occasion by Ignaz Seyfried.[108] At the end of the service, the coffin was carried in solemn procession out of the church and transferred to the state hearse.

Though some of the crowd dispersed after the religious ceremony, the majority followed the hearse to Währing. More than 200 carriages took part, while thousands followed on foot. The funeral cortege crossed the Alserbach by the Namentur, went by the almshouse and brick-kiln, crossed the Währing brook, and proceeded along the right bank to the parish church at Währing.

The parish priest, Father Johann Hayek, and his assistant priest were waiting there. The three altars of the little church were illuminated with candles, while the crowd was swelled by the presence of the parish schoolchildren and the local poor. The coffin was carried into the church before the main altar where it was blessed by the two priests. Then the parish choir sang the *Miserere* and the *Libera*.

Beethoven's coffin was carried in a solemn procession to the adjacent Friedhof Cemetery, where it was deposited before the main gate. Since, at that time, it was forbidden to deliver funeral orations on consecrated ground, actor Heinrich Anschütz delivered Grillparzer's moving address over the coffin in front of the cemetery gate[109]:

Standing by the grave of him who has passed away, we are in a manner the representatives of an entire nation, of the whole German people, mourning the loss of the one highly acclaimed half of that which was left us of the departed splendor of our native art, of the father-land's full spiritual bloom. There yet lives—and may his life be long!—the hero of verse in German speech and tongue; but the last master of tuneful song, the organ of soulful concord, the heir and amplifier of Händel and Bach's, of Haydn and Mozart's immortal fame is now no more, and we stand weeping over the riven strings of the harp that is hushed.

The harp that is hushed! Let me call him so! For he was an artist, and all that was his,

was his through art alone. The thorns of life had wounded him deeply, and as the cast-
away clings to the shore, so did he seek refuge in thine arms, O thou glorious sister and
peer of the Good and the True, thou balm of wounded hearts, heaven-born Art! To thee
he clung fast, and even when the portal was closed wherethrough thou hadst entered in
and spoken to him, when his deaf ear had blinded his vision for thy features, still did
he ever carry thine image within his heart, and when he died it still reposed on his breast.
He was an artist—and who shall arise to stand beside him?

As the rushing behemoth spurns the waves, so did he rove to the uttermost bounds of
his art. From the cooing of doves to the rolling of thunder, from the craftiest interweaving
of well-weighed expedients of art up to that awful pitch where planful design disappears
in the lawless whirl of contending natural forces, he had traversed and grasped it all. He
who comes after him will not continue him; he must begin anew, for he who went before
left off only where art leaves off. Adelaide—and Leonora! Triumph of the heroes of
Vittoria—and the humble sacrificial song of the Mass!—Ye children of the twice and
thrice divided voices! heaven-soaring harmony: "*Freude*, schöner Götterfunken," thou
swan-song! Muse of song and the seven-stringed lyre! Approach his grave and bestrew
it with laurel!

He was an artist, but a man as well. A man in every sense—in the highest. Because he
withdrew from the world, they called him a man-hater, and because he held aloof from
sentimentality, unfeeling. Ah, one who knows himself hard of heart, does not shrink!
The finest points are those most easily blunted and bent or broken! An excess of sensitiveness avoids a show of feeling! He fled the world because, in the whole range of
his loving nature, he found no weapon to oppose it. He withdrew from mankind after
he had given them his all and received nothing in return. He dwelt alone, because he
found no second Self. But to the end his heart beat warm for all men, in fatherly affection
for his kindred, for the world his all and his heart's blood.

Thus he was, thus he died, thus he will live to the end of time.

You, however, who have followed after us hitherward, let not your hearts be troubled!
You have not lost him, you have won him. No living man enters the halls of the im-
mortals. Not until the body has perished, do their portals unclose. He whom you mourn
stands from now onward among the great of all ages, inviolate forever. Return homeward
therefore, in sorrow, yet resigned! And should you ever in times to come feel the over-
powering might of his creations like an onrushing storm, when your mounting ecstasy
overflows in the midst of a generation yet unborn, then remember this hour, and think,
We were there, when they buried him, and when he died, we wept.[110]

After this stirring oration, which brought tears to many eyes, verses written
by Baron Francis Schlechta were distributed.[111] Then the coffin was carried to
the graveside where the priests consecrated the tomb and rendered the final
blessing of the corpse. The choir sang a Choral-Melody in D by Beethoven,
arranged by Seyfried, as a setting to a verse by Grillparzer: *Du, dem nie im
Leben*:

> Thou, to whom life vouchsafed nor home nor rest,
> Sleepest at length in peace and quiet gloom;
> O, if our hymn can reach thy spirit blest,
> List to thine own sweet song, within the tomb![112]

Three laurel wreaths were presented by Haslinger to Hummel, who placed them on the coffin. As twilight shadows began to fall, the casket was lowered into the grave. According to the local custom, those standing by the grave threw earth on the coffin while all the torches were extinguished.

The rumor was then prevalent that a substantial reward had been offered for Beethoven's head. As a precaution, the gravedigger covered the coffin with two thick layers of bricks and stones, and a watchman was engaged for the first few nights.

Many waited till the turf was smoothed over the coffin. So ended one of the most moving funerals in history.

After the funeral, Schubert went to the inn Zur Mehlgrube on the Neue Markt with his friends, Benedict Randhartinger and Franz Lachner. Raising his glass of wine, Schubert proposed a toast, "To the memory of our immortal Beethoven!" With his next glass of wine, Schubert proposed a second toast, "And now to the first of us to follow Beethoven!"[113] Little did he know that he himself would die the next year on 19 November 1828.

This anecdote, first reported in Kreissle von Hellborn's biography, has a ring of truth to it.[114] Otto Erich Deutsch, noting that Fritz von Hartmann wrote in his diary that on 29 March 1827 he remained at the Castle of Eisenstadt inn with Franz Schober, Schubert, and Moritz von Schwind until almost 1:00 A.M., pointed out the apparent contradiction.[115] However, it is possible, even likely, that Schubert visited both the Mehlgrube and the Castle of Eisenstadt on that sad evening.

On 3 April a Requiem Mass was offered for the repose of Beethoven's soul in the Augustinian Church, which was then the parish church of the Imperial Palace and the Habsburg court. The Italian singers gave an inspired performance of Mozart's *Requiem*, the highlight of which was the rendering of the *Dies irae* by renowned bass Luigi Lablache, who himself had paid 200 gulden to Barbaja to release the singers from their contract for this performance.[116] The *Miserere* and the *Libera me, Domine* were repeated at the end by popular request.

A second Requiem Mass was offered for Beethoven's soul on 5 April at the Karlskirche (the Church of St. Charles Borromeo), when Luigi Cherubini's *Requiem* was sung. By popular request a repeat performance for Beethoven was performed on 26 April by the Society of the Friends of Music.[117]

On 3 May 1827, at the Concert Spirituel in Vienna, the following verse by J. G. Seidl was recited by Heinrich Anschütz:

> Sounds were his colours, and the human heart
> The canvass upon which with highest art
> He drew his image—shrouded oft in sadness,
> And sometimes bright with more than mortal gladness.[118]

NOTES

1. TDR, V: 417–502; TK, III: 267–309; TF, 1012–51.
2. Schindler-Moscheles, II: 57–77, 318–24; Schindler-MacArdle, 318–32.

3. Breuning, *Memories of Beethoven*, 87–105.

4. L. Nohl, *Beethoven Depicted by His Contemporaries*, 323–54; L. Nohl, *Beethovens Leben*, ed. Paul Sakolowski, 3 vols. (Berlin: Schlesische Verlagsanstalt, 1909–1913), III: 491–533.

5. Stephan Ley, *Aus Beethovens Erdentagen* (Bonn: Glöckner, 1948), 204–23.

6. A. Leitzmann, *Ludwig van Beethoven: Berichte der Zeitgenossen, Briefe und persönliche Aufzeichnungen*, 2 vols. (Leipzig: Insel-Verlag, 1921), II: 357–402; Nettl, *Beethoven Encyclopedia*, 38–43; Sonneck, *Beethoven: Impressions*, 196–226; Landon, *Beethoven: A Documentary Study*, 366–93; T. K. Scherman and L. Biancolli, eds., *The Beethoven Companion* (New York: Doubleday, 1972), 1091–1101; Solomon, *Beethoven*, 285–93; M. Cooper, *Beethoven: The Last Decade 1817–1827* (Oxford: Oxford University Press, 1985), 81–85; Cooper, *Beethoven Compendium*, 138–40.

7. W. Schweisheimer, *Beethovens Leiden* (Munich: Georg Müller, 1922), 164–87; Forster, *Beethovens Krankheiten*, 28–34; Piroth, "Beethovens letzte Krankheit," 7–35; Dieter Kerner, *Krankheiten Grosser Musiker: Ludwig van Beethoven*, 2 vols. (Stuttgart: F. K. Schattauer Verlag, 1973), I: 89–146, 126–33; Gerhard Böhme, *Medizinische Porträts berühmter Komponisten: Ludwig van Beethoven*, 2 vols. (Stuttgart: Gustav Fischer Verlag, 1981), I: 73–78; Larkin, "Beethoven's Medical History," 445–47; Franz Hermann Franken, *Die Krankheiten grosser Komponisten: Ludwig van Beethoven*, 2 vols. (Wilhelmshaven, Germany: Florian Noetzel Verlag, 1986), I: 85–94; Bankl and Jesserer, *Die Krankheiten*, 45–66; J. G. O'Shea, "Medical Profile of Ludwig van Beethoven," *Music and Medicine: Medical Profiles of Great Composers* (London: J. M. Dent, 1990), 39–65, pp. 49–52; A. Neumayr, "Notes on the Life, Works, and Medical History of Ludwig van Beethoven," *Music and Medicine: Haydn, Mozart, Beethoven, Schubert*, trans. Bruce Cooper Clarke (Bloomington, Ind.: Medi-Ed Press, 1994), 225–346, cited from 288–303.

8. Breuning, *Memories of Beethoven*, 5–9; Schindler-MacArdle, 358, n. 250.

9. Dr. Andreas Ignaz Wawruch's retrospective report, *Ärztlicher Rückblick auf Ludwig van Beethovens letzte Lebensepoche*, dated 20 May 1827, trans. Erna Schwerin.

10. A-1541; LvBCB, X: 297, 10 v.

11. LvBCB, X: 298, 11 r.

12. Schindler-Moscheles, 11: 59–60; Schindler-MacArdle, 318; Breuning, *Memories of Beethoven*, 87. See Schindler's letter of 11 April 1827 to Moscheles in L. Nohl, *Beethoven Depicted by His Contemporaries*, 341–46; Albrecht, *Letters*, 478.

13. Medici and Hughes, *Mozart Pilgrimage*, 204.

14. See LvBCB, X: 298, 11 v, 12 r.

15. TDR, V: 419, n. 1.

16. Breuning, *Memories of Beethoven*, 90.

17. See LvBCB, X: 298–300, 314.

18. Forster, *Beethoven Krankheiten*, 33. 5.5 Mass, equivalent to 7.7 liters (5.5 quarts), was removed.

19. See conversation-book entries in Ley, *Aus Beethovens Erdentagen*, 207–8; Bankl and Jesserer, *Die Krankheiten*, 49.

20. See LvBCB, X: 302, 1 r.

21. Schindler-Moscheles, II: 61.

22. Schindler-MacArdle, 320.

23. Breuning, *Memories of Beethoven*, 87.

24. Werner E. Bunjes, *Medical and Pharmaceutical Dictionary: English-German*, 4th ed. (Stuttgart: Georg Thieme Verlag, 1981), 225.

25. P. B. Beeson and W. McDermott, eds., *Cecil-Loeb, Textbook of Medicine*, 12th

ed. (Philadelphia: W. B. Saunders, 1967), I: 150–53; K. J. Isselbacher et al., eds., *Harrison's Principles of Internal Medicine*, 2 vols. (New York: McGraw-Hill, 1994), I: 608.

26. P. J. Davies, "Beethoven's Nephropathy and Death," *Journal of the Royal Society of Medicine* 86 (1993): 159–61.

27. The receipt, dated 14 December 1826, is written in another hand. See Anderson, *Letters*, Appendix G, no. 19, p. 1433. See also A-1550. Samuel Arnold's first edition of Handel's works were published between 1787 and 1797. The forty volumes were sent by London harp maker Johann Andreas Stumpff via the firm of Johann Baptist Streicher in Vienna. In a lapse of memory, Gerhard von Breuning misdated the arrival of the books to mid-February 1827. See Breuning, *Memories of Beethoven*, 96. The Handel collection cost £45. For Stumpff's note of dedication see Albrecht, *Letters*, no. 435.

28. TF, 1025.

29. See TDR, V: 430ff; Ley, *Aus Beethovens Erdentagen*, 208–23; and Bankl and Jesserer, *Die Krankheiten*, 50–57.

30. I. von Seyfried, BS, Appendix, 16.

31. Tubera Salep, salep, or salep-root are the round or pear-shaped tubers of various orchids that grow in Germany and the East. Brownish-grey or yellow in color, they are hard and translucent, like horn. The main constituent is a mucilage named bassorin. Such vegetable mucilages swell up in water, forming a glutinous mass that is not readily absorbed by the intestines. In the form of a decoction, with 1–2 parts in 150 parts of water, and a little added sugar, it was used as a remedy for intestinal catarrh. See Binz, *Lectures on Pharmacology*, II: 384.

32. A-1547; B-2246.

33. TDR, V: 443–44.

34. Breuning, *Memories of Beethoven*, 92–93. Each bottle was subject to a refund of two kreuzer.

35. *Frankfurter Konversationsblatt*, 14 July 1842, trans. Erna Schwerin. See also TF, 1031.

36. Schindler-Moscheles, II: 61–62; Schindler-MacArdle, 320.

37. TF, 1029–30.

38. Schindler-MacArdle, 320; TF, 1031–32; Albrecht, *Letters*, no. 457.

39. TDR, V: 444, trans. Erna Schwerin; Albrecht, *Letters*, no. 454; TF, 1030.

40. TDR, V: 449, trans. Erna Schwerin. See also A-1565. Schindler dated the autograph 17 March 1827, but this seems incorrect—another forgery?

41. TF, 1033.

42. Breuning, *Memories of Beethoven*, 93–95.

43. Bankl and Jesserer, *Die Krankheiten*, 55.

44. Ibid., 56.

45. A-1553, 1558; B-2263, 2266.

46. A-1551; B-2257.

47. TF, 1037.

48. A-1550, 1554, 1555, 1559, 1563; B-2256, 2260, 2259, 2271, 2281.

49. Breuning, *Memories of Beethoven*, 98–99.

50. B-2261, trans. Erna Schwerin. See also Sonneck, *Beethoven: Impressions*, 214; Albrecht, *Letters*, no. 460.

51. TF, 1037–38; Breuning, *Memories of Beethoven*, 101.

52. TF, 1029.

53. Beethoven's bed was adjacent to the eastern wall. For a description, see Breuning, *Memories of Beethoven*, 89–90.

54. Ibid., 107.

55. A-1549, 1560, 1562, 1564, 1569, 1570; B-925 (22 April 1816), 2273, 2280, 2279, 2274, 2275 (7 March 1827).

56. TF, 1039.

57. TF, 1024, 1035.

58. A-1563; B-2281.

59. A-1566; B-2284.

60. Schindler-MacArdle, 321.

61. For an overview, see Maynard Solomon, "Schubert and Beethoven," *Nineteenth Century Music* 3 (1979–1980): 114–25. See also "Schubert und Beethoven in historischen Zeugnissen," *Schubertiade Journal* (Hohenems), February 1996, 2–7; L. Nohl, *Beethoven Depicted by His Contemporaries*, 301–4.

62. O. E. Deutsch, *Schubert: Memoirs by His Friends* (New York: MacMillan, 1958), 66.

63. Hiller's article, "Aus den letzen Tagen Ludwig van Beethovens," was published in the *Kölnische Zeitung*, 16 December 1870; reprinted, "Aus dem Ton-Leben unserer Zeit," in *Neue Folge* (Leipzig, 1871), pp. 169ff. The article is reproduced in TDR, V: 481–84. For English translations, see Sonneck, *Beethoven: Impressions* 214–19; TF, 1045–47; and *Monthly Music Record* 4 (1874): 82–84.

64. Sonneck, *Beethoven: Impressions*, 215.

65. Ibid., 215.

66. Ibid., 217.

67. Ibid., 218–19.

68. Landon, *Beethoven: A Documentary Study*, 385.

69. Breuning, *Memories of Beethoven*, 102–3.

70. TDR, V: 485; Bankl and Jesserer, *Die Krankheiten*, 59, trans. Erna Schwerin. The original autograph is in the Vienna State Archives.

71. For a discussion of Beethoven's last written words and signatures, see Unger, "Beethovens letzte Briefe," 153–58.

72. Schindler-Moscheles, II: 318–22.

73. *Cäcilia* 6, no. 24 (May 1827): 309.

74. L. Nohl, *Beethoven Depicted by His Contemporaries*, 347–49. See also Albrecht, *Letters*, no. 479.

75. Schindler-MacArdle, 324; Breuning, *Memories of Beethoven*, 101–2.

76. L. Nohl, *Beethoven Depicted by His Contemporaries*, 353–54.

77. TF, 1051.

78. For a discussion of the various "last words" attributed to Beethoven, see FRHB, I: 343–45.

79. L. Nohl, *Beethovens Leben*, III: 529; TF, 1049. Johann van Beethoven's report is in the Beethoven Haus in Bonn.

80. L. Nohl, *Beethoven Depicted by His Contemporaries*, 333–34.

81. The antiseptic properties of carbolic acid were discovered in 1860 by François Jules Lemaire. Joseph Lister in 1870 was the first doctor to apply antiseptic methods to manage wounds on the battlefield.

82. Trans. Erna Schwerin.

83. Breuning, *Memories of Beethoven*, 103–4.

84. L. Nohl, *Beethoven Depicted by His Contemporaries*, 351–53.

85. TF, 1050.

86. Breuning, *Memories of Beethoven*, 104.

87. Albrecht, *Letters*, no. 472.

88. Bankl and Jesserer, *Die Krankheiten*, 61.

89. This information was conveyed by Professor F. Steinhauser to Nicolas Slonimsky in 1959. See N. Slonimsky, "The Weather at Mozart's Funeral," *Music Quarterly* 46 (1960): 21.

90. Solomon, *Beethoven*, 292.

91. TDR, V: 579–83; T. von Frimmel, BS, 2 vols. (Munich: Georg Müller, 1905–1906), II: 171–99; TF, 1061–76.

92. Carl Danhauser's statement was dated 19 May 1891. See F. Kerst, *Die Erinnerungen an Beethoven*, II, 234; Landon, *Beethoven: A Documentary Study*, 396–97.

93. Schindler-MacArdle, 332; Breuning, *Memories of Beethoven*, 106.

94. See R. Bory, *Ludwig van Beethoven: His Life and Work in Pictures* (London: Thames and Hudson, 1966), 216.

95. Ibid., 228.

96. For a photograph of Danhauser's oil sketches of Beethoven's head and hands, see Schmidt-Görg and Schmidt, *Beethoven*, 31, 256.

97. Landon, *Beethoven: A Documentary Study*, 251–52. Ferdinand Hiller also cut a lock of Beethoven's hair on the day after his death, and he presented it to his son, Paul, as a birthday present on 1 May 1883 at Cologne. See BJ 10 (1995): 68.

98. Breuning, *Memories of Beethoven*, 108.

99. Seyfried, BS, Appendix, 42, translation amended by Erna Schwerin; S. Ley, *Beethovens Leben in authentischen Bildern und Texten* (Berlin: Bruno Cassirer, 1925), 145; Bankl and Jesserer, *Die Krankheiten* 66. The funeral invitation reproduced in 1832 in Seyfried's first edition shows minor discrepancies in the style of the typesetting by Anton Strauss's widow. See Ira F. Brilliant, "The Invitation to Beethoven's Funeral— The Second Version," BJ 13 (1998): 31–33.

100. It was written by the director of ceremonies, Andreas Zeller, and published in 1925: Robert Franz Müller, "Beethovens Begräbnis," *Reichspost* (Vienna), 26 March 1925, 2. The report was translated by Elliot Forbes: TF, 1052–55. See also the contemporary report in Landau's Beethoven-Album 1877, reprinted by Kerst, in Sonneck, *Beethoven: Impressions*, 226–29; and in Landon, *Beethoven: A Documentary Study*, 394–95. See also FRHB, I: 329–31.

101. The bouquets were attached to the left sleeve with white silk ties.

102. For English translations, see Seyfried, BS, Appendix, 46–47; Breuning, *Memories of Beethoven*, 110–12.

103. Weber's opera, composed in 1795, had antedated Schiller's drama of 1804.

104. L. Nohl, *Beethoven Depicted by His Contemporaries*, 359. See letter "Strange news from Vienna," by T. Hell (Winkler) and F. Hind in the Dresden *Abendzeitung* in April 1827. See also Seyfried, BS, Appendix, 39–41.

105. At Haslinger's request, on 26 March 1827, Seyfried set the penitential psalm to the music of Beethoven's "Equale for Four Trombones," WoO 30, no. 1, arranged for voices. The score is printed in Seyfried, BS, Appendix, 56–60; and in Schindler-Moscheles, II: 337–48.

106. Seyfried set it to Beethoven's "Equale for Four Trombones," WoO 30, no. 3. The score is printed in Seyfried, BS, 61–62; and in Schindler-Moscheles, II: 349–53.

107. The more conservative estimate of 10,000 was mentioned in *Der Sammler* of 14 April 1827.

108. The score is printed in Seyfried, BS, Appendix, 63–69; and in Schindler-Moscheles, II: 354–64.

109. Breuning, *Memories of Beethoven*, 109.

110. Sonneck, *Beethoven: Impressions*, 229–31. There are at least three versions of Grillparzer's funeral oration. The above version in Sonneck was taken from Grillparzer's *Collected Works*, as also were the versions in Nettl, *Beethoven Encyclopedia*, 77–78; TF, 1057–58; Breuning, *Memories of Beethoven*, 109–10 (with editorial comment, p. 141, n. 192). An earlier version, given by Grillparzer to Stephan von Breuning, was copied out by Gerhard, who then published it in his book, *Aus dem Schwarzspanierhause*. This earlier version was also published in TDR, V: 496–97. A third version was published in Schlosser, *Beethoven: The First Biography*, 113–18 (with editorial comment, pp. 179–81, n. 63). See also FRHB, I: 181–87.

111. The verses are reproduced in Seyfried, BS, Appendix, 46.

112. Seyfried, BS, Appendix, 45; the score is reproduced on pp. 70–73. The melody was Beethoven's "Equale in D," WoO 30, no. 2.

113. Breuning, *Memories of Beethoven*, 112.

114. Kreissle von Hellborn, *The Life of Schubert*, 2 vols. (London, 1869), I: 268–69.

115. O. E. Deutsch, *Schubert: A Documentary Biography* (New York: Da Capo Press, 1977), 623.

116. Breuning, *Memories of Beethoven*, 112–13.

117. Seyfried, BS, Appendix, 41.

118. Ibid., Appendix, 46.

5

The Autopsy

In Vienna, since the time of Dr. Gerhard van Swieten (1700–1772) and Dr. Anton de Haen (1704–1776), practicing clinicians were encouraged to perform postmortem examinations of their patients to ascertain the cause of the illnesses and death.[1]

THE PATHOLOGY MUSEUM IN VIENNA

One of Beethoven's physicians, Dr. Johann Peter Frank, who was especially interested in the postmortem procedure, was instrumental in the creation of a voluntary prosector's post in 1796 and in the foundation of the Pathologic Anatomy Museum. That post was filled in turn by Aloys Rudolf Vetter (from 1796 to 1803), and S. Hürtl (from 1803 to 1811). With the appointment in 1811 of Lorenz Biermayer (from 1811 to 1829), it became a salaried post, and in 1821 it was elevated to an associate professorship.

In 1826 Biermayer edited a catalogue of some 576 exhibits, and two years later his book on the museum was published.[2] Biermayer was succeeded by Johann Wagner (from 1829 to 1832), Carl von Rokitansky (from 1833 to 1874), and Richard Heschl (from 1875 to 1881).

In 1971 the museum was relocated on the first floor of the Narrenturm (Fool's Tower) in Courtyard VI of the old Vienna General Hospital. Since 1974 it has been called the Federal Pathologic-Anatomy Museum.[3]

BEETHOVEN'S POSTMORTEM EXAMINATION

Dr. Andreas Ignaz Wawruch was keen for an autopsy to be performed on his famous patient. Furthermore, Beethoven himself had expressed a wish that the true nature of his deafness and illnesses would be discovered. No doubt Johann van Beethoven and Stephan von Breuning would have given their consent.

On 27 March 1827, Dr. Wagner, Biermayer's assistant pathologist, performed a private postmortem examination in the Schwarzspanierhaus. According to the record in the archives of the Vienna Supreme Court, transcribed by Andreas Zeller, Dr. Wagner dissected the corpse on Tuesday morning.[4] The less reliable Gerhard von Breuning, writing in 1874, stated that the autopsy was performed in the evening.[5]

According to the local custom Dr. Wawruch also attended the postmortem examination. Medical writers have also concluded that Rokitansky attended; however, according to Gerhard von Breuning, "The autopsy was made by Dr. Johann Wagner, Rokitansky's predecessor."[6]

Professor Rokitansky (1804–1878) was the most famous pathologist of the Second Vienna Medical School. Following his studies in philosophy in Prague (1822–1824), he studied medicine in Vienna and graduated in 1828. He became a prosector in the pathology department on 1 November 1827, as an unpaid student-assistant under Dr. Wagner. While Rokitansky may have attended Beethoven's autopsy as a medical student, there is no record that he did so. His post was promoted in 1844 to a full professorship.

THE ORIGINAL MANUSCRIPT

In Ignaz von Seyfried's first edition, published in 1832 by Haslinger in Vienna, there appeared for the first time a German translation of Dr. Wagner's report. Presumably Seyfried obtained the original Latin text from Dr. Wagner and translated it into German.

Following Dr. Wagner's death in 1834 from tuberculosis, the original Latin report of Beethoven's autopsy vanished. Until recently all reports in the literature were based on Seyfried's German translation of the original. In 1853 Henry Hugh Pierson made an English translation of Seyfried's German text.[7]

Following the appointment of Professor J. Heinrich Holzner in 1969 as director, the old Vienna Pathology Museum was reorganized. All documents and specimens were carefully examined and catalogued. In 1970 Dr. Wagner's original autopsy report was rediscovered. A facsimile is reproduced in Illustration 11. It is clear that the report was written out by a secretary and only signed by Dr. Wagner.[8] Previous facsimiles appeared in 1986 and 1987.[9]

THE ORIGINAL LATIN TEXT

Protocollum
de sectione corporis Domini Ludwig van Beethoven
Corpus mortui imprimis in extremitatibus valde tabefactum ac petechiis nigris conspersum, abdomen nimis hydropice tumefactum contentumque. Cartilago auris magna et ir-

regulariter formata conspecta est, fossa scaphoidea praeprimis vero concha eiusdem amplissima atque dimidio altior solito erat; anguli diversi et sulci admodum elevati erant. Meatus acusticus externus imprimis ad membranam tympani occultam squamis cutis nitentibus obsessus apparuit. Tuba Eustachii valde incrassata eius membrana mucosa eversa ac ad partem osseam paululum angustata erat. Cellulae conspicuae processus mastoidei magni, qui incissura non insignitus, membrana mucosa sanginolenta obvelatae erant. Ubertatem sanguinis similem substantia cuncta ramis vasorum conspicuis pertexta ossis petrosi, imprimis regione cochleae, eius membrana spiralis paulum rubefacta conspecta, aeque demonstravit. Nervi faciei valde incrassati erant. Nervi acustici e contrario corrugati et sine medulla erant. Arteriae auditivae iuxta eos decurrentes ultra lumen calami corvini dilatatae et cartilaginosae erant. Nervus acusticus sinister multo tennior cum tribus lineis albidis tennuissimis, dexter cum crassiori candida linea e substantia multo consistentiori et sanguine abundantiori in hoc ambitu ventriculi quarti orti sunt. Sulci ceterum multo mollioris et aquatici cerebri, altero tanto profundi ac (ampliores) numerosiores quam solito visi sunt. Calvaria ex integro validam densitatem et crassitudinem fere dimidium pollicem metientem obtulit. Cavum thoracis itemque eius viscera indolem normalem demonstravit. Cavum abdominis quatuor mensuris albide—feruginosi liquoris repletum erat. Hepar in dimidium suis voluminis reductum corio simile, densum colore subviridicaeruleo conspicatum et in sua substantia nodis volumini fabae aequantibus pertextum; eius vasa omnia angustissima, incrassata atque sine sanguine erant. Vesica fellea fuscum liquorem hic inde multum sedimentum glarcae simile continuit. Lien amplius altero tanto major normali, solidus, colore nigricante in conspectum venit. Eodem modo pancreas majus et densum visum est, eius ductus excretorius lumini calami anseris pervius erat. Ventriculus una cum intestinis aere valde inflatus erat. Ambo renes in sua substantia pallide—rubri et relaxati textu cellulari unum pollicem metiente, qui turbido fusco liquore repletus obvelati erant. Unusquisque calix concremento calcareo, piso in medio secato aequante, obsessus erat.

Sectio privata die 27. Martii MCCMXXVII.

Doktor Joh. Wagner

Assistent beym pathologischen Musäum.

The following translation was made in Melbourne, in October 1987, by the late Dr. John Patrick Horan[10]:

Protocol

Concerning the post-mortem examination carried out on the body of Domini Ludwig van Beethoven.

The body of the dead man showed intense wasting[11] and scattered black petechiae especially in the extremities,[12] the abdomen was distended and swollen with fluid and its skin was stretched.[13] The cartilage of the external ear was seen to be large and irregularly shaped, its scaphoid fossa, in particular, was enlarged and its concha was very large and half again deeper than usual, its crura diverged and the sulci were very much deepened. The external auditory meatus appeared full of shining scales of skin and these extended right up to the tympanic membrane which was hidden behind them. The Eustachian Tube was considerably thickened, its mucous membrane was heaped up and in its osseous part it was a little narrowed.[14] The mastoid process was large but not remarkable for its incisura, its cells were seen to be covered by a blood-stained mucous

membrane. The whole of the petrous part of the temporal bone was covered with visible branches of blood vessels and also showed an abundance of material like blood especially in the region of the cochlea, the spiral membrane of which was seen to be a little reddened.[15] The facial nerves were very much thickened.[16] The acoustic nerves on the other hand were wrinkled and were without a medulla.[17] The auditory arteries running near them were dilated beyond the size of the lumen of a raven's quill and were cartilaginous.[18] The left acoustic nerve was much the thinner showing three very slender whitish roots, the right nerve had a much thicker white root, the brain substance in the region of the fourth ventricle was much denser in consistency and more vascular than these nerves which arose from it.[19] For the rest the sulci of the brain were much softer and more watery, twice as deep as usual and (much more) more numerous than is usually seen.[20] Again the calvaria was of normal density and thickness measuring nearly half the length of the terminal phalanx of the thumb.[21] The thoracic cavity and its contents were normal.[22] The abdominal cavity was filled with four measures of rust-coloured fluid.[23] The liver was reduced to half its normal size, was like leather, hard and in colour slightly bluish-green and throughout its substance were nodes each about the size of a bean.[24] All its vessels were greatly narrowed, considerably thickened and devoid of blood.[25] The gall-bladder contained a dark-coloured fluid and in this was a great deal of sediment like gravel.[26] The spleen was greater than twice the normal size, hard, and when it came into view blackish in colour.[27] In the same way the pancreas was found to be larger and firmer than normal, its excretory duct allowed the quill of a goose to be passed.[28] The stomach together with the intestines were greatly distended with air.[29] Both kidneys were pale red in colour and when opened out the cellular texture measured the length of the terminal phalanx of the thumb, it was covered with a dark turbid fluid which obscured the view. Every single calyx was filled with a calcereous concretion like a pea which had been cut across the middle.[30]
Private post-mortem carried out on
27th March 1827.

Dr. Joh Wagner
Assistant, Pathology Museum[31]

THE TWO ERRORS IN THE PIERSON-SEYFRIED TRANSLATIONS

1. There Were Not Scars Present in the Back of Beethoven's Throat

The Latin Text (J. Wagner) "Tuba Eustachii valde incrassata eius membrana mucosa eversa ac ad partem osseam paululum angustata erat."

Latin-German Translation (I. Seyfried) "Die eustachische Ohrtrompete war sehr verdickt, ihre Schleimhaut ausgewulstet und gegen den knöchernen Teil etwas verengert."[32]

German-English Translation (H. H. Pierson) "The Eustachian Tube was much thickened, its mucous lining swollen and somewhat contracted about the osseous portion of the tube. In front of its orifice and towards the tonsils some dimpled scars were observable."[33]

Latin-English Translation (J. Horan) "The Eustachian Tube was considerably thickened, its mucous membrane was heaped up and in its osseous part it was a little narrowed."

Comment

It must be emphasized that Dr. Wagner made no mention of scars adjacent to the tonsils. Such pharyngeal scars, resulting from healing of "snail-track ulcers" during the secondary phase, were a characteristic sign of previous syphilis. This mistranslation influenced early medical authors toward a diagnosis of syphilis.

2. Beethoven's Skull Was Not Abnormally Thickened

The Latin Text (J. Wagner) "Calvaria ex integro validam densitatem et crassitudinem fere dimidium pollicem metientem obtulit."

Latin-German Translation (I. Seyfried) "Das Schädelgewölbe zeigt durchgehends grosse Dichtheit und gegen einem halben Zoll betragende Dicke."

German-English Translation (H. H. Pierson) "The Calvarium exhibited throughout great density and a thickness amounting to about half an inch."

Latin-English Translation (J. Horan) "Again the calvaria was of normal density and thickness measuring nearly half the length of the terminal phalanx of the thumb."

Comment

While the Latin word *validam* might mean stout or strong, it also has an alternative meaning of healthy or sound. Seyfried assumed the former, writing *grosse Dichtheit*, which Pierson translated as "great density." However, Dr. Horan favored the healthy or sound alternative and translated "normal density and thickness." His conclusion was supported by the skull measurements at the second exhumation and the recent examination of the missing fragments (to be discussed in the next chapter). Even so, this mistranslation about the thickness of Beethoven's skull influenced some medical authors toward a diagnosis of pathological disorders of bone such as syphilitic osteitis and Paget's disease.

A MODERN EVALUATION OF THE POSTMORTEM REPORT IN THE LIGHT OF THE 2000s

In modern parlance, Dr. Wagner's findings can be translated into the following diagnoses:

Obstruction of the external ear canals

Meningo-neuro-labyrinthitis

Cerebral edema

Hepatic cirrhosis

Portal hypertension

Contaminated ascitic fluid (peritonitis)

Gallstones

Chronic pancreatitis

Renal papillary necrosis

Adynamic ileus

THE FATE OF THE TEMPORAL BONES

Dr. Wagner sawed out and removed both temporal bones with a view to further study and examination. No subsequent report was issued, however, and the bones later vanished. To this day their whereabouts remain unknown.

Dr. Joseph Hyrtl (1810–1894) was a medical student in Vienna from 1828 and graduated in 1835. Later, when he was a famous anatomist, he showed Wolfgang Amadeus Mozart's skull to Gerhard von Breuning.[34] He also informed Gerhard that as a medical student he remembered seeing Beethoven's hearing organs preserved in a sealed glass jar, in the possession of the mortuary orderly, Anton Dotter, but that they later disappeared.[35]

When Dr. Rokitansky succeeded Dr. Wagner in 1833 he also became the curator of the Pathology Museum. In his autobiography Rokitansky emphasized that Beethoven's temporal bones were missing. According to traditional rumors in Vienna, Dotter sold the bones to a foreign physician. There is no record of them in the extant official records.[36]

NOTES

1. Lesky, *Vienna Medical School*, 75–76. For a brief account of eighteenth-century medicine in Vienna, see Davies, *Mozart in Person*, 31–41.

2. K. A. Portele, "Festvortrag zur Feier 60. Geburtstages von Universitäts-professor Heinrich Holzner, Vorstand des Universitätsinstitutes für Pathologische Anatomie in Wien," *Mitteilungen des Pathologisch-anatomischen Bundesmuseums in Wien* 1(1986): 67–78. A facsimile of Biermayer's title pages are reproduced on pp. 70–71.

3. The Narrenturm was used as a lunatic asylum from April 1784 until 1866. See K. A. Portele, "Guide to the Federal Pathologic-Anatomy Museum," trans. J. Fiona Fuller in *Mitteilungen des Pathologisch-anatomischen Bundesmuseums in Wien* 1 (1987): 3–40.

4. TF, 1053.

5. Breuning, *Memories of Beethoven*, 106.

6. Ibid., 106.

7. I. von Seyfried, BS, Appendix, 43–44.

8. The original manuscript is now in the Federal Pathologic-Anatomy Museum in Vienna (M.N.21.297).

9. Hans Bankl and Hans Jesserer, "Die Krankheiten Ludwig van Beethovens," *Mit-*

teilungen des Pathologisch-Anatomischen Bundesmuseums in Wien 1(1986): 5–12; Bankl and Jesserer, *Die Krankheiten*, 84.

10. Dr. John Patrick Horan, MD, FRACP, FRCP (1907–1993) gained experience in performing postmortem examinations as a young postgraduate student. He was a Latin scholar and remained senior physician to inpatients at St. Vincent's Hospital in Melbourne until his retirement in 1969.

11. The multiple factors that contributed to Beethoven's protein-calorie malnutrition and extreme emaciation included reduced oral intake of nutrients, malabsorption owing to chronic pancreatitis, and possibly an enteropathy, the hypercatabolic state associated with prolonged illness caused by hepato-renal failure, chronic sepsis, and subacute diabetes mellitus, as well as disuse atrophy of his muscles.

12. Thrombocytopenic purpura caused by hepatic cirrhosis complicated by portal hypertension and hypersplenism, and probably also ecchymoses resulting from liver failure.

13. Ascites.

14. The obstruction of the external ear canal and eustachian tube would have contributed a significant degree of conductive deafness to Beethoven's hearing loss.

15. This suggests a labyrinthitis.

16. This is unlikely to be of pathological significance. Dr. Wagner was struck with the contrast of the quantitative comparison of the adjacent atrophy of the eighth cranial nerve.

17. Marked atrophy of both auditory nerves.

18. Dr. Wagner was describing definite pathological changes. The small arteries running in the internal auditory meatus are normally never thicker than one millimeter, whereas a raven's quill has a thickness of from four to five millimeters. Furthermore, he described cartilaginous thickening of these vessels. In the absence of a histological examination, it is impossible to differentiate with certainty from an arteriosclerosis, which is probable, or some other form of arteritis, or a combination thereof. See Bankl and Jesserer, *Die Krankheiten*, 86; P. J. Davies, "Beethoven's Deafness: A New Theory," *Medical Journal of Australia* 149 (1988): 648.

19. This thickening in the region of the floor of the fourth ventricle, considered in conjunction with the changes described in the auditory nerves and the labyrinthitis, strongly suggests thickening from a previous basal meningitis.

20. These changes suggest cerebral edema which is a well-recognized complication of liver failure and hepatic encephalopathy.

21. The length of the terminal phalanx of the thumb used to be a convenient measure for pathologists during a postmortem examination. It corresponded to one inch or one Viennese Zoll, equivalent to 2.6 cm. It must be emphasized that Dr. Wagner, in offering this measurement, stated that the thickness of the skull was normal. Many of the later proponents of syphilitic osteitis and Paget's disease have misinterpreted this point, partly influenced by a faulty translation.

22. The heart and lungs appeared normal. There was no pleural effusion present.

23. The unit of volumetric measure was a Mass or quart, equivalent to 1.4 liters. Four measures was equivalent to 5.6 liters. The presence of rust-colored ascitic fluid is an alteration from the usual straw-colored fluid, and it suggests a contamination resulting from an infection and/or altered blood.

24. This refers to a white bean of oblong shape that measures about 9 × 15 mm.

25. This probably refers to an arteriosclerosis, but in the absence of a histological

examination, it is not possible to exclude an arteritis. Dr. Wagner's description of the liver is characteristic of hepatic cirrhosis.

26. Multiple small gallstones.

27. Enlargement of the spleen occurs in portal hypertension complicating cirrhosis. The black color may relate to hemolysis, the deposition of iron pigments, and oxygen desaturation of the blood after death.

28. These are typical changes of chronic pancreatitis.

29. The greatly distended stomach and intestines suggest an ileus or bowel obstruction.

30. These changes are characteristic of renal papillary necrosis.

31. Davies, "Beethoven's Deafness," 646.

32. I. v. Seyfried, BS (1832 ed.), Appendix, 49; (1853 ed.), Appendix, 45; Schweisheimer, *Beethovens Leiden*, 185–86; Forster, *Beethovens Krankheiten*, 35–36; Bankl and Jesserer, *Die Krankheiten*, 86.

33. Seyfried, BS, Appendix, 43; TF, 1059.

34. For a discussion of Mozart's skull, see Davies, *Mozart in Person*, 171–74.

35. Breuning, *Memories of Beethoven*, 106.

36. Bankl and Jesserer, *Die Krankheiten*, 140, notes 60 and 61.

6

The Exhumations

Ludwig van Beethoven and Franz Schubert were both buried in traditional wooden coffins in the Währing Cemetery.[1] In 1873 the cemetery was closed, and in 1925 it was transformed into Schubert Park.[2]

At the suggestion of members Joseph Hellmesberger and Johann Krall, the board of directors of the Gesellschaft der Musikfreunde in Vienna decided to exhume the graves of Beethoven and Schubert to bury them again in metal caskets to prevent further decomposition of their remains. It was also decided that the resting places of these two famous composers should be established in a manner worthy of their greatness. At the time of the exhumation, a medical examination of their remains was to be undertaken.

THE FIRST EXHUMATION (1863)

This project was funded by the proceeds of a special concert given for this purpose. Two zinc caskets identified with oval metal plates—Beethoven, casket no. 1952, and Schubert, casket no. 1953—were supplied by the firm of A. M. Beschorner.

After the chief medical officer of the district of Klosterneuburg, Dr. August Grailich, had given his consent for the exhumation, the grave digger, Anton Zehrnpfennig, commenced digging on Monday, 12 October 1863, in the Währing Cemetery. Although Schubert's grave presented no difficulties, it took eight hours to excavate Beethoven's grave because of two thick layers of bricks adjacent to the coffin, even thicker toward the head. The original grave digger had been instructed to take these precautions because of the rumor that an attempt would be made to steal Beethoven's head from his grave.

Table 6.1
The Measurements of the Long Bones of Beethoven and Schubert at the First Exhumation in 1863

Bone	Beethoven	Schubert
Right humerus	12 Z. [31.64 cm.]	10 Z., 8 L. [27.61 cm.]
Right femur	16 Z., 3 L. [42.74 cm.]	15 Z. [39.45 cm.]
Right ulna	8 Z., 6 L. [22.35 cm.]	7 Z., 10 L. [20.60 cm.]
Right radius	8 Z., 8 L. [22.79 cm.]	7 Z., 6 L. [19.72 cm.]
Left tibia	13 Z. [34.19 cm.]	12 Z., 4 L. [32.44 cm.]

1 Zoll = 2.63 cm.
1 Linie = 2.19 mm.

Following these preliminary diggings, two guards were posted to guard the tombs during the nights of 12 and 13 October.[3]

On the morning of Tuesday, 13 October at 9:45 the exhumation commenced. The first few of the yellowish-white bones to appear were from the upper extremities, followed by one of the thigh bones, the sacrum, and a piece of the pelvis. The highlight was the examination of the skull which was found to have fragmented into nine pieces. It was confirmed that both petrous portions of the temporal bone, housing the inner ears, had been sawed out. It was also noted that part of the parietal bone was missing.

The anatomist, Professor Carl von Patruban, who had been invited to attend, and the director of the board, Dr. Standthartner, pieced together the fragments of the skull with difficulty owing to the gaps caused by splinters of bone lost during Dr. Wagner's sawing and other missing parts. Only five teeth were in situ in the upper jaw; four healthy teeth had fallen out since the burial, and four teeth were missing. On the other hand, in the lower jaw, only the left second molar and the right wisdom tooth were missing. The left lower wisdom tooth was capped with gold. The nasal septum was found as a separate piece.

Dr. Gerhard von Breuning also assisted in the examination of the remainder of Beethoven's skeleton, which was mostly in a state of good preservation. The long bones of the upper and lower extremities were complete, but the left patella, some of the carpal bones of the wrist, and some of the tarsal bones of the ankle could not be found.

The spine was complete from the neck to the coccyx, and all of the individual vertebrae were intact, except one which had disintegrated into two parts. Both collarbones, shoulder blades, and the pelvic bones were intact, but some of the ribs could not be found. Remarkably, part of the ossified larynx was discovered.[4]

Professor Patruban took the following measurements of some of the long bones of Beethoven and Schubert, which were recorded by Dr. Standthartner (see Table 6.1). The right humerus was measured from the head to the internal protuberance (medial epicondyle), the right ulna from the coronoid process to the lower articular surface, the right radius from the upper to the lower articular surface, the right femur from the greater trochanter to the internal protuberance (medial epicondyle), and the left tibia from the center of the upper articular surface to the center of the lower articular surface.

In addition, parts of Beethoven's clothing and shoes, fragments of the coffin, and the adjacent soil were removed for further examination, although some were given as souvenirs to a few present. Schubert's hair, which was found to be detached from his scalp, was given over to his brother.

The committee gave serious consideration as to whether the skulls of Beethoven and Schubert should be reburied, thereby forever precluding their accessibility for scientific study. A committee meeting was set for 15 October to consider these matters.

Meanwhile it was decided to seal both caskets temporarily with locks. On 13 October the bones of the skeletons, excluding the skulls, were laid out in the new metal caskets in as natural a sequence as possible. Beethoven's vertebral bones, being complete, were fastened together with twine. The reburial procedure was temporarily interrupted by a shower of rain. The caskets were then locked and transferred to the Chapel of the Cemetery, where they were placed next to the altar—Beethoven on the Epistle (right) side and Schubert on the Evangelist (left) side.

The skulls of Beethoven and Schubert were handed over to Breuning and Standthartner, and the other remains to be examined were deposited in the office of the directors of the society.

At the board meeting held two days later, it was decided to rebury the skulls after they had been photographed and cast in plaster, and scientific measurements had been taken. Beethoven's clothing and the fragments of the coffin were to be reburied in a separate zinc box to be specially constructed by A. M. Beschorner to avoid any further decomposition of the skeleton. Schubert's hair was not to be reburied.

Accordingly the photographer, J. B. Rottmayer, took photographs, full face and in profile, on 16 and 20 October, at about noon, of the skulls of Beethoven and Schubert.[5] From noon on 17 October until the forenoon of 19 October, the sculptor Alois Wittman made a cast of Schubert's skull in a special studio, especially provided for the purpose. From 19 to 21 October, Wittman made a casting of Beethoven's skull, after having used a clay base to combine the different fragments as naturally as possible. Only a copy made by K. Stolarzyk survives today in the Federal Museum of Pathologic-Anatomy in Vienna.

During the evening hours of 20 and 21 October, Dr. Franz Romeo Seligmann (1808–1892) took precise measurements and made detailed drawings of both skulls. A dentist, Dr. Carl Faber, made accurate dental impressions.

Meanwhile, a detailed examination of Beethoven's clothing and the adherent soil disclosed several additional remains and bone splinters: the lower end of the left shinbone, the lower end of the left pelvic bone, a rib fragment, the hyoid bone, seven smaller parts of the tarsal bones, and other fragments of bones belonging to the fingers and ribs. All of these remains were reburied in the zinc casket on the evening of 22 October. In the forenoon of Friday, 23 October 1863, the earthly remains of Beethoven and Schubert were reburied in newly established vaults in the Währing Cemetery.

Gerhard von Breuning's Memoirs (1886)

In his memoirs of the first exhumation, Gerhard von Breuning provided additional information.[6] Beethoven's skeleton, which rested in drier earth, was of a lighter texture than that of Schubert, which rested in moister earth, and was almost a black-brown color. Schubert's detached hair contained a comb and fragments of a floral wreath. The contrast between the firm opaqueness and thickness of Beethoven's skull compared to the feminine delicacy of Schubert's raised great interest among both phrenologists and lay people.[7]

While the committee of the Gesellschaft der Musikfreunde agreed to have photographs and castings of gypsum made of the skulls of Beethoven and Schubert, it was stipulated that such were not to be displayed in windows of art shops. Dr. F. R. Seligmann went to Breuning's house to make a gypsum cast of the base of Beethoven's skull.[8]

A noted anthropologist from Bonn, Professor Hermann Schaaffhausen, was excited by Dr. Wagner's description that the convolutions of Beethoven's brain were twice as deep and numerous as usual. After a study of photographic enlargements of Klein's life mask, Schaaffhausen concluded, "The gigantic, serious face of Beethoven below the mighty forehead shows an expression full of strength and defiance, as is reflected in his works."[9]

When, in 1885, the professor of anatomy at the University of Vienna, Carl Langer Ritter von Edenberg (1819–1887), asked Gerhard von Breuning to assist him in making gypsum models of the skulls of Beethoven and Schubert, the photographs by Rottmayer and the busts by Wittman could not be located.[10] Breuning was of the opinion that at the time of transfer of the remains of Beethoven and Schubert to the Central Cemetery in Vienna, the skulls should be retained in a museum, allowing access for future scientific study.[11]

At a meeting of the Viennese Anthropological Society held on 19 April 1887, there was discussion of the comparative anatomy of the skulls of Joseph Haydn, Beethoven, and Schubert, with input from Langer von Edenberg, Schaaffhausen, and a famous neuroanatomist, Theodor Meynert (1833–1892).[12]

Rottmayer's Photograph

The publication of Rottmayer's photograph misled several authors to suggest that the apparent swelling in the right temporal region was clear evidence of bone pathology such as syphilitic osteitis or Paget's disease. Yet Dr. Wagner made no mention of any such swelling in his report, nor is such a prominence visible in any of the authentic masks, busts, or portraits. Indeed, a detailed comparative study of Rottmayer's photograph with the authentic busts, masks, and portraits, made by noted anthropologists Schaaffhausen and Professor Mandylzewski of Vienna, led to an agreement that the apparent right temporal bulge in the photograph was an artifact related to the difficulty of piecing the skull fragments together with clay.[13]

THE SECOND EXHUMATION (1888)

Sixty-one years after Beethoven's death, in 1888, the board of directors of the Friends of Music decided to transfer the remains of Beethoven and Schubert to graves of honor in the composers' plot at the Central Cemetery in Vienna. At the time of the second exhumation, the opportunity was taken to open Beethoven's coffin a second time for a further study of his skull. The following report was issued by Dr. A. Weisbach, Dr. C. Toldt, and Dr. T. Meynert:

Report on the examination of 21 June 1888 on the remains of Ludwig van Beethoven, on the occasion of the transfer from the Währing to the Central Cemetery of the City of Vienna

(Supplement to the reports of the sittings of the Vienna Anthropological Society, no. 4–6, 1888):

It must be noted in this connection, that only a period of about 20 minutes was available for this examination and, in addition, the external circumstances were highly unfavorable. The examination had therefore to be limited to the available parts of the skull. Regarding the skeletal parts of the sacrum and limbs, it should be noted that they seemed to have retained the condition, number and order in which they had been placed in the casket during the first exhumation in 1863, as recorded in the earlier report. We identified the following parts of the skull and examined them:

1. The well preserved skeleton of the upper part of the face with the greater part of the frontal bone. The latter seemed to have been sawed horizontally above the region of the frontal boss. Both maxillary bones are completely preserved; the lower most edges of the nasal bones had crumbled. The walls of both orbits are completely preserved, except for small deficiencies in the paper plate of the ethmoid, the lacrimal bones, and the roof of the left orbit. Only small parts of the zygomatic process are lacking, as are small parts of the posterior border of the hard palate. Furthermore, the damaged body, the small wing, and parts of the large and descending wings of the mandible, and finally the anterior part of the squamous section of the zygoma have been preserved on this part of the skull. There is still a part of the tuberosity of the mandibular joint present on the last named, and particularly on the left side.

From among the teeth, the upper jaw contains on the right side the canine and the second premolar, and on the left side the medial incisor, the canine, both premolars, and the anterior two molars. The roots of the absent incisors are well preserved.

2. The mandible in intact condition provided with all the teeth with the exception of the right wisdom tooth and the second left molar.

3. The occipital bone with attachments on both sides of the tuberosity of the temporal bone and the parietal bones. The base and the apex of the squamous portion are missing.

Table 6.2

Measurements of Beethoven's Skull at the Second Exhumation in 1888 Compared to the Plaster Cast of 1863

Measurements in mm.	From the Bone	From the Plaster Cast
Smallest diameter of the forehead	107	109
Width of the face (between the lowest points of the zygoma-maxillary suture)	109	105*
Width of the cheek bones	129	137*
Interorbital width	28	28
Total height of the face	110	114
Height of the upper part of the face	64	67
Height of nose	49.2	47.5
Distance of the border of the alveolar margin from the root of the nasal spine	14	15
Maximum width of the nasal opening	26.5	26.3
Maximum width of the right orbit	43	44
Maximum height of the right orbit	36	36
Maximum width of the left orbit	41	40
Maximum height of the left orbit	36	36
External width of the maxilla (at the level of the two premolars)	58	59
External width of the maxilla at the head	121	121
External width of the maxilla at the angle	99	100

*It was not possible to make precise measurements of these parameters from the cast.

4. The anterior part of the cranial vault, consisting of the upper sawed-off part of the squamous part of the frontal bone, and the anterior half of both parietal bones.

5. Two pieces of the posterior part of the cranial vault, i.e., of the parietal bones, one of which, the larger part, is recognizable as the apex of the squamous portion of the occipital bone.

It could not be ascertained whether additional, minute fragments of the skull were present in the casket, because of the limited time available. Only the parts of the facial skeleton designated under paragraphs 1 and 2 were suitable for measurement. The results of these are collected in the following table [see Table 6.2].

The following comments are offered about the facial skeleton:

Above the deeply sunken root of the nose, the sharply defined and approximating frontal ridges curve upwards in such a way, that a glabella is actually not present. Above it rises the squamous part of the frontal bone without any suggestion of frontal bossing, flat, and falling away posteriorly. The exterior compact table of the squamous part of the frontal bone is in parts somewhat flattened but clearly demonstrable. The diploë is strongly developed. The squamous part of the frontal bone, above the region of the frontal bosses, has a thickness of 7.5 mm on the left side, and 7 mm on the right side. There is no evidence of a frontal suture.[14] The orbital inlets, from the point of view of their measurement, are greater than the usual size, and demonstrate a most striking asymmetry of outline.[15]

The inlet of the left orbit shows an almost straight and horizontal upper border which becomes angular at the lateral and medial border; in the same way there appears to be a rather sharp angle between the lateral and the inferior border, while the medial border is inclined obliquely, backwards and outwards, without a sharp line of demarcation with the lower border. All in all, therefore, the entry to the left orbit appears angular, its greatest average height being vertical, and its greatest width horizontal.

The entry to the right orbit is broader, as a consequence of marked bowing of the zygomatic margin, its longest diameter is from the lower outer to the upper inner margin (against the Foveola *trochlearis*), the greatest vertical diameter lying at right angles to the former. The lower border (as well as the whole floor of the orbit) is very markedly inclined to a lower and outer direction. The transition from the lateral to the upper and the lower border describes a flat arch. The entrance to the right orbit appears therefore to be quite markedly oblique, its outline rounded but widened.

The relationships of the alveolar part of the maxilla are worthy of note. Its intermediate portion, due to the consequence of the marked prominence of the *Juga alveolaria* of both canine teeth, is flattened in a frontal direction and markedly inclined towards the front. By the same token the strong central incisor projected forward at an angle. The degree of angulation could not be determined at the level of the bone itself. The lower anterior nasal spine is markedly developed. Praenasal fossae are not present. In the immediate relationship with the obliqueness of the anterior part of the alveolar process, is the complete flattening of the hard palate in a sagittal plane. But also in the horizontal plane the latter is only slightly arched, in spite of the well preserved sockets for the premolars and molars. The mandible is small in relationship to the upper part of the face; its alveolar part and the part corresponding to the incisors are markedly inclined forward. The mental protuberance shows on its lower margin a shallow depression, while on the left coronoid process there is a small accessory spur.

In addition, the following should be noted:

The inner surface of the available fragments of the cranial vault show only moderately developed *Juga cerebralia*. This applies especially to the orbital processes of the frontal bone and the wing of the sphenoid. To the last mentioned is attached the part of the skull mentioned under paragraph 1, to such an extent that also the condition of the middle cranial fossa can to some extent be gaged. It appears in no way to be particularly deep, but rather quite shallow and flat.

The cribriform plate of the ethmoid bone is quite depressed between the orbital processes of the frontal bone, i.e., the inner surface of the latter fall away on both sides from the incisura ethmoidalis.

The squamous part of the occipital bone, in the horizontal plane, is curved in a circular, not parabolic fashion, which does not permit a very marked overhang of the occiput.

In the parts of the cranial vault, designated under paragraph 4, the flattening of the squamous part of the frontal bone is not very noticeable. The saw cut of the latter approximates reasonably well to the corresponding part of the underneath section of the frontal bone. In these, and in the remaining fragments, the suture lines on the outer surface are reasonably clearly recognizable, even though they are in part obliterated by senile fusion. On the other hand there was no sign of a suture line on the inner surface of the skull bones. One could determine this from the coronal suture, the sagittal suture, and the lambdoid suture, the spheno-parietal, spheno-frontal, and the spheno-temporal sutures. Even the suture lines of the facial bones are only partly obliterated, and to a large extent well preserved.

From these findings the following conclusions can be drawn:

1. The plaster cast of Beethoven's skull, prepared by the sculptor Alois Wittman in the year 1863, can, from the point of view of the parts of the face, be considered completely accurate, and therefore a reliable basis for further investigations of the latter. This is based on a close agreement of all important measurements [see Table 6.2], and in particular, through a study of the visible characteristics of the form of the facial skeleton, comparing the original and the mould. The good state of preservation, and the intact relationships of all parts, would make a good mould easily obtainable.

With regard to the accuracy, on the other hand, of the relationships within the cranial vault and in particular those relating to length, breadth, height and contour of the occipital region, serious reservations have been raised about the plaster cast. Deterioration of the cranial vault in several of the fragments, so that the opposing margins no longer coincide, and total interruption of relationships in the ear region and the base of the skull, as a consequence of deficiencies within the large bony pieces, makes it appear quite impossible that the overall shape of the skull indicated by the cast cannot be redefined with any certainty, whereby it should be emphasised that the condition of the cranial bones, as judged by the official record which we have from 1863, was no better than at present. What the plaster cast does definitely indicate however is the highly developed flattening of the forehead region as far up as the vertex, which the surviving skull fragments cannot indicate with any certainty.

2. There can be no real objection to the authenticity of the skull fragments found in the coffin. They bear the unmistakable stamp of those reports emanating from contemporaries and based on Professor Wagner's examination of Beethoven's body and relative to their state of preservation they conform fully to the skeletal parts which remain.

3. It is an undeniable fact that Beethoven's skull agrees in no way with our concepts of beauty and harmony of form. The hitherto quite pathetic quibbling and fault finding which we have seen from time to time lack any basis in fact.

The pronounced slope of the forehead cannot be attributed either to prior loosening of the suture lines or post-mortem changes in the bones. As mentioned above, all the cranial fragments do in fact show changes of senile synostosis which corresponds with the great artist's advanced age; the major proportions are still quite clearly recognisable. The characteristics by which senile fusion can be distinguished from earlier changes are so well marked that the validity of their assessment can be assured.[16]

It can be considered even less likely that the flatness of the forehead could be attributed to compression of the skull fragments in the grave or degeneration of their superficial layers by decay. Against the first proposition it can be stated unequivocally that the sawn off upper table portion of the frontal bone matches exactly the shape of the under portion left attached to the facial bones which would have been quite impossible if the fragments lying apart from each other in the coffin had through pressure of earth suffered a substantial change in dimensions. The second assumption is refuted by the above-mentioned finding in which the outer table of the frontal bone shows only minimal superficial desquamation of the compact outer table and the thickness of the frontal bone at the level of the sawcut approximates the considerable figure of 7.0 to 7.5 mm.[17] Beethoven's skull is distinguished by a high degree of alveolar prognathism. As the degree of this cannot be determined entirely by the bone itself, and as it seemed desirable to be able to define it more exactly, we sought additional help from the plaster cast. From it, it appears that the angle which the anterior alveolar process makes with the horizontal near the central point approximates 54 deg.[18] This means naturally that the position of the trans-sectional line can be quite considerably influenced. To determine this point more accurately we used the plaster cast. Assuming that the hypothetical horizontal plane is correct, this shows the angle of profile to be 78.5 deg.

It is clear that this latter measurement may prove to be considerably smaller were the alveolar process to possess average height. The unusual shortness of the latter, considering that all the incisor alveoli are present—the extent to which these can be attributed to ageing changes may be left undecided—as well as the striking prominence of the inferior nasal spine or the prominence of the root line of the upper lip linked to it can suffice, in order to explain that the markedly prognathous jaw may not have been so striking in life. The last mentioned condition is also, in any case, applicable to the shape of the lower part of the nose which appears quite flat on the death mask.

4. Regarding the interior of the cranium and the quality of the inner surface of the cranial bones we have no significant findings to report. Just the same we are able to state that the *Juga cerebralia* and the *Impressiones digitatae* are only moderately developed. This is also apparent in the plaster cast of the left half of the anterior cranial fossa which Professor Romeo Seligmann prepared on the occasion of the first exhumation of Beethoven's mortal remains in 1863 and which he kindly made available to us. We do not wish to attribute any value to this fact in the event that one may possibly draw conclusions about the number and arrangement of the gyri or even the depth of the sulci on the surface of the cerebrum. Professor Joh. Wagner has made the observation after autopsy examination of Beethoven's body that the cerebral gyri were only as deep and numerous as is usual,[19] hence according to our view the condition in the inner surface of the skull would certainly not be in agreement. Just the same, out of respect for this worthy anatomist we must state our conviction that one can ascribe only limited value to multiple experiments culminating in results of this nature if not supported by direct facts and figures, and that in general any utterance concerning the depth of the sulci is an over-statement. It was quite impossible to prepare a cast of the cranial cavity or express any opinion concerning the cranial capacity because of the state of the skull fragments.[20]

THE MISSING FRAGMENTS FROM BEETHOVEN'S SKULL

In the report of the first exhumation, it was established not only that both petrous portions of the temporal bone had been sawed out by Dr. Wagner, but also that part of the parietal bone was missing. Furthermore, in the report of the second exhumation, it was also noted that part of the occipital bone could not be accounted for.

Anthropologist Felix von Luschan used the assistance of a Lucae apparatus to draw a plaster cast of Beethoven's skull. In the left lateral view there was a suggestion that parts of the occiput were missing.[21] T. von Frimmel also noted that Beethoven's left parietal bone was missing.[22] Furthermore, Professor Schaaffhausen, after a study of Wittman's cast, wrote, "The plaster cast lacks a part behind the knob of the left parietal bone, and a part of the one above the occipital squama."[23]

In 1985 the jigsaw puzzle was solved when three fragments, allegedly from the vault of Beethoven's skull, were handed over to Professor H. Jesserer and Professor H. Bankl in Vienna for a medical examination. It transpired that these three fragments had been confiscated by Seligmann at the time of the first exhumation. The three fragments were safely preserved in a zinc box which passed on into the estate of his son, Albert F. Seligmann, and subsequently to a great-grand nephew who handed them over for a medical examination.[24]

After detailed studies and consultations, Jesserer and Bankl concluded confidently that the three fragments were indeed almost certainly from the skull of Ludwig van Beethoven. The larger solitary fragment, measuring 7.8 × 6.1 cm, was assigned to the occipital bone; while the other two adjacent fragments, measuring together 8.2 × 6.7 cm, were assigned to the left parietal bone.[25]

The appearance of the three fragments was unremarkable: each was of normal thickness, and the clearly recognizable diploë was anatomically regular. Special x-rays of the three fragments revealed a normal appearance conforming with Beethoven's age of fifty-six years.[26] There was no evidence of Paget's osteodystrophy or any other bone pathology.

The solitary fragment from the occipital bone had a thickness of 4.0–8.5 mm, increasing to 16.4 mm at the site of a natural protuberance. The thickness of the adjacent fragments from the left parietal bone measured 4.0–8.2 mm, increasing to 10 mm at the region of a bone crista on the internal surface. The internal and external tables measured 1 mm, and the diploë displayed the usual cancellous porous structure.[27] These measurements of thickness are within the normal range of 3.0–12.9 mm for the adult German population.[28]

NOTES

1. Following his death on 19 November 1828, Schubert was buried on 21 November, only three graves distant from Beethoven's burial site.

2. O. E. Deutsch, *Schubert: A Documentary Biography* (London: J. M. Dent, 1946), 622.

3. The official report, in three parts, of the first exhumation, between 13 and 23 October 1863, is preserved in the archives of the City of Vienna. The excerpts pertaining to Beethoven were extracted in Bankl and Jesserer, *Die Krankheiten*, 89–95. I am grateful to Erna Schwerin for her translation.

4. Ossification of three of the cartilages of the larynx (i.e., the thyroid, cricoid, and the arytenoid) commences about the twenty-fifth year, and by the age of sixty-five conversion into bone may be complete. See *Gray's Anatomy: Descriptive and Applied*, ed. T. B. Johnston and J. Whillis, 29th ed. (London: Longmans, Green, 1947), 1276.

5. Rottmayer's photograph in profile of Beethoven's skull has not survived.

6. "Die Schädel Beethovens und Schuberts" was first published in *Feuilleton of the Neuen freien Presse* on 17 September 1886. It was reprinted as an appendix in Alfred C. Kalischer's edition of *Aus dem Schwarzspanierhause* (Berlin: Schuster and Loeffler, 1907; New York: Georg Olms Verlag, 1970), 209–21.

7. Ibid., 213–14, trans. Erna Schwerin.

8. Ibid., 215.

9. Ibid., 218. Breuning misspelled it Schaffhausen.

10. Ibid., 220.

11. Ibid., 220–21.

12. Hofrath Professor Dr. C. Langer von Edenberg, "Die Cranien dreier musikalischer Koryphäen," *Mittheilungen der Anthropologischen Gesellschaft in Wien* 17 (1887): 33–36.

13. Frimmel, BS, I: 153–57; F. A. Schmidt, "Noch einmal: 'Beethovens Gehörleiden und letzte Krankheit,' " *Deutsche Medizinische Wöchenschrift* 54 (1928): 284; H. Gattner, "Zu Beethovens Krankheit und sein Tod," *Münchener Medizinische Wöchenschrift* 100 (1958): 1009–10.

14. A frontal (metopic) suture is present in only 7 to 12.3 percent of the German population. See Johannes Lang, *Clinical Anatomy of the Head*, trans. R. R. Wilson and D. P. Winstanley (Berlin: Springer-Verlag, 1983), 11. I am grateful to neurosurgeon Dr. J. Keith Henderson for this information.

15. The maximum height of both of Beethoven's orbits was 36 mm, and this is within the normal range of from 31.8 to 38.5 mm. The maximum width of his right orbit was 43 mm, which was 2 mm greater than on the left side. In the German population the right orbit is on an average 1.72 mm broader than the left. However Beethoven's interorbital width, measured from the meeting point on either side of the frontal bone, the frontal process of the maxilla, and the lacrimal bone, was 28 mm, which is wider than normal (19–25.6 mm). See Lang, *Clinical Anatomy of the Head*, 2–3.

16. Welcher, *Investigations of the Growth and Structure of the Human Skull* (Vienna, 1962), 15 (cited in the report).

17. The normal range of the thickness of the squamous part of the frontal bone in German adults is from 3.2 to 12.5 mm on the left side and from 3.2 to 12.6 mm on the right. See Lang, *Clinical Anatomy of the Head*, 14.

18. This angle cannot be determined with the desired accuracy because the extrnal auditory meatus is lacking on both sides. Nevertheless the place at which the upper border of same should exist can be determined approximately by using the zygoma.

19. See Schaaffhausen's address to the Sixteenth Assembly of the German Anthropological Society, *Proceedings of the German Society of Anthropology, Ethnography and Pre-history*, October 1885, p. 147. The three examiners were inaccurate on this point. Dr. Wagner stated, "the sulci of the brain were much softer and more watery, twice as deep as usual and (much more) more numerous than is usually seen."

20. A. Weisbach, C. Toldt, and Th. Meynert, "Bericht über die an den Gebeinen Ludwig van Beethoven's gelegentlich der Uebertragung derselben aus dem Währinger Orts-Friedhofe auf den Central-Friedhof der Stadt Wien am 21.Juni 1888 vorgenommene

Untersuchung," *Mitteilungen der Anthropologischen Gesellschaft in Wien* 18 (1888): 73–76, trans. Dr. Andrew C. Newell and Erna Schwerin.

21. It is reproduced in Frimmel, BS, I: 168.

22. Frimmels *Nachlass*, M 43, in the Beethoven Haus in Bonn, is reproduced in Bankl and Jesserer, *Die Krankheiten*, 113.

23. Schaaffhausen, "Correspondenz-Blatt der deutschen anthropologischen Gesellschaft," 1887, 160, cited in H. Jesserer and H. Bankl, "Ertaubte Beethoven an einer Pagetschen Krankheit?" *Laryngology, Rhinology, Otology* 65 (1986): 595, trans. Erna Schwerin.

24. The three fragments are illustrated in Schaaffhausen, "Correspondenz," 593; and Bankl and Jesserer, *Die Krankheiten*, 107.

25. Jesserer and Bankl, "Ertraubte Beethoven," 592–96; Bankl and Jesserer, *Die Krankheiten*, 106–9.

26. The x-rays of the three fragments are illustrated in Jesserer and Bankl, "Ertraubte Beethoven," 596.

27. Bankl and Jesserer, *Die Krankheiten*, 106.

28. Lang, *Clinical Anatomy of the Head*, 14.

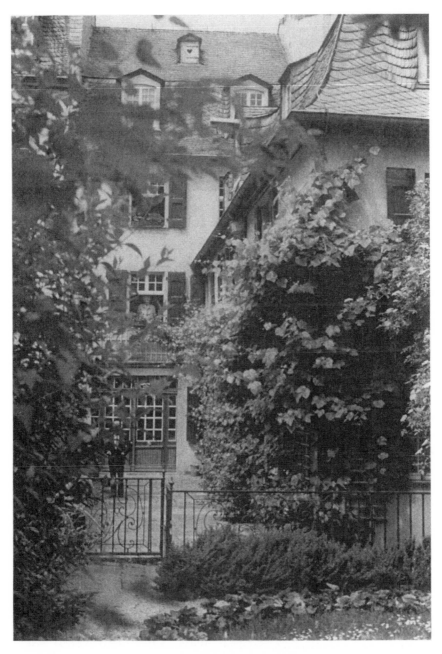

Beethoven's birth house, a view from the garden. The highly probable date of his birth was 16 December 1770. He was christened Ludovicus the next day, at the baptismal font in the Church of St. Remigius. Author's photograph, courtesy Mario Cotela.

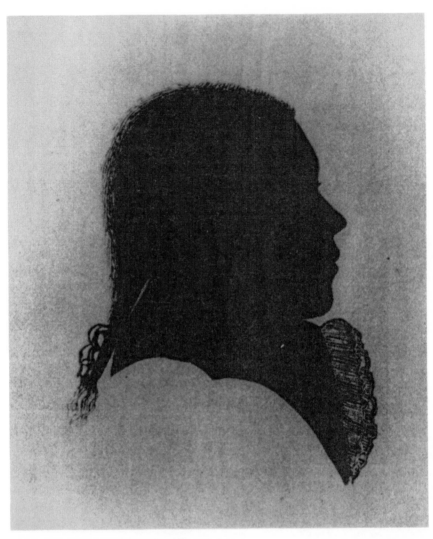

Beethoven at the age of sixteen. Silhouette, 1786, attributed to Joseph Neeson. The pigtail and jabot were typical of the period. Note the central vaulting of the forehead, the protruding lips, the powerful chin, and short neck. From Stephan Ley, *Beethovens Leben in authentischen Bildern und Texten* (Berlin: Bruno Cassirer, 1925), courtesy Mario Cotela.

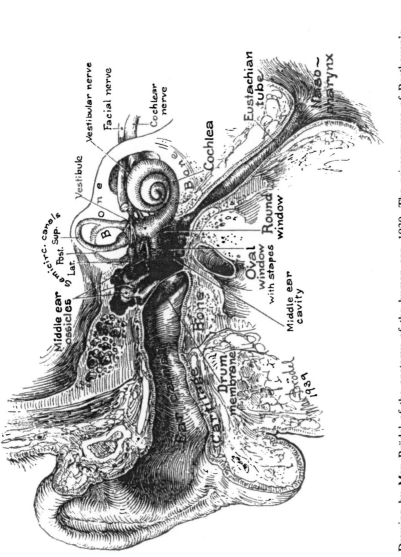

Drawing by Max Brödel of the anatomy of the human ear, 1939. The primary cause of Beethoven's deafness was a meningo-neuro-labyrinthitis, contracted during a bout of typhus fever. There was also obstruction of the ear canal with debris, but the middle ear appeared normal. From J. Nolte, ed., *The Human Brain: An Introduction to Its Functional Anatomy*, 4th ed. (St. Louis: Mosby-Year Book, Inc., 1999), courtesy Mario Cotela.

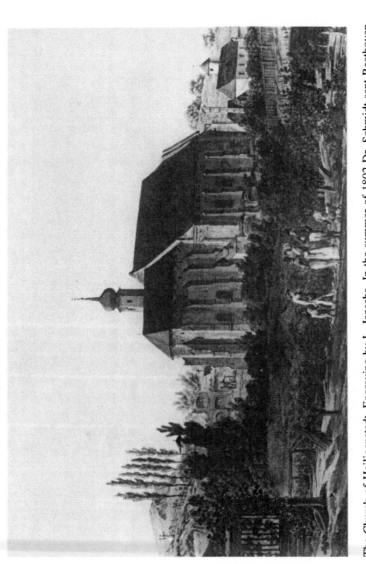

The Church of Heiligenstadt. Engraving by L. Janscha. In the summer of 1802 Dr. Schmidt sent Beethoven to the secluded country town of Heiligenstadt, to spare the effort of his hearing mechanism and to take the spa cure. During his suffering reaction Ludwig was inspired to compose his Oratorio, and after an altercation with his favorite younger brother, Carl, during a period of despair on 6 October, he wrote the famous *Heiligenstadt Testament*. By permission of Historisches Museum der Stadt, Wien.

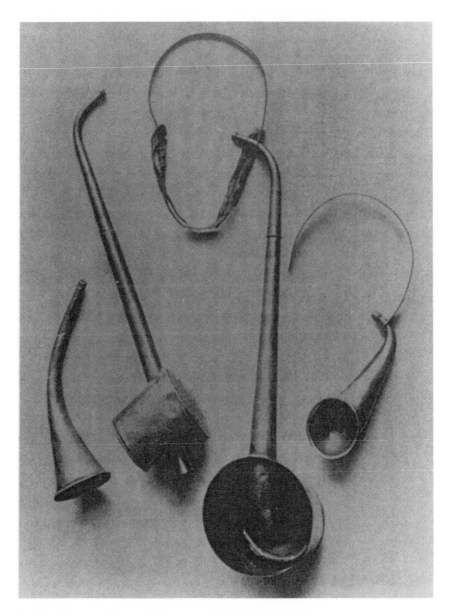

Beethoven's ear trumpets. These were manufactured by Mälzel during 1812–1814. The most useful of the four was the smallest one, which was taken on outings. The two with headbands were designed for use at the keyboard. No doubt the acoustic trauma generated by these devices contributed to the progression of his deafness. From Stephan Ley, *Beethovens Leben in authentischen Bildern und Texten*, courtesy Mario Cotela.

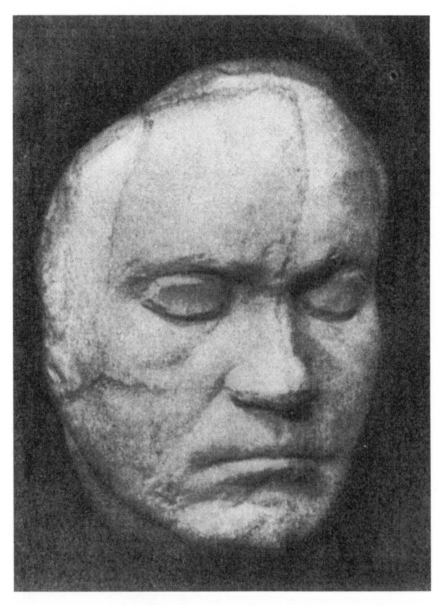

Beethoven's life-mask by Franz Klein. Klein made the casting at a solitary session in 1812. Cotton wads cover the eyes. Note the forced grimace of annoyance as Beethoven reacted to the discomfort and sense of impending suffocation. He violently tore the mask from his face, hurled it aside, and charged out of the room in a huff. Although the negative mold broke into pieces, Klein was able to join them together to reconstitute the cast. This most authentic image reveals exceptional fine details of scars, individual skin pores, and lines on the lips. From Stephan Ley, *Beethovens Leben in authentischen Bildern und Texten*, courtesy Mario Cotela.

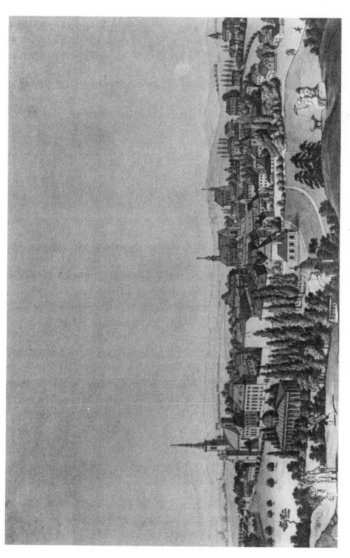

The thermal spa town of Baden near Vienna. Engraving by Vincenz Grüner after V. Grimm. The thermal sulphur springs at Baden attracted large crowds. There was reputed benefit, especially for rheumatic complaints, chronic skin disorders, and hemorrhoids. Beethoven attended in 1804, 1807, 1809–1810, 1813–1816, and 1821–1825. By permission of Historisches Museum der Stadt, Wien.

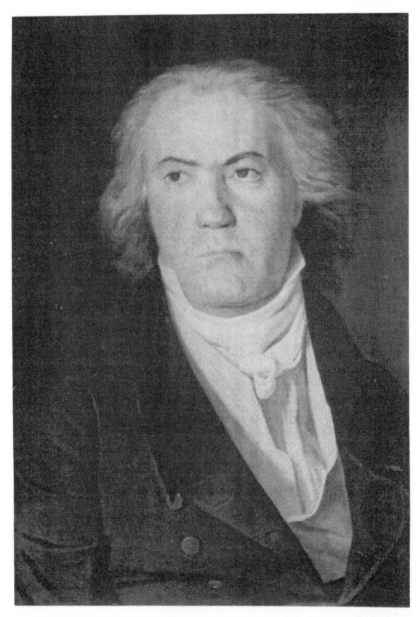

Beethoven. Oil painting by Ferdinand Georg Waldmüller, 1823. Following its commission by Gottfried C. Härtel, Beethoven reluctantly gave the gifted portraitist just one sitting, during which the preoccupied composer would sometimes leave his seat to register his inspiration on paper at his writing table next door. At the time Ludwig was suffering from uveitis, and when the artist asked him to sit facing the window, his eye discomfort was aggravated by the glare. This austere portrait bristles with Ludwig's hostile reaction of anger and resentment, which resulted in his driving out the artist before he had finished. A second sitting was refused so that Waldmüller had to complete the portrait from memory. From Robert Bory, *Ludwig van Beethoven: His Life and Work in Pictures* (London: Thames & Hudson, 1966), courtesy Mario Cotela.

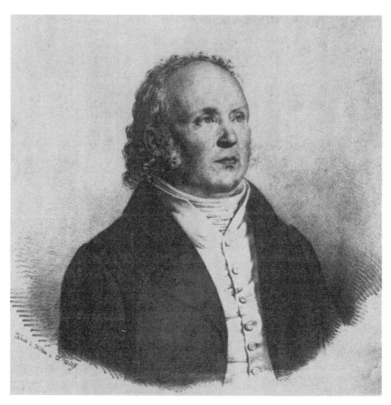

Dr. Andreas Ignaz Wawruch (1773–1842). Lithograph by Franz Wolf. From 1819 Wawruch was Director of the Medical Clinic in Vienna, while also Professor of Special Pathology and Therapy of Internal Medicine. Dr. Wawruch treated Beethoven throughout his final illness. His "Medical Review of L. v. Beethoven's Last Days" was first published on 30 April 1842 in the *Wiener Zeitschrift*. The criticisms of Dr. Wawruch's treatment of Beethoven by Schindler and Gerhard von Breuning were unfounded. By permission of Historisches Museum der Stadt, Wien.

Beethoven's last written words: The codicil to his will on 23 March 1827. While his brother Johann and Schindler propped up and supported the sick composer, Stephan von Breuning kept the pen moistened with ink while supervising Beethoven to copy out the prepared text. The tremulous script, errors, repetitions, and omissions reflect Ludwig's state of stupor due to hepatic encephalopathy. From Stephan Ley, *Beethovens Leben in authentischen Bildern und Texten*, courtesy Mario Cotela.

The autograph of Beethoven's autopsy report. The original Latin report was rediscovered in 1970 by Professor Holzner. The autograph was written by a secretary and signed by Dr. Wagner, who performed the post-mortem examination on the morning of Tuesday, 27 March 1827. Two errors in the Pierson-Seyfried translations misled early medical scholars. Beethoven's temporal bones have disappeared. Courtesy of the Federal Pathologic-Anatomy Museum in Vienna and Mario Cotela.

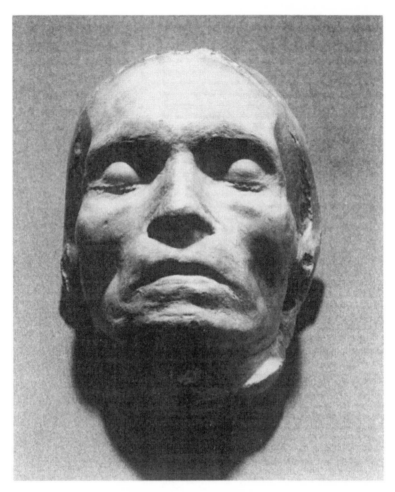

Beethoven's death mask by Joseph Danhauser. View from the front. It was cast on 28 March 1827. The distortion of the right side of the face and the sagging cheek followed Dr. Wagner's removal of the temporal bones. This mask was given by Danhauser to Franz Liszt in 1840, and it was acquired by the museum from Princess Marie von Hohenlohe. By permission of Historisches Museum der Stadt, Wien.

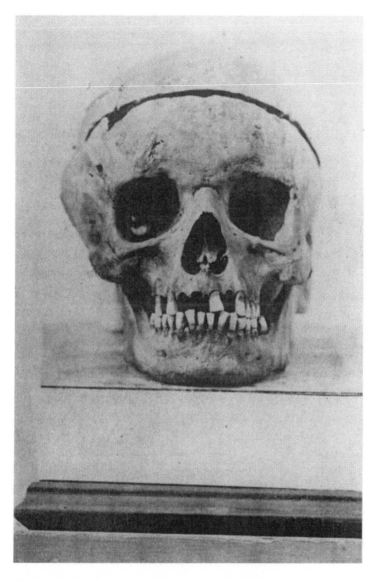

J. B. Rottmayer's photograph of Beethoven's skull at the first exhumation in 1863. Beethoven's skull was found to have fragmented into nine pieces. It was difficult to reunite the fragments because of missing parts and gaps due to splinters of bone lost during the sawing process. The molding of the parts together with clay was especially difficult in the right temporal region, giving rise to a prominent bulge there. His left lower wisdom tooth was capped with gold. Rottmayer took photographs of the skulls of Beethoven and Schubert on 16 and 20 October. The artefact in the right temporal region was misdiagnosed by early scholars as a disease of the bony skull such as syphilitic osteitis or Paget's Disease of bone. By permission of Historisches Museum der Stadt, Wien.

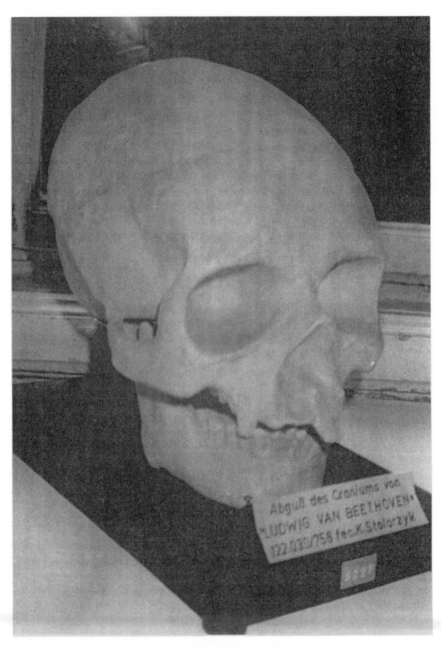

K. Stolarzyk's plaster cast of Beethoven's skull. Alois Wittman's cast, molded during the first exhumation between 19 and 21 October 1863, has vanished. Only this copy survives today. Author's photograph, courtesy of the Federal Pathologic-Anatomy Museum in Vienna and Mario Cotela.

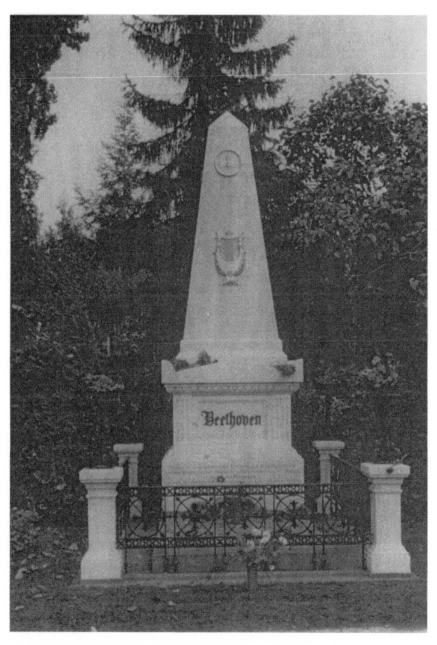

Beethoven's grave of honor in the Central Cemetery of Vienna. Beethoven's grave in the Währing Cemetery was opened a second time on 21 June 1888, sixty-one years after his death. After a brief further examination of his skull his remains were transferred to the section devoted to the honor graves of the composers in the Central Cemetery of Vienna. Author's photograph, courtesy Mario Cotela.

7

The Question of Venereal Disease: A Critical Reevaluation

The notion that Beethoven suffered with a syphylitic affliction received its initial impetus in 1879 with the influential entry of George Grove.[1] Authoritative medical rebuttals were made in 1921 by the Italian otologist G. Bilancioni, who favored a diagnosis of otosclerosis involving the cochlea as the cause of Beethoven's deafness,[2] and in 1922 by the German otologist Waldemar Schweisheimer, who asserted that it was an acoustic neuritis of the inner ear.[3] The lack of agreement between these two medical authorities cast a further shadow over the issue.

During the centenary year of 1927, the syphilitic hypothesis was rekindled in the biographies of André de Hevesy[4] and Ernest Newman.[5] Newman's work inspired a vitriolic counterattack by Carl Engel.[6]

There was further controversy over J. B. Rottmayer's photograph of the exhumed skull, but the alleged defamatory prescriptions were never published. Most recent medical authors remain opposed to a luetic diagnosis.[7]

GEORGE GROVE'S ENTRY

In 1879 Grove wrote that Beethoven probably suffered from syphilis:

The post-mortem examination showed that the liver was shrunk to half its proper size, and was hard and tough like leather, with numerous nodules the size of a bean woven into its texture and appearing on its surface. There were also marks of ulceration of the pharynx, about the tonsils and Eustachian tubes. The arteries of the ears were [atheromatous], and the auditory nerves—especially that of the right ear—were degenerated and to all appearance paralysed. The whole of these appearances are most probably the result of syphilitic affections at an early period of his life. This diagnosis, which I owe to the kindness of my friend Dr. Lauder Brunton, is confirmed by the existence of two prescriptions, of which, since the passage in the text was written, I have been told by Mr. [Alexander Wheelock] Thayer, who heard of them from Dr. Bertolini.[8]

We have seen that Dr. Brunton was influenced by a mistranslation in the Seyfried-Pierson report of the autopsy. Brunton also misinterpreted the report of the liver disease as indicative of syphilis, mistaking the bean-sized nodules of macronodular cirrhosis for syphilitic gummata. With the hindsight of medical knowledge today, Brunton's misdiagnosis then is understandable.

In 1838 Phillippe Ricord (1800–1889) first proved that syphilis and gonorrhea are distinct venereal diseases, and he defined the specific character of syphilis, which he divided into the three stages of primary, secondary, and tertiary infection.[9] Confusion developed in the medical literature concerning the terminology of late luetic liver disease and its relationship to cirrhosis. The variety of descriptive terms included gummatous hepatitis, hepar lobatum, syphilitic nodular cirrhosis, tertiary syphilis of the liver, late syphilis of the liver, or even syphilitic cirrhosis.[10] This confusion was largely resolved by R. D. Hahn's article in 1943[11] and S. S. Lichtman's chapter in *Diseases of the Liver, Gall Bladder and Bile Ducts* in 1949.[12]

Although the Wassermann serological test for syphilis was introduced in 1906, the more sensitive and specific treponemal antibody tests became available only between 1957 and 1967.[13]

THE ALLEGED DEFAMATORY PRESCRIPTIONS

Although Thayer made no specific mention of them in his biography, it is implied from Grove's statement that prescriptions were among Beethoven's letters and notes burned by Dr. Joseph Andreas Bertolini in 1831.[14] Otto Jahn visited Dr. Bertolini twice in Vienna in 1852, and he took notes each time.

It is also implied, as pointed out by Newman, that Dr. Bertolini was under the impression that he was treating Beethoven for a venereal disease.[15] Need it be emphasized that the prescriptions could not exist today if they were burned in 1831?

It has been assumed that the defamatory prescriptions were concerned with mercury. Even if that were true, would it prove beyond any doubt that Beethoven was being treated for syphilis? No, it would not.

Prior to Ricord's publication in 1838, there was confusion about the nature of syphilis and gonorrhea. Furthermore, by the middle of the nineteenth century, there was a tendency for physicians to prescribe mercury as a panacea for many illnesses. Even in the 1890s mercury was recommended not only for syphilis but also for intestinal obstruction, the early stages of typhoid fever, and certain forms of intestinal catarrh. Mercury was also used as a laxative, a diuretic, and a cholagogue to stimulate the flow of bile from the liver.[16]

WHAT DID THAYER COMMIT TO PRINT?

Those who have had occasion and opportunity to ascertain the facts, know, that he had not [puritanic scruples on moderate gratification of the sexual], and are also aware that he did not always escape the common penalties of transgressing the laws of strict purity.[17]

In response to Dr. Alois Weissenbach's comment about the absolute purity of Beethoven's morals, Thayer added the adjoinder, "which, unfortunately, is not true."[18]

Thayer also wrote about how Dr. Bertolini had, in 1831, burned the letters and notes of Beethoven "because a few were not of a nature to be risked in careless hands."[19]

It would appear that Thayer was under the impression that Dr. Bertolini treated Beethoven for a venereal disease.

THE THAYER-FRIMMEL-JACOBSOHN-DE HEVESY CORRESPONDENCE

Thayer was approached directly on this sensitive issue not only by Grove, but also by T. von Frimmel. In response to Frimmel, Thayer wrote on 29 October 1880 that Beethoven's venereal disease "was well known to many persons" and went on to state "that his ill health and his deafness perhaps come from some common cause."[20]

In 1912 Frimmel added the ominous lues to the list of possible infections that could cause deafness due to atrophy of the auditory nerves.[21] Leo Jacobsohn was influenced by Frimmel's communication, and also by the apparent right temporal swelling in Rottmayer's photograph of the exhumed skull. Although in his article in 1910 Jacobsohn had favored a chronic middle-ear suppuration following typhus fever as the cause of Beethoven's deafness,[22] in his centenary article he diagnosed congenital syphilis as the cause.[23] Jacobsohn added,

After Frimmel's communication I do not feel I am committing any indiscretion when I say that in the private possession of a man of culture in Berlin there is an as yet unpublished note in Beethoven's own hand referring to a cure that leaves no doubt as to the specific nature of his malady.[24]

In a footnote E. Newman linked this with de Hevesy's discovery of Beethoven's intention to purchase a book on venereal disease.[25] Earlier in his book, de Hevesy had stated, "Thayer, in a letter to Dr. Frimmel, declares that Beethoven, in his youth, had been attacked by syphilis."[26]

In April 1819 Beethoven noted in a conversation-book the title of a book by L. V. Lagneau on the recognition, cure, and prevention of venereal disease.[27] It comes as no surprise to learn that Beethoven expressed his interest in venereal diseases, which were then rampant in Vienna. Nor does such interest offer proof that he himself was afflicted with a venereal disease, although he may have been. Perhaps he considered buying the book to assist in his instruction of his nephew, who was then thirteen years old. After all he had written to the Magistracy in February 1819, "I confess that I feel myself better fitted than anybody else to incite my nephew to virtue and industry by my own example."[28]

Mention of the alleged defamatory prescription continued to appear in the literature. In 1913 it was in the possession of the illustrious first professor of otology in Vienna, Adam Politzer.[29] Politzer's son-in-law, a well-known music journalist, informed Dr. E. Prieger, the Beethoven enthusiast in Bonn, "There is no doubt about it."[30]

According to Dieter Kerner, the document was deposited in the United States:

The Beethoven researcher Max Unger wrote in no. 10/1958 of the *Neue Zeitschrift für Musik* that the musicologist Max Friedländer informed him verbally some time after the First World War about a prescription for syphilis, which was made out in the name of Beethoven, and which was included in the collection of Friedländer's documents. But Friedländer did not under any circumstances want to publicize it; for he was of the opinion that the memory of the immortal [Beethoven] would thus be dimmed. Later on he is supposed to have made a gift of the document to a museum after his emigration to the United States—thus obscuring a valuable source.[31]

Maynard Solomon assured me that the whereabouts of these prescriptions, if they exist at all, has never been established.[32]

PROSTITUTES?

Vienna's girls for amusement catered to all strata of society. There were only a few high-class mistresses, who in exchange for living in style in their own fine residences, with their own horses and carriages, could charge from 2,000 to 3,000 gulden a year.

The more common situation was for two or three mistresses to live together in a matron's house, and they would charge from 500 to 600 gulden a year. Sometimes such a mistress was shared by a group of friends who visited her in rotation.

The wealthier prostitutes, who could afford fine dress, appeared on the streets at noon or in the evening to solicit wealthy clients. The poor street nymphs appeared only at night between darkness and ten o'clock on such avenues as the Graben, the Kohlmarkt, and the Hof. Whores frequented the suburban beer houses where they serviced soldiers, coachmen, and manual laborers.

During the reign of Emperor Joseph II, convicted prostitutes were treated harshly. Their hair was shaved off, and they were sent to work in gangs as street cleaners, or made to launder the linen for the General Hospital. While there was talk of strict medical supervision of brothels to control the spread of venereal diseases, no agreement was reached.[33]

Beethoven made a few references to prostitutes. In his letter from Prague on 19 February 1796, he warned his brother Johann, "Be on your guard against the whole tribe of bad women" in Vienna.[34] Admittedly this reference to prostitutes may have been inspired by a recent encounter with a prostitute in Prague, but even if such speculation were correct, it would not prove that Beethoven had sought sexual favors with such a woman. On the contrary, the warning tone of the letter is more likely to have been prompted by a disgust of such illicit sensual gratification.

Early in 1809, after his quarrel with Countess Erdödy, Beethoven moved out of his rooms in her apartment to new lodgings for a short time on the second floor of no. 1087 Walfischgasse, where there was a brothel. It seems likely that this was an act of spite against the countess. Beethoven became angry with his friend Baron Ignaz von Gleichenstein not only because he did not acknowledge his dedication of the Opus 69 Cello Sonata, but also because he had not been to visit him since his return to Vienna.[35] Poor Gleichenstein was probably too embarrassed to visit him at such a house of ill repute. If Beethoven had intended to consort with prostitutes at this brothel, he would hardly have taken lodgings at the same address.

Editha and Richard Sterba pointed out that the word "fortresses," in some of Beethoven's letters to Zmeskall, was a coded reference to prostitutes.[36] Solomon concluded that Zmeskall was in the habit of patronizing prostitutes, and that perhaps Beethoven also did so from c. 1811.[37] Harry Goldschmidt referred to the ignored fact that Beethoven made use of prostitutes,[38] and M.-E. Tellenbach argued against such an unsubstantiated hypothesis.[39]

Let us examine the relevant parts of Beethoven's letters to Zmeskall:

Be zealous in defending the fortresses of the Empire which, as you know, lost their virginity a long time ago and have already received several assaults.[40]

Enjoy life, but not voluptuously—Proprietor, Governor, Pasha of various rotten fortresses!!!!![41]

I need not warn you any more to take care not to be wounded near certain fortresses. Why, everywhere there is profound peace!!!!![42]

Keep away from rotten fortresses, for an attack from them is more deadly than one from well preserved ones.[43]

In all four instances Beethoven was consistent in warning Zmeskall to take care because of the risk of contracting a venereal disease. On another occasion, in keeping with his own strict moral beliefs, he explicitly informed Zmeskall that he himself was not interested:

In regard to the fortresses, I fancy that I have already given you to understand that I do not want to spend any time in marshy districts.[44]

However, in two other passages, the meaning is far from clear:

Yes! and include me too, even if it's at night.[45]

I have seen nothing—I have heard nothing—Meanwhile I am always ready for it. The time that I prefer most of all is at about half past three or four o'clock in the afternoon.[46]

In the first instance the meaning is too vague to permit an accurate deduction. In the second note, is Beethoven expressing annoyance at the failure of another party to keep an appointment with him? He liked to run his errands at about four o'clock.

In the now lost *Boldrini* pocket sketchbook, which G. Nottebohm examined in Artaria's shop, Beethoven made the entry: "34 × r. am Lusthaus."[47] On this occasion, the word *Lusthaus* did not refer to a brothel, but to the round, free-standing pavilion at the southeastern end of the Prater, where Beethoven had a meal for 34 kreuzer.

At the Artist's Ball in February 1816 Beethoven accused his sister-in-law Johanna (that "Queen of Night") of behaving like a prostitute: "exposing not only her mental but also her bodily nakedness—it was whispered that she—was willing to hire herself—for 20 gulden! Oh horrible!"[48]

Two years earlier, he made the following entry in his Tagebuch, "From today on never go into that house—without shame at craving something from such a person."[49]

This passage implies that he had visited that house previously and that he was disgusted with himself for having craved to have sex with that woman. Beethoven was harsh with himself when he deviated from his high moral standards. Perhaps this entry implied that the woman was not a prostitute, but rather someone known to him, with whom a sexual liaison would have been forbidden? Indeed, could the woman have been his sister-in-law Johanna? Her identity remains unknown.

In 1817 Beethoven made the following entry in his Tagebuch, "Sensual gratification without a spiritual union is and remains bestial, afterwards one has no trace of noble feeling but rather remorse."[50]

Once again Beethoven expressed his disgust of lust for sexual gratification out of wedlock. He found spiritual consolation in the exercise of the rational control of his reason over the passions of his body, "The frailties of nature are given by nature herself and sovereign Reason shall seek to guide and diminish them through her strength."[51]

At some time between 8 and 15 February 1820, Janschikh wrote in a conversation-book, "Where were you going today around 7:00 o'clock walking the streets [*auf dem Strich gegangen*] near the Haarmarkt?"[52] The details of

Beethoven's spoken reply to this question are unknown, but in response, Janschikh wrote in Latin, *"Culpam transferre in / alium"* (To transfer the blame to another).[53] The precise meaning of this dialogue between Beethoven and Janschikh is unclear, and to draw definite conclusions from it, concerning Beethoven's relations with prostitutes, if any, is sheer speculation.[54] Furthermore, it has been pointed out more recently that it was probable that at that time Beethoven was visiting Mathias Tuscher, Carl's guardian of the previous year, who resided at 682 Haarmarkt.[55]

The case for his having consorted with prostitutes remains unproven.

COULD SYPHILIS HAVE CAUSED BEETHOVEN'S DEAFNESS?

The syphilitic advocates have argued either that Beethoven contracted the disease after sexual exposure as a young man, or that he was infected in utero by his mother. A chronological survey of the literature is summarized in Table 7.1.

The Nature of Luetic Deafness

A common cause of deafness in the nineteenth century, syphilis caused the affliction by involvement of the middle ear or the inner ear, either separately or in combination.

An oto-labyrinthitis resulted from the spread of middle-ear infection into the labyrinth. A primary inner-ear involvement was caused either by a spread from a basal meningitis early in the disease, resulting in a meningo-neurolabyrinthitis, or a direct involvement of the labyrinth in the tertiary phase, due to an obliterative endarteritis causing a gummatous osteomyelitis or periostitis, or a nongummatous osteitis. The onset of the deafness could be either early or late in both the congenital and acquired varieties of lues.[56]

Compatibility with the Autopsy Report

Dr. Johann Joseph Wagner's report, suggestive of a meningo-neurolabyrinthitis, associated with atrophy of the auditory nerves and thickening of the auditory arteries is quite compatible with the sequela of an early syphilitic meningitis.[57] Dr. Wagner made no mention of a focal macroscopic anomaly to suggest a tertiary gummatous labyrinthitis, but unfortunately Beethoven's temporal bones are missing. D. Kerner and others have argued that the apparent right temporal swelling in Rottmayer's photograph of the exhumed skull was suggestive of syphilitic osteitis, but we have seen that this was artefact.

Table 7.1
Chronological Survey of the Literature Advocating a Syphilitic Cause for Beethoven's Deafness

Year of Publication	Author*
Acquired Syphilis	
1879	T. L. Brunton (in G. Grove, *Beethoven*, 1896)
1879	G. Grove
1912	T. v. Frimmel
1926	B. Springer
1927	A. de Hevesy
1927	E. Newman
1927	W. Wallace
1930	M. P. Bertein and N. R. Appercé
1937	P. Squires
1938	W. Biechteler
1949	E. Hoffmann
1950	W. H. Becker
1958	B. F. McCabe
1965	T. Antonini
1966	P. H. Bergfors
1989	P. Sandblom
Congenital or Conatal Syphilis	
1927	F. Kahn
1927	L. Jacobsohn
1931	Dr. Werther
1934	J. G. Canuyt
1957	D. Kerner
1973	D. Kerner

*Publication details are listed in the bibliography.

DID BEETHOVEN CONTRACT SYPHILIS AS A YOUNG MAN?

The mysterious, dangerous, febrile illness contracted during the summer of 1796 provides the vital clue to the cause of Beethoven's deafness. In the *Fischhof* manuscript it is clearly stated that, during his convalescence from this illness, his deafness commenced, and from this time it steadily increased.[58]

This illness is presumably the "terrible typhus" referred to by Dr. Weissenbach, and it seems probable that it caused the meningo-neuro-labyrinthitis described by Dr. Wagner. It was characteristic of Beethoven that he made reference to his illnesses in his letters and correspondence. Only four or five of his letters written in 1796 have survived, but in none of them is there any reference to this serious illness.[59]

Presumably he was fully recovered by November since there is no mention then of ill health in Stephan von Breuning's letter to his brother, Lenz, and Franz Gerhard Wegeler.[60] Six months later, Beethoven informed Wegeler that he was well and that his health was steadily improving.[61] There is no reference to illness in any of the other five surviving letters from 1797.

Even in his first reference to his deafness in the summer of 1801, in his letters to Wegeler and Carl Amenda, there is no reference to this preceding serious illness. Why were the details of it suppressed? Could it be that Beethoven suffered with syphilitic meningitis within the context of the following reconstructed scenario? Was it the appearance of a primary chancre, after an indiscreet sexual contact, that prompted his letter of warning to his brother Johann? Then after his return to Vienna did Beethoven develop during the summer of 1796 secondary syphilis which caused meningo-neuro-labyrinthitis?

That would be most unlikely because of the subsequent course of his deafness. After a sudden onset, the deafness caused by syphilitic meningitis, associated with atrophy of the auditory nerves, usually runs a rapid fulminating course over days, weeks, or months and often leads to early complete hearing loss, as in the case of the composer Bedrich Smetana (1824–1884). Smetana's hearing loss was associated with constant severe tinnitus, diplacusis (the hearing of a single tone as if it were two tones of different pitch), and episodic vertigo.[62]

Associated vestibular symptoms, such as vertigo, vomiting, or staggering gait, are of variable severity; they would dominate the clinical course in some patients, but in others, be mild or absent.

Other associated cranial neuropathies are sometimes present, involving the seventh, second, sixth, third, fifth, ninth, tenth, or the twelfth cranial nerves.[63] There was no such involvement in Beethoven.

Admittedly other manifestations of secondary syphilis, such as the skin rash, lymphadenopathy, and mucous patches in the throat, are sometimes mild, and they might easily be missed. However, the absence of the development of neurosyphilis or other tertiary manifestations in Beethoven's later life argues against a diagnosis of acquired early syphilis as the cause of his deafness.

Meningitis also occurs as a sequela of congenital syphilis; however, it should be noted that it occurs early, usually from nine months to two years of age,[64] a scenario incompatible with Beethoven's history.

SYPHILITIC LABYRINTHITIS

The more common cause of deafness than meningitis, in both the congenital and acquired forms of syphilis, is a specific labyrinthitis caused by tertiary lesions of the temporal bone. While a rapid loss of hearing could develop after a

sudden onset, especially in children, the more usual course in adults is a more
gradual progressive deafness with characteristic fluctuations in the hearing.
Loudness recruitment is associated with early loss of bone conduction and poor
voice discrimination. This affliction would mimic Ménière's disease when the
complication of endolymphatic hydrops developed, with the addition of episodic
vertigo, tinnitus, and auditory fullness.[65] Aside from tinnitus, such characteristic
symptoms were absent from Beethoven's medical history.

CONCERNING CONGENITAL SYPHILITIC DEAFNESS

About one in ten patients with conatal lues contracted in utero would develop
deafness, which was most commonly due to a specific labyrinthitis, as outlined
above. The age of onset of the hearing loss varied from four years to the late
forties, most usually between eight and fifteen.

While the hearing loss was occasionally a unique, solitary manifestation, it
was usually associated with other stigmata such as interstitial keratitis, frontal
bossing (the hot cross bun skull), Hutchinson's teeth (peg-shaped, notched incisors), mulberry molars, saddle-nose deformity, saber shins, perforated nasal
septum, Clutten's joints, stunted stature, or rhagades. Naso-pharyngeal lesions
or scars were present in one third.

The most common stigma was interstitial keratitis which usually preceded the
deafness by several years (average, 3–6 years; range 1–31 years).[66]

COULD BEETHOVEN HAVE SUFFERED FROM
CONGENITAL SYPHILIS?

The advocates in favor of conatal lues are listed in Table 7.1. Kerner concluded that congenital syphilis caused not only Beethoven's deafness, but also
his liver disease and pancreatic disorder.[67] Kerner's arguments were convinc-
ingly refuted by H. Gattner.[68]

Even though Beethoven's deafness was associated with tinnitus, there was no
evidence of luetic hydrops, in so far that, in his history from 1798, there was
no suggestion of characteristic fluctuations in hearing, or vertigo, or auditory
fullness.

Kerner concluded that the root of Beethoven's nose was deeply recessed,
indicative of a saddle-nose deformity, one of the stigmata of congenital syphilis.
Such a flattening resulted from failure of normal development of the bones of
the nasal cavity due to "syphilitic snuffles" early in life. But Kerner's conclusion
is incorrect. The profile of Beethoven's nose is especially well defined in Neeson's silhouette, in which there is not a trace of a saddle-nose deformity. Nor
is there any evidence of such a deformity in the authentic masks and portraits.

Kerner also argued that the right temporal bulge in Rottmayer's photograph
and Beethoven's thickened skull bones were indicative of syphilitic osteitis.
However, we have seen that such apparent changes were related to a mistrans-

lation of the autopsy report and artefact. Furthermore, there was no evidence of bone pathology detected in the recent scientific examination of the three fragments from the exhumed skull.

There is no mention in the literature that either of Beethoven's parents ever suffered with syphilis. Furthermore women with luetic infection of the uterus are prone to suffer recurrent miscarriages or give birth to stillborn infants. After Beethoven's birth, his mother was delivered of five healthy, viable infants, though three died in infancy of illnesses contracted after birth. Nor was there any evidence of luetic affliction in either of Beethoven's surviving brothers.

In view of all this, there is convincing evidence that Beethoven was not afflicted with congenital syphilis.

WAS DR. BERTOLINI MISTAKEN?

If Beethoven's alleged venereal disease was well known to many persons during his lifetime, then why has it remained a secret? If Dr. Bertolini was under the impression that he was treating Beethoven for a venereal infection, then how can this be reconciled with the above negative appraisal against syphilis?

The answer remains unknown because Beethoven did not make a pronouncement on the matter. It remains possible that he contracted another venereal infection such as gonorrhea, as suggested by E. Larkin,[69] but there is no history of dysuria, urethral discharge, or obstructive symptoms. It seems more probable that Dr. Bertolini was simply mistaken about the diagnosis of Beethoven's complaints. Another possibility is that the attack of typhus fever in 1796 was contracted coincidentally soon after a sexual exposure, so that it was misdiagnosed as a venereal infection.

CONCLUSION

In the absence of a specific serological test, and microscopic sections from the diseased organs, it is not possible to exclude syphilis with absolute certainty; however, the balance of all the available evidence does not favor a syphilitic diagnosis to account for Beethoven's deafness or other illnesses.

NOTES

1. G. Grove, *Beethoven Schubert Mendelssohn* (London: Macmillan, 1951), 31 n. 4.

2. G. Bilancioni, "La sordità di Beethoven," *Giornale di medicina militaire* 69 (1921): 531–41; G. Bilancioni, *La sordità di Beethoven: Considerazioni di un otologo* (Rome: A. F. Formiggini, 1921).

3. Schweisheimer, *Beethovens Leiden*, 12–97.

4. De Hevesy, *Beethoven The Man*, 162.

5. E. Newman, *The Unconscious Beethoven* (London: Victor Gollancz, rev., 1968), 37–51.

6. C. Engel, "Views and Reviews," *Music Quarterly* 13 (1927): 646–62; C. Engel, *Discords Mingled* (New York: Alfred Knopf, 1931).

7. Forster, *Beethovens Krankheiten*, 62; Böhme, *Medizinische Porträts*, I: 82–83; Larkin, "Beethoven's medical history," 449–53; Bankl and Jesserer, *Die Krankheiten*, 118–19; J. G. O'Shea, "Medical Profile of Ludwig van Beethoven," *Music and Medicine*, 48, 53; A. Neumayr, "Notes on the Life, Works, and Medical History of Ludwig van Beethoven," *Music and Medicine*, 312–17. See also T. G. Palferman, "Letter to the Editor," *Physicians of London* 26 (1992): 112–14.

8. Grove, *Beethoven Schubert Mendelssohn*, 31, n. 4.

9. Garrison and Morton, *A Medical Bibliography*, nos. 2381, 5202.

10. P. J. Davies, "Review Article: Hepatic Syphilis: An Historical Review," *Journal of Gastroenterology & Hepatology* vol. 3 (1988): 287–94.

11. R. D. Hahn, "Syphilis of the Liver," *American Journal of Syphilis, Gonorrhea, and Venereal Diseases* 27 (1943): 529–62.

12. S. S. Lichtman, "The Role of Syphilis in Cirrhosis of the Liver," in *Diseases of the Liver, Gall Bladder and Bile Ducts* (London: Henry Kimpton, 1949), 541–42.

13. Garrison and Morton, *A Medical Bibliography*, nos. 2402, 2419: 1–4.

14. TK, II: 87.

15. Newman, *The Unconscious Beethoven*, 42.

16. Binz, *Lectures on Pharmacology*, II: 127, 144; Brunton, *Lectures on the Action of Medicines*, 471, 608–11.

17. TK, I: 253.

18. TK, II: 294.

19. Ibid., 87.

20. L. Jacobsohn, "Beethovens Gehörleiden und letzte Krankheit," *Deutsche Medizinische Wöchenschrift* 53 (1927): 1610–12; D. W. MacArdle, *Beethoven Abstracts* (Detroit: Information Coordinators, 1973), 299 (F); T. von Frimmel, *Wiener Abendpost*, 1911, no. 283.

21. T. von Frimmel, "Beethovens Taubheit," *Beethoven-Forschung* 1 (1912): 82–99.

22. L. Jacobsohn, "Ludwig van Beethovens Gehörleiden," *Deutsche Medizinische Wöchenschrift* 36 (1910): 1282–85.

23. Jacobsohn, "Beethovens Gehörleiden," 1610–12.

24. Newman, *The Unconscious Beethoven*, 43.

25. Ibid., n. 1.

26. De Hevesy, *Beethoven The Man*, 130, n. 1.

27. The book, *Die Kunst, alle Arten der Lustseuche zu erkennen, zu heilen, und sich dafür zu sichern*, published in Erfurt, was available at Carl Gerold's bookshop for 5 fl. 54 kr. W.W. The advertisement appeared in the *Intelligenzblatt*, no. 84, on 14 April 1819, p. 750. See LvBCB, I: 55, 41 r; Schünemann, *Beethovens Konversationshefte* I: 47, 41 a. De Hevesy translated the title into French (*Beethoven The Man*, 162). See also R. Specht, *Beethoven As He Lived* (New York: Harrison, Smith, and Robert Haas, 1933), 43; Kerner, *Krankheiten grosser Musiker*, I: 104; Solomon, *Beethoven*, 262.

28. TF, 721.

29. Forster, *Beethovens Krankheiten*, 54, n. 1.

30. F. Schultze, "Die Krankheiten Beethovens," *Münchener Medizinische Wöchenschrift* 75 (1928): 1041.

31. Kerner, *Krankheiten grosser Musiker*, I: 104–5, trans. Erna Schwerin.

32. Personal communication, 11 May 1988.

33. See Johann Pezzl, "Sketch of Vienna, 1786–90," in *Mozart and Vienna*, ed. H.C.R. Landon (London: Thames and Hudson, 1991), 84, 136, 151, 152, 170.

34. A-16; B-20.

35. A-213; B-428 (February 1810).

36. E. Sterba and R. Sterba, *Beethoven and His Nephew: A Psychoanalitic Study of Their Relationship*, trans. W. R. Trask (London: D. Dobson, 1957), 110.

37. Solomon, *Beethoven*, 220–21, 262–63; A. Tyson, BS 3 (Cambridge: Cambridge University Press, 1982), 268; M. Solomon, *Beethoven Essays* (Cambridge: Harvard University Press, 1988), 283–84.

38. H. Goldschmidt, *Zu Beethoven* (Berlin: Verlag Neue Musik, 1979), 1: 220.

39. M-E. Tellenbach, *Beethoven und seine 'Unsterbliche Geliebte' Josephine Brunswick* (Zurich: Atlantis, 1983), 285–88.

40. A-407; B-625.

41. A-562; B-841.

42. A-653; B-970.

43. A-681; B-1014.

44. A-715; B-1008 (November-December 1816).

45. A-597; B-881.

46. A-846; B-490 (Spring 1811).

47. G. Nottebohm, *Zweite Beethoveniana* (New York: Johnson Reprint, 1970), 353.

48. A-611; B-904.

49. *Tagebuch-28.*

50. *Tagebuch-122.*

51. *Tagebuch-138.*

52. LvBCB, I: 254, 54 v.

53. Ibid., trans. Aldo Rebeschini.

54. W. Meredith, "Editor's note," BJ, 12 (1997):49.

55. Barry Cooper, "Letter to the Editor," BJ 14 (1999): 102; LvBCB, I, 420, note 71.

56. See A. Politzer, *Politzer's Text-book of the Diseases of the Ear and Adjacent Organs*, 3rd ed., ed. W. Dalby, trans. Oscar Dodd (London: Baillière, Tindall and Cox, 1894), 409–10, 645–49; C. Ernest West, "Aural Syphilis," in *A System of Syphilis in Six Volumes* (London: Oxford Medical Publications, 1910), V:234–87; O. Mayer and J. S. Fraser, "Pathological Changes in the Ear in Late Congenital Syphilis," *Journal of Laryngology & Otology* 51 (1936): 683–714; D. Nabarro, *Congenital Syphilis* (London: Edward Arnold, 1954), 362–69; C. S. Karmody and H. F. Schuknecht, "Deafness in Congenital Syphilis," *Archives of Otolaryngology* 83 (1966): 18–27.

57. B. F. McCabe, "Beethoven's Deafness," *Annals of Otology, Rhinology, and Laryngology* 67 (1958): 192–206.

58. TF, 187–88.

59. A-16, 18; B-20, 22, 23. See also Albrecht, *Letters*, nos. 21, 22, 23. The original autograph of no. 22 is incomplete. Two letters assigned by Anderson, *Letters of Beethoven*, to 1796 (A-15, 19) have been assigned by S. Brandenburg to other years (B-19, 1795; B-414, November 1809). S. Brandenburg, *Ludwig van Beethoven: Briefwechsel Gesamtausgabe*, 7 vols. (Munich: G. Henle, 1996–1998).

60. Letter dated 23 November 1796. See Wegeler and Ries, 156.

61. A-20; B-30.

62. H. Feldmann, "Acute Hearing Loss in the Early Stage of Acquired Syphilis; a Report of One Historical and One Recent Case," *Laryngology, Rhinology, and Otology*

65 (1986):16–20; Y. F. Cudennec, G. Gruselle, and P. de Rotalier, "Bedrich Smetana, L'autre grand sourd et la controverse sur sa maladie," *Histoire des Sciences Médicales* (Paris) 22 (1988):133–40; G. Dean Beaumont, "The Deafness of Bedrich Smetana, 1824–1884," *Australian Journal of Otolaryngology* 1 (1992): 173–77.

63. J. H. Lloyd, "Syphilis of the Eighth Nerve," *Archives of Neurology and Psychiatry* 5(1921): 572–79.

64. Nabarro, *Congenital Syphilis*, 368–69.

65. G. D. Becker, "Late Syphilitic Hearing Loss: A Diagnostic and Therapeutic Dilemma," *The Laryngoscope* 89 (1979): 1273–88.

66. A. Keidel and J. E. Kemp, "Deafness in Late Congenital Syphilis," *Southern Medical Journal* 16 (1923):647–51; Dalsgaard-Nielsen, "Correlation between Syphilitic Interstitial Keratitis and Deafness," *Acta Ophthalmologica* (Copenhagen) 16 (1938):635–47; Nabarro, *Congenital Syphilis*, 365.

67. Kerner, *Krankheiten grosser Musiker*, 89–146.

68. Gattner, "Zu Beethovens Krankheit," *Münchener medizinische Wöchenschrift*, 100 (1958), 1009–10.

69. Larkin, "Beethoven's Medical History," 453.

8

The Cause of Beethoven's Deafness

Much of the considerable literature on Beethoven's health is devoted to hypothesizing about the cause of his deafness. With the hindsight of medical knowledge in the year 2000, it is fascinating to recall the earlier theories.

In 1816 Dr. Alois Weissenbach presented the vital clue that Beethoven's hearing impairment followed a dreadful attack of typhus fever, and Ludwig Nohl linked this with the severe illness suffered during the summer of 1796, noted in the *Fischhof* manuscript.[1]

In the *Stuttgart Morgenblatt* in 1823 it was stated, "[Beethoven] finds it injurious to live in a house with a northerly aspect, or exposed to strong winds, for he is very subject to rheumatism, to which he attributes his deafness."[2]

Dr. T. Lauder Brunton's diagnosis of acquired syphilis was discussed in chapter 7, and in 1880 T. von Frimmel proposed a traumatic aetiology, quoting Charles Neate's anecdote about a fall noted in chapter 2.

Then came several articles in the French literature. In 1900 Dr. Paul Garnault supported Weissenbach's theory when he advocated an acoustic neuritis following typhus in 1796.[3] Two years later, W. Nagel[4] supported the diagnosis of otitis media made by Dr. Buss.[5]

In his thesis written in 1905, Fernand Vieille favored a dry otosclerosis (*une otite scléreuse*).[6] Later that year Dr. G. Baratoux was more precise in his diagnosis of otosclerosis (*l'affection designée sous le nom de spongiosité progressive de la capsule labyrinthique, avec ankylose de l'etrier*).[7] In the second part of the same letter, Marcel Natier argued against middle-ear infection and advocated that the atrophy of the auditory nerves was related to a chronic enteritis following typhus, associated with a similar degeneration of the auditory center in the brain.[8]

In 1905 the learned Parisian physician Dr. Klotz-Forest proposed that, following the attack of typhus in 1796, Beethoven was subject to recurrent bouts of middle-ear infection which caused his deafness.[9] However, Klotz-Forest used Anton Schindler's first edition as his source for the autopsy report, which was incomplete, describing only the atrophy of the auditory nerves and the thickening of the floor of the fourth ventricle. Schindler omitted Dr. Johann Joseph Wagner's description of the external ear canal, the eustachian tube, the mastoid process, and the temporal bone.[10] In response, Dr. Pierre Bonnier disagreed, pointing out the absence of a history of ear discharge, and he proposed an acoustic neuritis following typhus.[11]

In a penetrating article published in the centenary year of 1927, Viennese otologist Heinrich Neumann included Paget's disease of the skull among the possible causes of the acoustic neuritis.[12] More recently various hypotheses have included mercury poisoning,[13] brucellosis,[14] autoimmune sensorineural deafness,[15] sarcoidosis,[16] and meningo-neuro-labyrinthitis.[17] Several scholars maintain that the cause remains unknown or idiopathic. A chronological survey of the literature is given in Table 8.1.

One reason for the controversy and disagreement is the lack of a medical record. In any event the science of otology was then in its infancy. Not only must the astute modern physician extract the natural history and clinical course of Beethoven's deafness from a meticulous search of the original sources, but the proposed provisional diagnosis must pass the test of compatibility with the reports of the exhumations and the rediscovered original autopsy report. The complex cause of Beethoven's deafness is to be found in the borderlands of clinical medicine, medical history, otology, neuroanatomy, neurophysiology, and neuropathology. It should not be assumed that one solitary cause was responsible.

THE ONSET

Although Beethoven's deafness is among the most famous illnesses of all composers, the precise details of the onset of the problem remain unknown.

In the *Heiligenstadt Testament* Beethoven wrote that he had been hopelessly afflicted for six years. That would imply an onset in 1796. Also, in the *Fischhof Manuscript*, it was stated that the hearing loss commenced in 1796 after the dangerous summer illness.

Yet in his letter of 29 June 1801 to Franz Gerhard Wegeler, Beethoven stated that his hearing had grown steadily worse over the previous three years. Five months later he informed Wegeler that the hearing impairment, which started in the left ear, was associated with buzzing and singing. Though there was lessening of the tinnitus, the hearing loss had increased.

In his medical report Dr. Andreas Ignaz Wawruch stated, "In the beginning of his thirtieth year he began having problems with hemorrhoids and with annoying whistling and rushing in both ears. He soon became hard of hearing,

Table 8.1
Chronological Survey of the Literature Concerning the Cause of Beethoven's Deafness

Acoustic Trauma
1935: I. Frank
1958: H. Gattner
1996: P. J. Davies*

Alcoholism
1921: G. Gradenigo
1938: B. Pincherle

Amyloidosis
1994: A. J. Richards

Arteriosclerosis
1905: F. Vieille*
1908: J. Niemack-Charles

Autoimmune
1988: P. J. Davies
1995: Y. F. Cudennec

Brucellosis
1977: H. Scherf*

"Cerebral Congestion"
(Functional)
1863: A. B. Marx
1929: R. Rolland
1930: M. Semenoff

Drug-Induced Ototoxicity
1967: W. Scheidt
1970: R. W. Gutt
1977: H. Scherf*
1996: P. J. Davies*

Head Injury
1880: T. v. Frimmel
1970: J. W. Miller
1977: H. Scherf*

Hereditary
1922: W. Schweisheimer*
1925: R. Quenouille
1927: M. Grünewald

Idiopathic
1907: J. Ermoloff
1914: J. F. Rogers
1922: W. Möllendorff
1928: H.L.F.A. Boyle
1930: M. Sorsby
1932: E. Tremble
1936: C. K. Carpenter
1960: V. Brandt
1971: Editorial: *New England Journal of Medicine*
1973: D. Baker
1974: S. L. Sellars; M. Schachter
1983: Y. F. Cudennec et al.
1986: F. H. Franken; H. Jesserer and H. Bankl*

Otitis Media
1902: Dr. Buss; W. Nagel
1905: Klotz-Forest
1908: J. Niemack-Charles
1910: L. Jacobsohn
1911: M. Menier
1927: J. Bokay
1942: A. Peyser
1982: K. Aterman et al.

Otosclerosis
1905: F. Vieille*; G. Baratoux
1921: G. Bilancioni
1926: T. v. Frimmel*
1927: G. Ernest; R. Loewe-Cannstadt; W. J. Turner; C. Engel
1928: J. Berberich
1933: J. Pfuhl
1934: J. G. Canuyt*
1935: I. Frank*
1936: T. J. Harris
1942: E. Brünger
1951: E. H. Coon
1960: T. Cawthorne
1961: P. Reading
1965: N. Asherton*; P. H. Beales
1970: K. M. Stevens and W. J. Hemenway
1971: J. Archimbaud
1978: M. Landsberger
1980: N. I. Chalat
1983: J. H. Leavesley
1985: E. Larkin
1987: P. C. Adams; H. Bankl and H. Jesserer
1990: J. G. O'Shea
1996: A. K. Kubba and M. Young*

Paget's Disease of the Skull
1927: H. Neumann*
1965: N. Asherton
1970, 1971, 1972: V. S. Naiken
1971: D. Golding
1975: R.T.R. Wentges
1977: A. Czeizel
1985: H. Bankl
1989: P. Sandblom*

Presbycusis
1964: A. Laskiewicz*
1994: A. Neumayr*
1996: P. J. Davies*

Rheumatism
1823: *Stuttgart Morgenblatt*

Sarcoidosis
1990, 1992, 1993: T. G. Palferman

Sensorineural
(Acoustic Neuritis)
1816: A. Weissenbach
1900: P. Garnault
1905: M. Natier; P. Bonnier
1920, 1922, 1944: W. Schweisheimer
1921: Editorial: *Lancet*
1923: F. v. Lepel
1927: W. Behrend; H. Neumann*
1928: R. Blondel; G. Marage; F. Schultze
1934: A. Braun
1936: I. W. Voorhees; Editorial: *Medical Journal of Australia*
1937: C. Magenau
1956: W. Forster
1958: H. Gattner*
1960: M. Piroth
1963: L. M. Sellers
1964: L. A. Adams; A. Laskiewicz*
1970: H. Neuman
1977: J. D. Hood
1981: G. Böhme
1988: P. J. Davies; I. Teply
1994: A. Neumayr*
1996: A. K. Kubba and M. Young*; P. J. Davies*

Tuberculosis
1938: P. Bodros

Typhus Fever
1816: A. Weissenbach
1900: P. Garnault
1905: M. Natier; P. Bonnier
1927: H. Neumann*
1964: A. Laskiewicz*
1977: J. D. Hood
1994: A. Neumayr*
1996: P. J. Davies*

Whipple's Disease
1994: O.M.P. Sharma

*Author advocates more than one cause.

and in spite of remissions lasting for months, the malady increased to total deafness. All attempts at relief were fruitless."[18]

An unsubstantiated anecdote written by Johann Peter Lyser (alias Ludwig Peter August Burmeister), in the *Wiener Zeitschrift* of 16 September 1845, would appear to be unreliable, since it is in conflict with the composer's own remarks about his earlier hearing acuity. According to Lyser, Beethoven's deafness first became manifest in Bonn prior to his mother's death in 1787 when he was listening to fairy tales one evening in Nikolaus Simrock's household.[19]

THE COURSE AND NATURAL HISTORY

Although initially there were fluctuations in the hearing loss, it was persistent from 1798 and slowly progressive too, so that by 1814 the use of ear trumpets became necessary. On 25 January 1815 Beethoven made his last appearance as an accompanist, and according to Simrock he was in 1816 completely deaf in the right ear. The conversation-books came into usage in 1818, while Gerhard von Breuning established that Beethoven in 1826 was stone deaf.

The natural history would appear to be that, after an insidious onset in 1796, there was apparent improvement or fluctuation until 1798, when persistent hearing loss developed initially on the left side, but soon involving both ears. The slowly progressive course resulted in total right-sided deafness in eighteen years, although it was more prolonged in the left ear.

THE MECHANISM OF BEETHOVEN'S DEAFNESS

The loss of high tones, the loud voice in speech, the early loss of speech discrimination, and especially the loudness recruitment phenomenon all indicate that the predominant mechanism was a sensorineural loss.

During the visit of Baron de Trémont in 1809, Beethoven informed the baron that, although he was hard of hearing, if he spoke slowly, Beethoven would understand him. In sensorineural deafness poor voice discrimination occurs especially during rapid speech, when the softened, high-pitched consonants are swamped by the louder, low-pitched vowels. In conductive deafness caused by affections of the external auditory canal, or the middle ear cleft, or the labyrinthine windows, hearing by air conduction is reduced while bone conduction remains normal. Therefore a person with conductive deafness might hear his or her own voice relatively better by bone conduction, compared to air conduction, and might be deceived into thinking that he or she was shouting when, in fact, he or she was talking normally. Because the otosclerotic lowers his or her voice he or she may be almost inaudible, especially in noisy surroundings.

On the other hand, in sensorineural or perceptive deafness, owing to affections of the cochlea (sensory) or the auditory nerve (neural), the reduced hearing by bone conduction is associated with a lesser loss by air conduction. Because the person with perceptive deafness hears his or her own voice less well by bone conduction, the person is deceived into thinking that he or she is not talking loudly enough and raises his or her voice. Constanze von Breuning was embarrassed by Beethoven's loud voice and ringing laugh.

The tuning fork tests used today by the physician in the functional examination of hearing were not available to Beethoven's doctors. Ernst Heinrich Weber of Leipzig described his test in 1834, and Friedrich Heinrich Rinne of Göttingen introduced his test in 1855. Arthur Hartmann invented the audiometer in 1878.

LOUDNESS RECRUITMENT

A person with normal hearing develops loudness discomfort when subjected to between 90 and 105 decibels of noise; a deaf person can often tolerate much higher levels. In 1936 E. P. Fowler described the loudness recruitment phenomenon in which a relatively slight sudden increase in the intensity of a noise is accompanied by an unexpected, exaggerated increased sensation of loudness, causing distortion and ear discomfort. The presence of loudness recruitment is of localizing value in a deaf patient, since it occurs mainly in lesions of the organ of Corti in the cochlea, and never in conductive deafness.[20]

Let us now consider six examples of apparent loudness recruitment in Beethoven's history. Beethoven informed the organist Karl Gottfried Freudenberg that although he played the organ a good deal in his youth, he was forced to quit playing it because "[m]y nerves could not stand the power of the gigantic instrument."[21]

In his letter of 29 June 1801 to Wegeler, he referred to his poor voice discrimination and recruitment: "Sometimes too I can scarcely hear a person who speaks softly; I can hear sounds, it is true, but cannot make out the words. But if anyone shouts, I can't bear it."[22]

During the French occupation of Vienna in May 1809, Beethoven took refuge in the cellar of his brother Caspar Carl's house and covered his head with pillows to escape the noise of the cannon.[23] The recruitment induced by the battery of twenty howitzers would have caused agonizing pain in his ears. During his visit five years later, Dr. Weissenbach noted that Beethoven was "painfully sensible to discordant sounds."[24]

In March 1820 Schindler made the following entry in a conversation-book:

It seems that the little machine, too, will no longer perform its duties properly / so I shall also have to take to writing, like the others / the Archduke has a very faint voice hence the sound [is] not so loud / I'm careful to talk softly into the horn and yet it offends your ear.[25]

The Archduke Rudolph was the only member of Beethoven's intimate circle never to appear in the conversation-books. It would appear that he was able to converse with Beethoven by speaking into the small ear trumpet because he was able to regulate the loudness of his voice without inducing recruitment. On the other hand, when Schindler shouted into the trumpet, Beethoven could not tolerate the distortion and pain of the induced recruitment.

When suffering with earache during the winter of 1822, Beethoven excused himself from attending the concert of cellist Bernhard Romberg because "even your playing would only cause me pain today."[26] The loud acoustic vibrations of the cello would have aggravated the earache through recruitment.

When Beethoven was seated at the keyboard, with one of the larger ear trumpets attached by a headband, he was also utilizing bone conduction to hear the piano. The obstruction of the external auditory canals with debris, described by Dr. Wagner, would certainly have produced a significant component of conductive deafness. Such debris, which no doubt would have accumulated from the successive instillations over the years of ear drops, infusions, and potions, would have effectively blocked out air conduction by way of this vehicle.[27]

Likewise, intermittent obstruction of the eustachian tubes during corhyza or other upper-respiratory tract infections may have not only caused earache, but also contributed a conductive element to the hearing loss.

The evidence then from the original sources leads to the conclusion that, while the mechanism of Beethoven's deafness was predominantly sensorineural, there was also a lesser conductive element to the hearing loss. In other words, it was a mixed deafness.[28]

SUMMER OF 1796: A DANGEROUS TYPHUS

In the *Fischhof-Manuskript*[29] in Berlin there is a reference to a serious illness:

In 1796 Beethoven returned home on a very hot summer day, tore open doors and windows, took off his outer clothing, and cooled off at the open window in the cross ventilation. The consequence was a dangerous illness (*gefährliche Krankheit*), which during his convalescence, affected his organs of hearing, and from which time on his deafness increased.[30]

During the Congress of Vienna in 1814, Beethoven became acquainted with Salzburg surgeon, writer, and poet Dr. Weissenbach (1766–1821). Beethoven set Weissenbach's text for his cantata *Der glorreiche Augenblick* (the Glorious Moment), Op. 136, which was given its premiere in the large Redoutensaal hall on 29 November 1814.[31]

Beethoven and Weissenbach became friendly and often lunched together at the Römischer Kaiser (Roman Emperor) tavern, at the corner of Freyung and Renngasse, in whose spacious hall the performances of Schuppanzigh's quartet were given. Weissenbach, himself deaf, took the opportunity to discuss at length Beethoven's ill health and hearing impairment. Weissenbach's memoirs, *Meine Reise zum Kongress in Wien. Wahrheit und Dichtung*, were published in Vienna in 1816. Consider now the following extract:

Beethoven has greater bodily vigour and robustness than usually fall to the lot of men of high intellect. The whole man is visible in his countenance. If M. Gall, the phrenologist, is right in the position he has assigned to the faculties, musical genius may be grasped with the hand on Beethoven's head. His strength extends, however, only to flesh and bones, his nervous system being in the highest degree weakly. How often has it grieved me to see the spiritual strings of this harmonious organism so easily snapped and put out of tune. He once had a dreadful attack of typhus fever (*einen furchtbaren Typhus bestanden*), and from that time may be dated the decay of his nervous system, and, in all probability, his painful loss of hearing. I have often had long talks with him about this deprivation, which is a far greater misfortune to him than to most people.[32]

It seems probable that the dangerous illness mentioned in the *Fischhof* manuscript and the dreadful typhus described by Dr. Weissenbach were one and the same bout, contracted during the summer of 1796, as proposed by Ludwig Nohl in 1876.[33]

Alexander Wheelock Thayer hypothesized that the attack of typhus took place in Bonn during 1784 or 1785, which would account not only for the serious illness mentioned above by Beethoven to Fanny Giannatasio del Rio, but also offer origin and continuity to the subsequent recurrent bouts of gastrointestinal disorder.[34] But there is no documentary evidence to support such a hypothesis, which is unlikely.

In fact, as Thayer pointed out, there is a complete hiatus in biographical details from late June until November 1796. Earlier that year, on 19 February, in the letter from Prague to his brother Johann, Beethoven stated that he was well. The last piece of information about that tour referred to an improvisation at the pianoforte at the Singakademie in Berlin on 28 June. Then there is no further information until his excursion to Pressburg (now Bratislava) and Budapest in November 1796.[35]

Elliot Forbes has argued that Beethoven's fitness to travel to Pressburg in November precluded the likelihood of a serious illness earlier that summer, and he proposed that the illness occurred the following year during the summer of 1797.[36] However, that objection is not valid. Although in cases of typhoid fever there is persistent fever for from four to eight weeks in untreated patients, the debility is shorter in typhus fever.[37] The fever in cases of endemic murine typhus fever usually lasts from nine to fourteen days and, after defervescence, there is rapid recovery.[38] Even so, such apparent rapid recovery does not preclude the sequela of deafness.

Beethoven presumably returned to Vienna from Berlin in early July 1796, and he presumably suffered the serious febrile illness during either July or August. Travelers are at risk of contracting an endemic disease since they lack the immunity of the local population, and he may have contracted an illness during his travels. The incubation period of endemic murine typhus fever is from eight to sixteen days, so that if Beethoven were bitten by an infected flea during his return journey, he would have suffered the onset of illness within two weeks of his arrival back in Vienna.

Wegeler had returned to Bonn in the middle of 1796,[39] so that Beethoven probably would have turned to his intimate friend Lenz von Breuning for help. He was a pupil of Dr. Johann Nepomuk Hunczowsky, who might have been consulted. Alternatively, Beethoven was also friendly with Dr. Joseph Frank and his father, Johann Peter Frank. There is no record of events until 19 November 1796, when Beethoven wrote to Johann A. Streicher from Pressburg.[40] He was in good form then and looking forward to his concert four days later. In his letter of 23 November Stephan von Breuning wrote to Wegeler and Christoph von Breuning that through travel Beethoven had become more staid and appreciative of the value of friendship.[41]

In his letter of 29 May 1797 to Wegeler, Beethoven informed his friend that he was well and that his health was steadily improving.[42] In that letter Beethoven admitted that he owed Wegeler a letter. That letter from Wegeler to Beethoven, which has not survived, may have made reference to the recent serious illness.

Beethoven wrote a farewell note to Lenz von Breuning on 1 October 1797, "Continue to be my friend; you will always find me the same."[43] Little did he then know that Lenz would die unexpectedly at the age of twenty-one on 10 April 1798. The lack of documentary evidence concerning the dangerous typhus in 1796 is surprising. The absence of Wegeler from Vienna at that time, and the premature demise of von Breuning, probably contributed to the hiatus of information about it.

MENINGO-NEURO-LABYRINTHITIS

Dr. Wagner's description of the thickening of the brain substance and increased vascularity, in the region of the floor of the fourth ventricle, together with bilateral atrophy of the auditory nerves and reddening of the spiral membrane of the cochlea, is indicative of a meningo-neuro-labyrinthitis.[44] Such pathology results from the spread of inflammation from a basal meningitis of the base of the brain into the auditory nerves and the labyrinth of the inner ear. The atrophy of the auditory nerves is a sequela of septic inflammation causing neuronal destruction.

Before checking for compatibility with Beethoven's scenario, let us discuss first the possible causes and then the clinical features of meningo-neuro-labyrinthitis. The causes of meningo-neuro-labyrinthitis are listed in Table 8.2. It is important to note at the outset that there is considerable variation in the prognosis with regard to survival in the absence of specific treatment. While survival was usual in murine typhus and viral meningitis, there was an appreciable mortality in pyogenic meningitis. Even in 1986 the case fatality rate in the United States for bacterial meningitis was in the range of from 3 to 22 percent.[45] The proposal of P. Bodros that Beethoven's deafness was due to tuberculosis is untenable because tuberculous meningitis without specific treat-

Table 8.2
The Causes of Meningo-Neuro-Labyrinthitis

Pyogenic Meningitis: meningococcal (cerebro-spinal fever), pneumococcal, *Haemophilus influenzae*, tuberculous, congenital and acquired syphilis, streptococcal, staphylococcal, Gram-negative bacilli, brucellosis, *Listeria* sp., *Acinetobacter* sp., oto-labyrinthitis.

Infectious Diseases: typhus fever, typhoid fever, scarlet fever, rheumatic fever, pneumonia, whooping cough, erysipelas, HIV/AIDS, influenza, measles, mumps, maternal rubella, smallpox.

Miscellaneous: penetrating wounds, infective endocarditis, sarcoidosis, amyloidosis, immune deficiency states, leukemia, malignancy, Behçet's disease, uveomeningitic syndromes.

ment is invariably fatal.[46] Nor was there evidence of active tuberculosis in the lungs, intestines, or elsewhere.

TYPHUS FEVER

Murine typhus fever, transmitted by rat fleas infected with *Rickettsia typhi*, was endemic in Europe during Beethoven's life. It was prone to occur in urban areas during the late summer and autumn. The febrile illness with a duration of from nine to fourteen days was associated with headache, a skin rash, myalgia, and some alteration of consciousness by way of stupor, prostration, delirium, agitation, or coma. The lungs and alimentary tract were often affected, and there was occasional involvement of the heart and kidneys. A rapid recovery after defervescence was usual.

Though uncommon, deafness was a well-recognized complication, often with an onset toward the end of the first week. After a short rapid course, there was often improvement during convalescence. There was also sometimes a conductive element due to otitis media.

Adam Politzer described the tendency to recovery:

Secondary purulent inflammations of the labyrinth have been occasionally observed in meningitis and with epidemic cerebro-spinal meningitis. . . . That inflammatory changes may become quite resolved, is apparent from the clinical observation of cases of typhus, scarlatina, etc., in which deafness occurring during the disease disappears again during convalescence, the function of hearing returning to its normal state.[47]

On the other hand, epidemic louse-borne typhus fever was at times a much more severe illness with a high mortality of up to 60 percent, especially in the elderly or debilitated. Notable epidemics occurred during the Thirty Years' War and the Napoleonic wars. Deafness was a rare complication of typhoid fever.

There is confusion in the terminology in German: murine typhus—*Ratten-*

flecktyphus; epidemic typhus—*Fleckfieber*; typhoid fever—*Typhus abdominalis*, *Unterleibstyphus*, and *Bauchtyphus*.

MENINGITIS

Pyogenic meningitis today accounts for 6 percent of all cases of severe deafness in childhood. Hearing loss was more commonly observed in epidemics of cerebro-spinal meningitis, and it is fascinating to recall that the incidence of hearing disturbances varied from low to very high in individual epidemics.

Politzer's description of the pathology is compatible with Dr. Wagner's autopsy report:

Softening or thickening of the ependyma of the fourth ventricle, purulent infiltration and softening of the auditory nerve (described by Knapp), embedding of the latter in meningeal exudation (described by Schwartze), shrivelling of the nerve stem, and lastly purulent inflammation of the membranous labyrinth, the origin of which can be traced to transmission of the inflammation either along the sheath of the auditory nerve (neuritis descendens) or through the aqueducts.[48]

However, in such cases of hearing loss after cerebro-spinal meningitis, there were commonly associated vestibular disturbances, such as staggering gait, in half to two thirds of cases. Such ataxia tended to persist for a few months to a year or longer. In adults, tinnitus was usual; in some cases, there were disturbances of vision or speech or some other palsy.[49]

It also needs to be emphasized that Politzer described a latent period preceding progression of the deafness in some cases: "Some time after convalescence a considerable improvement sets in, which, however, is followed in the course of months, or even years, by a progressive deterioration."[50]

COMPATIBILITY WITH BEETHOVEN'S HISTORY

The meningo-neuro-labyrinthitis described by Dr. Wagner is compatible with a sequela of typhus fever or some form of meningitis. Likewise, the serious febrile illness in the summer of 1796 referred to in the *Fischhof* manuscript, and the "terrible typhus" described by Dr. Weissenbach, are compatible with typhus fever or some other form of meningitis. Furthermore, the apparent recovery during convalescence, followed by recurrence and slow progression from 1798, is compatible with the natural history of Beethoven's hearing loss, as described above by Politzer.

Viennese otologist Heinrich Neumann, in 1927, favored an acoustic neuritis following typhus, although he felt that such deafness would have been aggravated by recurrent upper-respiratory infections and intestinal catarrh, and he raised the additional possibility of Paget's disease of the temporal bone or some rare atypical otosclerosis.[51]

Dr. J. D. Hood also proposed that Beethoven's deafness was a sequela of typhus.[52] Dr. Anton Neumayr also diagnosed meningitis as the initial cause of Beethoven's hearing loss, resulting from either typhus or *Haemophilus influenzae*. Neumayr, however, favored an earlier onset, in 1787, in keeping with J.P.T. Lyser's anecdote, which he was inclined to accept. He suggested that the deafness continued to progress because of repeated attacks of otitis media related to his many head colds and his frequent intestinal disorders.[53]

Other causes of Beethoven's deafness have been proposed in the literature.

BRUCELLOSIS

In his book Horst Scherf proposed that, during the return to Bonn from Vienna in 1787, Beethoven contracted a *Brucella abortus* infection from the ingestion of infected milk. This gave rise to chronic relapsing brucellosis, which would account for Beethoven's fevers, abdominal complaints, and liver disease.[54]

Scherf also hypothesized that neuro-brucellosis would have caused Beethoven's melancholy, depression, headaches, and irritability. Furthermore, he advocated that involvement of the auditory nerves in association with a granulomatous vasculitis of the auditory arteries caused a nerve deafness. The hearing loss was aggravated by the head injury sustained during the fall described by Neate. Possibly further aggravation was caused by the drugs administered to the composer.[55]

In 1896 Bernhard Bang (1848–1932), a physician and veterinarian in Copenhagen, described a form of chronic brucellosis contracted from infected cattle.[56] Cattle handlers, such as farmers, abbatoir workers, and veterinarians, are at risk of infection through occupational contact with infected animals. Human infection also results from the ingestion of infected milk or milk products.

However, the highest prevalence of brucellosis is in the Mediterranean countries, Asia, and Central and South America. Furthermore, *Brucella abortus* usually causes mild disease with noncaseating granulomatous lesions in lymph nodes, liver, and spleen. Even before the availability of effective antibiotics such as streptomycin and tetracyclines, only 15 percent suffered an illness exceeding three months in duration.

Neurologic involvement, though uncommon, includes meningoencephalitis, myelitis, radiculitis, and peripheral neuritis. Involvement of the auditory nerve is not a well-recognized entity.[57] Brucellosis is an unlikely cause of Beethoven's deafness.

SARCOIDOSIS

Sarcoidosis is worthy of serious consideration because it is a recognized, albeit rare, cause of basal meningitis and nerve deafness. The involvement of the nervous system in about 5 percent of cases gives rise to granulomatous affliction of the meninges, especially at the base of the brain, and local deposits of sarcoid granulomas in the substance of the brain or spinal cord.

The resulting neuropathies include cranial nerve palsies and peripheral neuropathies. Those cranial nerves whose roots are grouped together at the base of the brain tend to be involved together, resulting in multiple cranial nerve palsies. An obstructive hydrocephalus may develop, while epileptiform convulsions are not infrequent. Hypothalamic symptoms such as rapid weight gain, somnolence, polydipsia, and polyuria may dominate the clinical picture. Meningeal sarcoidosis may run a prolonged course over five years or longer.[58]

The most commonly involved cranial nerves are the seventh, resulting in unilateral or bilateral facial palsy, which usually resolves spontaneously, and the second, resulting in various degrees of blurred vision and blindness. The ninth and tenth cranial nerves are the next most commonly involved, producing symptoms of difficulty in swallowing, hoarseness, and a nasal voice.

The auditory nerve is the fourth most frequently affected, and the hearing loss, which may be an early presenting feature, is commonly associated with tinnitus and vertigo. Fluctuations in severity are characteristic, and spontaneous resolution is well documented.[59]

Dr. Tom Palferman cleverly applied Occam's razor to propose sarcoidosis as the possible single explanation for all aspects of Beethoven's diseases, including the deafness.[60] The probability of a diagnosis of neurosarcoidosis would be enhanced by a history of associated involvement of the parotid or lacrimal glands, or erythema nodosum, but such characteristic features are absent from Beethoven's history, as are other neuropathies or hypothalamic symptoms.[61]

Likewise, the absence of mention of lymphadenopathy by Beethoven's physicians or Dr. Wagner argues against a diagnosis of sarcoidosis. In 1774 William Hewson gave the first complete account of the anatomical features of the lymphatics.[62]

Furthermore, sarcoid-related hearing loss runs a rapid course without any tendency to a slowly progressive involvement. On the contrary, there is a tendency in the natural history of sarcoid-related deafness toward spontaneous improvement. Such recovery in modern times is often enhanced by the administration of corticosteroids.

The absence of characteristic concurrent symptoms in Beethoven's history also supports arguments against sarcoidosis as the cause of his hearing loss. In the case reports to 1970 of sarcoid-related deafness, the majority (86.6 percent) suffered concurrent or preceding uveitis; Beethoven's eye disorder commenced twenty-seven years after the onset of his hearing loss. The following concurrent symptoms, all absent in Beethoven's history, were also reported in the literature: vestibular symptoms in 61.5 percent, facial paralysis in 61.5 percent, and parotid swelling in 46.2 percent.[63]

Sarcoidosis is discussed again in the appropriate sections elsewhere, and it will emerge that the case for sarcoid involvement of Beethoven's lungs, kidneys, and skin is not convincing. Sarcoidosis is a less likely cause of Beethoven's deafness.

WHIPPLE'S DISEASE

Whipple's disease is a rare multisystem disorder caused by infection with the bacillus *Tropheryma whippeli*. Affecting predominantly males during the fourth and fifth decades, it involves the small intestine, liver, lymph nodes, heart, central nervous system, eyes, kidneys, joint synovium, lungs, and pancreas.[64]

Professor O. P. Sharma also applied Occam's razor to hypothesize Whipple's disease as the cause of most of Beethoven's medical problems.[65]

However, Whipple's disease is invariably fatal unless prolonged treatment with the appropriate antibiotics is administered.[66] Furthermore, involvement of the central nervous system, which occurs in about 10 percent of cases, is a serious sequela with a poor prognosis. The manifestations include confusion, memory loss, dementia, focal cranial nerve palsies, nystagmus, ophthalmoplegia, and facial myoclonus.[67] A slowly progressive deafness is not a recognized feature.

The notion that Beethoven survived over thirty years with untreated Whipple's disease that involved his central nervous system is too remote to remain within the realm of possibility. Whipple's disease is a most unlikely cause of Beethoven's deafness.

THE CENTRAL OR FUNCTIONAL THEORIES OF ROLLAND AND MARAGE

Influenced by his study of the writings of Ramakrishna and his disciple Vivekananda, Romain Rolland proposed his esoteric yoga theory:

These exercises [of Beethoven's genius] in passionate and boundless concentration always conducted to the brink of cerebral apoplexy or of mental alienation. . . . Such [cerebral] congestions [were further aggravated by Beethoven's habitual practice of douching his head] brutally with ice-cold ablutions. . . . Could not the otitis have been brought on by this cerebral régime, in truth that of a genius, but a murderous régime, the natural psycho-physiological dispositions thus provoking the catastrophe? And could this, in its turn, have reinforced tenfold the dispositions of Nature?[68]

While there is no doubt that Beethoven's hearing loss contributed to his bouts of depression and aggravated his paranoia, Rolland's yoga theory does not account for the atrophy of both auditory nerves or the deafness.

The research of French otologist Dr. G. Marage resulted in three communications which were presented at the sittings of the French Académie des Sci-

ences on 9 and 23 January 1928 and on 2 December 1929, and later published
in the reports of this learned society.

In his first paper, Marage used clinical arguments to discredit the diagnosis
of otosclerosis, syphilis, and head injury, concluding that the deafness was
caused by a labyrinthitis of the inner ear.[69] In his second paper, he discussed
the effect of deafness on musical composition.[70]

In his third paper, Marage discussed the causes and consequences of Beethoven's deafness. He made reference to his protracted correspondence with Romain Rolland who was then correcting the proofs of the first volume of his
biography. With regard to the probable cause of the otitis interna, Marage concluded, "An intensive overworking of the auditory centers which finished by
destroying an organ of exquisite sensibility."[71]

In addition to this central cerebral congestion, Dr. Marage postulated that an
intestinal factor was responsible. He suggested that a long-standing membranous
colitis could have acted as a focus for the spread of infection to remote structures
such as the central nervous system.[72]

INTESTINAL AUTOINTOXICATION

Even in the late nineteenth century it was believed that toxins were contin-
uously produced in the human body from four sources: metabolic reactions in
the tissues, in the secretions of bile from the gall bladder, from the consumption
of contaminated food, and from the putrefaction of intestinal contents. However,
the presence of toxins and poisons in the blood did not usually cause diseases
because they were either eliminated in the urine or feces, or neutralized in the
liver. Intestinal stasis gave way to autointoxication, resulting from an over-
production of toxins which caused diseases of varying kinds and severity.[73]

Beethoven and his physicians believed that his hearing loss was, in some
way, related to his chronic gastrointestinal ailment. Several medical researchers
have also shared this view, proposing that some form of chronic intestinal toxemia was responsible.[74]

Recently, autoimmune mechanisms have been described to account for that
rare form of nerve deafness associated with inflammatory bowel disease.[75]

AUTOIMMUNE SENSORINEURAL HEARING LOSS

In 1979 B. F. McCabe described a new form of hearing loss—autoimmune
sensorineural deafness—which responds to treatment with corticosteroids and
immuno-suppressive drugs such as cyclophosphamide.

The bilateral hearing loss, which usually progresses rapidly over a period of
weeks or months, is associated with poor discrimination scores and sloping
audiometric curves. Vestibular symptoms are present unless there is symmetrical
involvement of both the auditory and vestibular divisions of the eighth cranial

nerve. There is no family history of hearing disorders, and in some cases, there develop facial paralysis or necrotic changes in the middle ear and mastoid.[76]

Autoimmune sensorineural hearing loss may rarely be associated with inflammatory bowel disease, and it has been proposed that it may have contributed a major component to Beethoven's deafness.[77]

Admittedly, this form of hearing loss usually progresses rapidly unless appropriate treatment is administered. However the initial damage to Beethoven's inner ear resulted from meningitis, and it is possible that autoimmune mechanisms contributed to the slow progression of his deafness.[78]

It has been pointed out that in the autopsy report Dr. Wagner described pathological changes of thickening and cartilaginous consistency in the auditory arteries. In the absence of a histological examination it is impossible to differentiate arteriosclerosis from some form of arteritis, such as autoimmune vasculitis, or even a combination of the two.

There is no convincing clinical evidence that Beethoven suffered with a collagen vascular disorder such as polyarteritis nodosa, Wegener's granulomatosis, Cogan's syndrome, rheumatoid arthritis, Sjogren's syndrome, or mixed connective tissue disease, though admittedly the detection of serological autoantibodies features prominently in the modern diagnosis of these disorders. The question of systemic lupus erythematosis will be considered in the next chapter.

HEAD INJURY

Trauma to the head may result in conductive, perceptive, or a mixed hearing loss. In cases of severe concussion, deafness may result from a fracture of the base of the skull that causes direct injury to the auditory nerve, or damage to the ossicles of the middle ear, or a bloody effusion into the middle ear.

It has been proposed that Beethoven's deafness was caused by the beatings inflicted on him by his father during his childhood.[79] If that were true, the hearing loss would have commenced during his childhood.

Quoting the heavy fall described to Charles Neate, T. von Frimmel proposed that Beethoven's deafness resulted from traumatic injury to the auditory nerves.[80] This story, however, is at variance with other accounts, and Dr. Wagner's description of meningo-neuro-labyrinthitis is not compatible with post-traumatic atrophy of the auditory nerves.

While it is unlikely that such a fall was the primary cause of Beethoven's hearing loss, it is well known that nerve deafness may be aggravated by trauma to the head. Such temporary aggravation caused by a hemorrhage was suggested by Scherf.[81]

ACOUSTIC TRAUMA

Following the initial affliction caused by meningo-neuro-labyrinthitis, the chronic acoustic trauma of noise undoubtedly added insult to injury.[82] Those basal turns of the cochlea, situated near the labyrinthine windows, are most susceptible to acoustic trauma.[83]

Throughout his life in Vienna, Beethoven's ears were subjected not only to the appreciable noise of his musical life but also to significant acoustic trauma from horses, carts, and carriages, not to forget the occasional sharp outbursts from guns and cannons during the wars.

Beethoven informed Herr Sandra that his use of ear trumpets had aggravated his deafness, and that his sparing use of such devices had preserved a little hearing in his left ear. Furthermore Beethoven advised Herr Sandra that conversation-books were to be preferred to ear trumpets as a means of communication, so as to preserve the hearing.

It must also be emphasized that those extraordinary amplifying devices that were fitted to Beethoven's pianos would have generated colossal noise and further acoustic trauma.

PRESBYCUSIS

It should also be noted that the degenerative changes in the inner ear that are associated with aging are enhanced by previous injury and prolonged exposure to noise.[84] Aging results in the atrophy of hair-cells and auditory nerve fibers in the cochlea.[85] Presbycusis was undoubtedly a secondary or aggravating factor in the deafness.

DRUG-INDUCED OTOTOXICITY

It has been proposed that mercury poisoning was responsible for Beethoven's deafness.[86] Although organic mercury poisoning with methyl mercury, present for example in industrial waste, may cause hearing disorders, such do not occur in isolation and are associated with other neurologic defects.

In any event, if Beethoven were treated with mercury, it would have been in an inorganic form. There is no evidence in his history of the characteristic intention tremor or of mercurial erethism (short-term memory loss, timidity, insomnia, excitability, or delirium).[87]

Admittedly, the fluid retention during Beethoven's final illness may conceivably have been caused by a nephrotic syndrome resulting from mercury nephrotoxicity; however, more convincing alternative explanations will be advanced.

Though Peruvian bark was introduced into Spain in 1632, its active ingredient, quinine, was not isolated till 1820. During Beethoven's life it was a popular remedy for malaria and fevers.

Tinnitus and high-tone hearing loss, which are characteristic symptoms of cinchonism, are usually transient, rarely permanent.[88]

Other ototoxic drugs such as salicylates and aminoglycosides were not in use during Beethoven's life, but unfortunately the precise details of the drugs prescribed by his physicians are unknown.

Although ototoxic drugs or chemicals may have contributed a minor role, it is unlikely that they played a major part in the pathogenesis of Beethoven's deafness.

PAGET'S DISEASE OF THE SKULL

In his outstanding paper during the centenary year, Neumann proposed for the first time that the apparent thickening of the right temporal bone, evident in J. B. Rottmayer's photograph, may have been caused by Paget's disease.[89]

N. Asherton pointed out that otosclerosis was sometimes associated with Paget's disease of the skull, and he hypothesized a rare malignant type of diffuse otosclerosis associated with Paget's disease of the temporal bones. Illustrating his article with Lyser's drawing, Asherton argued that Beethoven's unusually large head for his short height, with his hat tilted to one side, were suggestive of Paget's disease of the skull.[90]

Further arguments were elaborated upon by V. S. Naiken who hypothesized a diagnosis of "Paget's disease of bone, localized to the vault and base of the skull, including the temporal bones, and possibly involving the face, axial skeleton, and the extremities."[91] Naiken argued that the diagnosis of Paget's disease was suggested by the "unusual physical characteristics of the composer," as evident from 1815 onward.

Naiken proposed that Paget's disease accounted for several features which are well illustrated in the drawings of Lyser and Böhm—the oversized asymmetrical head, the large Olympian forehead, the overhanging brows, the protruding lower jaw, the prominent cheeks and teeth, the short legs in proportion to his height, the large hands with thick fingers, and the wide shoulders.

Was it not Paget's disease, Naiken argued, that accounted for such contemporary descriptions as simian ugliness, fantastic gargoyle, Gorgon-headed totem, original cave man, leonine, and leper-like countenance? Paget's disease would also account, Naiken suggested, for the right temporal bulge and apparent enlargement of his skull which caused Beethoven to wear his hat back on his collar.

It was critical to Naiken's argument that such characteristic physical features were absent in Beethoven's youth, as evident, he stated, in Gerhard von Kügelgen's portrait and contemporary accounts. The absence of these features in Beethoven's earlier life would support the proposed presence of an evolving pathological process in the bones such as Paget's disease.[92]

Other causes of osteodystrophy, such as leontiasis ossea, acromegaly, and Van Buchem's disease (hyperostosis corticalis localisata, or generalisata), were dismissed in favor of Paget's disease.

It was also argued that the autopsy findings "of a markedly and uniformly dense skull vault, approximately a half inch thick, as well as the vascularized petrous bone" were compatible with Paget's disease.[93] Furthermore, it was pointed out that thickening of the superficial substance of the base of the brain, caused by the thickening of the pia-arachnoid leptomeninges adherent to the base of the skull, had been described in Paget's disease.[94]

Dismissing syphilis and otosclerosis, Naiken proposed that Paget's disease of the skull was the cause of Beethoven's headaches and deafness. Hearing loss in Paget's disease is usually due to circumferential bony overgrowth in the region of the internal auditory meatus, which causes compression of the seventh and eighth cranial nerves, leading in severe cases to pressure atrophy of the nerve trunks. Less commonly, a fracture of the labyrinthine capsule causes injury to the cochlea. However, Paget's disease may also result in a conductive hearing loss by encroachment of, or deposition of, new bone into the middle-ear ossicles, or fibrotic changes in the annular ligament.[95]

Admittedly, an onset at the age of twenty-six is rare; deafness usually starts after the age of forty-five. This diagnosis would otherwise account for a slowly progressive nerve deafness, associated with tinnitus, with initial loss of the high frequencies, and eventual atrophy of both auditory nerves.

CONTRA PAGET'S DISEASE

The above characteristic physical features of Beethoven were not confined to his last eleven years, but were present earlier in his life. A critical comparison of the authentic busts, masks, and portraits reveals no dramatic change in these characteristic features.

Frimmel emphasized that the essential feature of Beethoven's forehead was not so much its exceptional height, but rather its unusual width, and especially the striking vaulting of its central part, extending to the frontal eminences.[96]

Such prominent central vaulting is visible in the anonymous half-length oil portrait of the thirteen-year-old composer given by Beethoven to Zmeskall, Joseph Neeson's silhouette of 1786, the oval engraving by Johann Neidl in 1801, and in Klein's mask and bust of 1812.

It comes as no surprise to find no evidence of Beethoven's characteristic physical features in the miniature portrait formerly attributed to Kügelgen in 1791, since Frimmel established that the subject was not Beethoven, but rather the poet Max von Schenkendorf.[97]

We have seen that the report that "the calvarium exhibited throughout great density and a thickness amounting to about half an inch" was an error in the Seyfried-Pierson translation of the autopsy record. Furthermore, it has been pointed out that the apparent bulge in Rottmayer's photograph was an artefact.

During the first exhumation in 1863, all of Beethoven's bones were carefully examined, and measurements of the long bones were recorded. There was no report of thickening of any of his bones, such as would have been apparent were Paget's disease present.

The skull was examined a second time at the second exhumation in 1888, and measurements were recorded. There was neither any record of abnormal thickening, nor of obliteration of any of the sutures that would have been expected in the presence of Paget's disease. Nor was there any history of the characteristic symptom of an increasing hat size.

Although Paget's disease, affecting both the temporal bones and the base of the skull, might account for a nerve deafness associated with an appearance of meningo-neuritis, there was no history of facial spasms, or atrophy of the facial nerves. Dr. Wagner described thickening of the facial nerves, though this is of doubtful pathological significance.

Finally, the absence of bone abnormality in the recent examination and x-ray of the three fragments from Beethoven's occipital and left parietal bones offers decisive evidence against Paget's disease, as pointed out by Dr. H. Bankl, who himself had earlier advocated that diagnosis.[98]

Admittedly Paget's disease cannot be excluded with absolute certainty because the temporal bones are not available for study. However monostotic Paget's disease, confined to the temporal bones, without involvement of other parts of the skeleton, is extremely rare.[99] Furthermore, the proposal that Paget's disease might remain isolated to the temporal bones for over thirty years is far too remote a possibility.

Despite the superficial attractiveness of the Paget's disease hypothesis, it is an unlikely cause of Beethoven's deafness. Nor did Beethoven show evidence of other osteodystrophies that may be associated with deafness, such as osteogenesis imperfecta, achondroplasia, osteopetrosis, or enchondromatosis.

OTITIS MEDIA

In the earlier discussion of the mechanism of Beethoven's deafness, it was suggested that the conductive component would be accounted for by a combination of chronic obstructive otitis externa and intermittent obstruction of the eustachian tubes complicating upper-respiratory tract infections. The latter would also account for Beethoven's winter earaches.

Hearing by bone conduction is reduced in perceptive deafness, though it remains normal in conductive hearing loss. Klotz-Forest overemphasized the significance of Rattel's dubious anecdote, arguing erroneously that Beethoven would have been unable to utilize such bone conduction if he was afflicted with a nerve deafness.[100] In response, Dr. Pierre Bonnier pointed out that, though in cases of nerve deafness hearing by bone conduction was diminished, Beethoven's utilization of bone conduction, through the head bands attached to his ear trumpets, in no way excluded a diagnosis of nerve deafness.[101]

L. Jacobsohn and M. Menier proposed that, following the attack of typhus in 1796, Beethoven developed a chronic middle-ear infection of the type resembling otosclerosis, or chronic adhesive otitis media.[102]

CONTRA OTITIS MEDIA

There was an absence in Beethoven's history of that characteristic symptom of chronic middle-ear infection: an aggravation of the hearing loss during exacerbations of infection. Furthermore, the deafness of otitis media tends to be associated with early loss of high and low pitch, with preservation of the middle scale.[103]

Not only was there an absence of a history of discharge from the ear, but Dr. Wagner carefully inspected both tympanic membranes and reported no abnormality in either.

Total deafness complicating otitis media is usually associated with the direct spread of infection to the inner ear, usually during an exacerbation of a long-standing chronic infection of the middle-ear cleft, and almost invariably in association with cholesteatoma.[104] Dr. Wagner dissected both mastoids and reported no abnormality in their air-containing cells, "which were seen to be covered by a blood-stained mucous membrane." He would not have missed the soft, putty-like consistency of a cholesteatoma.

M. Sorsby pointed out that the absence of a cholesteatoma was conclusive evidence against chronic suppurative otitis media, but that it did not exclude the chronic adhesive type.[105] The degree of hearing loss in this variety is determined mainly by the extent of damage to the middle-ear ossicular chain. Dr. Wagner described no abnormality in the middle ear.

Otitis media is an unlikely cause of Beethoven's deafness.

OTOSCLEROSIS

Since first proposed in 1905 by Vieille and Baratoux, otosclerosis has been considered by many scholars to be the likely cause of Beethoven's deafness because it is a common cause of slowly progressive hearing loss, associated with tinnitus, following an onset in young manhood (see Table 8.1).

Otosclerosis (or otospongiosis) is a hereditary disorder of collagen metabolism, characterized by the deposition of abnormal bone at certain sites in the temporal bones. Conductive deafness occurs when the involvement of the stapedial footplate encroaches upon the oval window.[106] Involvement of the cochlea, which occurs in 35 percent of cases, may give rise to a slowly progressive sensorineural deafness associated with loudness recruitment.[107] Though uncommon, a severe subtotal hearing loss may occur.

It is clear from Dr. Wagner's autopsy report that he was fully conversant with the anatomy of the ear. Gabriele Fallopius had described the tympanic membrane in 1561; three years later, the eustachian tube was described by Bartolommeo Eustachius. In 1645 Cecilio Folius had given an accurate description of the anatomy of the ear with clear delineation of the three ossicles, the round and oval windows, the semicircular canals, and the cochlea.[108]

Although, during the eighteenth century, there were sporadic autopsy reports by Antonio Valsalva and others of ankylosis of the stapes in deaf people, the first detailed study was conducted by the father of British otology Joseph Toynbee of London, who in 1857 detected the presence of stapes ankylosis in 39 of 1,959 dissections of temporal bones.[109] In 1894 Politzer introduced the term otosclerosis and described its histopathology.

A detailed study conducted by Italian otologist G. Bilancioni proposed that Beethoven was afflicted with the mixed form of involvement of the stapes and the cochlea, and the theory soon gained support.[110] However, to account for a slowly progressive sensorineural deafness associated with loudness recruitment, four authors have advocated the less common cochlear otosclerosis, in which the disease is confined to the cochlea.[111]

CONTRA OTOSCLEROSIS

An impressive array of authors, headed by Marage,[112] I. W. Voorhees,[113] Waldemar Schweisheimer,[114] W. Forster,[115] A. Laskiewicz,[116] and G. Böhme,[117] have argued persuasively against a diagnosis of otosclerosis in favor of an acoustic neuritis. Beethoven's loud raucous voice, his noisy ringing laugh, and his early loss of speech discrimination do not support a diagnosis of otosclerosis.[118]

In 1672 Thomas Willis of London first described the paradoxical phenomenon of paracusis where the deaf person has a better hearing in noisy, as opposed to quiet, surroundings. Though paracusis occurs in other forms of conductive deafness, it is characteristic of stapedial otosclerosis.[119] There was no suggestion of paracusis in Beethoven's history, rather the opposite, for early on he had trouble hearing the actor in the theater,[120] while in 1814 he conversed better with Dr. Weissenbach in a small room in the Zur rose inn in the Wollzeile.[121]

Although a family history of deafness was documented in from 54 to 80 percent of cases of otosclerosis, there was no such history recorded in Beethoven's family.[122]

As a young pathologist, Dr. Wagner probably tried to keep up with recent advances by reading the medical literature. In his *History of Otology*, Politzer listed the various treatises, dissertations, and otological studies published between 1810 and 1826.[123]

Those cases of otosclerosis, which are complicated by advanced subtotal hearing loss, are usually associated with advanced immobilization of the stapes and obliteration of the oval and round windows.[124]

In his excellent article, Maurice Sorsby argued persuasively, "Against otosclerosis it may be urged that in the post-mortem examination the cochlea was inspected; to have done so the region of the stapes must have been looked at and bony fixation of the stapes could hardly have escaped observation."[125]

It must also be emphasized that the marked degree of atrophy of both auditory nerves, and the thickening of the brain substance over the floor of the fourth ventricle, described by Dr. Wagner, cannot be accounted for by otosclerosis. Even in those rare cases of otosclerosis, as proposed by Asherton, with extensive involvement of the cochlea, resulting in invasion of the scala tympani, or rupture of the cochlear duct, or even destructive lesions involving the internal auditory canal, marked atrophy of the auditory nerves is not a feature, and the neuronal degeneration is most pronounced in the basal turn of the cochlea.[126]

It has also been proposed that Beethoven's hearing loss was caused by a degree of otosclerosis combined with an independent nerve deafness, both unrelated to his other medical conditions.[127] This is unlikely. Surely, in that situation, the slow progressive course of the former would have been hastened by the latter.

In conclusion, although otosclerosis would account for the slowly progressive course of Beethoven's deafness, associated with loudness recruitment, that diagnosis is discredited by other clinical features and the autopsy findings.

MISCELLANY

A Sudden Chill

Carl Czerny attributed Beethoven's deafness to a sudden chill induced when Maximiliane Brentano emptied a bottle of ice-cold water over his head, while he was teasing her when he was overheated.[128] Such a chill in 1812 could not have caused the hearing loss because his impairment was then already well established, and the human hearing mechanism is well insulated and protected from sudden fluctuations of environmental temperature.

Alcohol-Related Damage

Though the interaction of alcohol toxicity and vitamin B deficiencies may give rise to such diverse neurological sequela as Wernicke's disease, Korsakoff's psychosis, cerebellar degeneration, polyneuropathy, pellagra, and nutritional optic neuropathy (tobacco-alcohol amblyopia), hearing loss is not an established complication.[129]

Arteriosclerotic Heart Disease

Although ischemic heart disease associated with atrial fibrillation may be complicated by cerebral embolism, causing cerebral infarction, leading to sudden hearing loss, such a scenario is not applicable to Beethoven's case.

Hereditary Taint

Inspired by C. Lombroso's now discredited degeneration theory, Dr. Schweisheimer proposed that Beethoven's hereditary taint contributed to the atrophy of his auditory nerves.[130]

In the 1841 oil portrait of Johann van Beethoven painted by Leopold Gross,

now in the State Museum of Vienna, the sixty-five-year-old brother of the deceased composer shows evidence of a right-sided oculomotor nerve palsy, by
way of a ptosis and external strabismus.[131] It is not possible to ascertain the
cause without further clinical information. However, such a lesion, if isolated,
may be congenital. Even so there is no evidence in Beethoven's case of any
progressive sensorineural deafness of an hereditary nature, nor of retinitis pig-
mentosa.[132]

Immune Deficiency

It has also been proposed that Beethoven's hearing loss was due to a chronic
otitis media, related to IgA deficiency, complicated further by spread into the
inner ear (oto-labyrinthitis).[133] However the case for middle-ear infection has
been discredited.

Amyloidosis

Systemic amyloidosis is a multisystem disorder in which the characteristic
fibril proteins may be deposited in the brain, causing disruption of function.
However, in such cases, the cranial nerves are usually spared, apart from those
concerned with the pupillary reflexes. Isolated deafness is not a recognized feature of systemic amyloidosis, which will be considered further in the next chapter.[134]

Lead Poisoning

Sensorineural deafness may rarely develop either in the acute phase or during
the aftermath of lead encephalopathy, especially in children with very high blood
levels of lead. Lead encephalopathy is rare in adults when it occurs only after
rapid intense absorption of the metal. The condition usually presents after a
period of impaired health lasting weeks or months. As the encephalopathy develops, worsening intense headaches, associated with projectile vomiting are
accompanied by excitement, confusion, delirium, grand mal convulsions, visual
impairment caused by optic neuritis, lethargy, and coma.

One patient in four dies with cerebral edema and renal failure; about 40
percent of the survivors suffer with neurological sequela such as mental retar-
dation, seizure disorders, cerebral palsy, blindness resulting from optic atrophy,
or dystonia.[135]

Such a scenario is not evident in Beethoven's case, neither before the onset
of deafness, nor during his final illness, so that lead poisoning is an unlikely
cause of his deafness or death. Admittedly, cerebral edema and proliferative
meningitis have been noted at autopsy in fatal cases, but Dr. Wagner made no
mention of other characteristic changes such as punctuate hemorrhages, gliosis,
or areas of focal necrosis.[136]

Lead poisoning will be considered again in the discussion of Beethoven's gastrointestinal complaint, headaches, eye disorder, and kidney disease.

SUMMARY AND CONCLUSIONS

The accounts of Beethoven's deafness from original sources suggest a mixed mechanism with a predominant sensorineural loss associated with a lesser conductive element. The precise details of the onset remain unknown.

Although otosclerosis is a common cause of slowly progressive deafness commencing in young manhood, there is no family history of it. Furthermore, Dr. Wagner's findings are inconsistent with otosclerosis, but rather are indicative of meningo-neuro-labyrinthitis. An infectious disease such as typhus fever is a more likely cause than pyogenic meningitis or sarcoidosis.

The advocates inclined toward a diagnosis of syphilis or Paget's disease were misled by errors in the translation of Dr. Wagner's autopsy report and the publication of Rottmayer's photograph of Beethoven's exhumed skull.

When the absence of a history of auricular discharge is considered together with the description of healthy ear drums, the diagnosis of middle-ear infection is unlikely. However, there is no doubt that the obstruction of both external ear canals with debris would have contributed a significant component of conductive hearing loss.

No doubt Beethoven's deafness was aggravated by such secondary factors as acoustic trauma, aging, and possibly ototoxic drugs such as quinine. Autoimmune mechanisms may also have contributed.

NOTES

1. L. Nohl, *Beethoven Depicted by His Contemporaries*, 144, n. 2.
2. Ibid., 243–44.
3. P. Garnault, "La surdité de Beethoven," Letter to the editor, *La Chronique Médicale* 12 (1905): 522–24.
4. W. Nagel, "Beethovens *Heiligenstadter Testament*," *Die Musik* 1(1902): 1050–58.
5. FRHB, 11:306.
6. F. Vieille, "Etat mental de Beethoven," *Thèse de Lyon*, M.D. thesis, 1905, 23. It remains unclear whether he was referring to a chronic adhesive otitis media.
7. G. Baratoux and M. Natier, "A propos de la surdité de Beethoven," Letter to the editor, *La Chronique Médicale* 12 (1905): 492–96.
8. Ibid., 493–96.
9. Klotz-Forest, "La surdité de Beethoven," 321–31.
10. Schindler-Moscheles, 11:78–79.
11. P. Bonnier, "La surdité de Beethoven," Letter to the editor, *La Chronique Médicale* 12 (1905): 521–22.
12. H. Neumann, "Beethovens Gehörleiden," *Wiener Medizinische Wöchschrift* 77 (1927):1015–19.

13. W. Scheidt, "Quecksilbervergiftung bei Mozart, Beethoven und Schubert?" *Med. Klin.* 62 (1967): 195–96.

14. H. Scherf, *Die Krankheit Beethovens* (Munich: Eigenverlag, 1977), 70–71.

15. Davies, "Beethoven's Deafness," 644–49.

16. Palferman, "Classical Notes," 640–45; T. G. Palferman, "Beethoven's Medical History: Themes and Variations," BN 7 (1992): 2–9; T. G. Palferman, "Beethoven: A Medical Biography," *Journal of Medical Biography* 1 (1993):35–45.

17. P. J. Davies, "The Cause of Beethoven's Deafness," in *Aflame with Music: 100 Years of Music at the University of Melbourne*, ed. Brenton Broadstock et al., (Melbourne: Centre for Studies in Australian Music, 1996), 143–51. It was first presented in his lecture delivered at the University of Melbourne on 6 June 1995.

18. Dr. Wawruch's retrospective medical report, trans. Erna Schwerin.

19. A. Neumayr, "Notes on the life, works, and medical history of Ludwig van Beethoven," 322; Bankl and Jesserer, *Die Krankheiten*, 10.

20. J. Ballantyne and J.A.M. Martin, *Deafness*, 4th ed. (Edinburgh: Churchill Livingstone, 1984), 53–62.

21. TF, 956.

22. A-51; B-65.

23. Schindler-Moscheles, I:123.

24. TF, 595.

25. Schünemann, *Beethovens Konversationshefte*, I: 371; LvBCB, I:377, 18 v, trans. Peter Stadlen in "Schindler's Beethoven Forgeries," MT 118 (1977): 551.

26. A-1072; B-1457.

27. Davies, "Beethoven's Deafness," 647.

28. Ibid., 647.

29. The *Fischhof Manuscript*, an unusual document in the Deutsche Staatsbibliothek, Berlin, is made up of transcripts by Joseph Fischof of various documents from a collection of Anton Gräffer. These were intended for a projected, though abandoned, biography of Beethoven. The original text is discussed by Clemens Brenneis in H. Goldschmidt, ed., *Zu Beethoven*, vol. 2, *Aufsätze und Documente* (Berlin: Verlag Neue Musik, 1984).

30. TDR, II:19; Bankl and Jesserer, *Die Krankheiten*, 11, trans. Erna Schwerin; TF, 187–88. For a description and transcription of the *Fischhof Manuscript* see Clemens Brenneis, "Das Fischhof-Manuskript in der Deutschen Staatsbibliothek," in Goldschmidt, *Zu Beethoven 2*, 27–87.

31. KHV, 411–17.

32. L. Nohl, *Beethoven Depicted by His Contemporaries* 144–45.

33. Ibid., 144, n. 2.

34. TK, I:263.

35. For details of Beethoven's excursion to Pressburg, see Frimmel, BS, II: 33–8.

36. TF, 188.

37. Isselbacher, *Harrison's Principles*, 672. For an account of Mozart's bout of typhoid fever in the Hague in 1765, see Davies, *Mozart in Person*, 22–23.

38. Isselbacher, *Harrison's Principles*, 752–53.

39. Wegeler and Ries, *Remembering Beethoven*, 5.

40. A-17; B-23. A facsimile of this letter was first published by Oscar G. Sonneck, *Beethoven Letters in America* (New York: G. Schirmer, The Beethoven Association, 1927), 182–83.

41. TF, 187.

42. A-20; B-30.

43. A-21; B-8.

44. Davies, "The Cause of Beethoven's Deafness," 147–48.

45. Isselbacher, *Harrison's Principles*, II: 2296.

46. P. Bodros, "La surdité et la maladie de Beethoven," *Presse Médicale* 48 (1938): 949–50.

47. Politzer, *Politzer's Text-Book*, 637.

48. Ibid., 685–86.

49. Ibid., 687–88.

50. Ibid., 685.

51. H. Neumann, "Beethoven's Gehörleiden," 1015–19.

52. J. D. Hood, "Deafness and Musical Appreciation," in *Music and the Brain*, ed., M. Critchley and R. A. Henson (London: W. Heinemann, 1977), 341.

53. Neumayr, "Notes," 322–23.

54. Scherf, *Die Krankheit Beethovens*, 65–66.

55. Ibid., 70–75.

56. The other three species of brucella that cause infection in humans are *B. melitensis* (sheep and goats), *B. suis* (swine), and *B. canis* (dogs).

57. Isselbacher, *Harrison's Principles*, I:685–87.

58. J. G. Scadding, *Sarcoidosis* (London: Eyre and Spottiswoode, 1967), 272–90; Om. P. Sharma, *Sarcoidosis: A Clinical Approach* (Springfield, Ill., Charles C. Thomas, 1975), 97–102; Isselbacher, *Harrison's Principles*, II: 1679–84.

59. P. Delaney, "Neurologic Manifestations in Sarcoidosis," *Annals of Internal Medicine* 87 (1977): 336–45.

60. Palferman, "Classical Notes," 640–45; Palferman, "Beethoven's Medical History," 2–9; Palferman, "Beethoven: A Medical Biography," 35–45.

61. J. Colover, "Sarcoidosis with Involvement of the Nervous System," *Brain* 71 (1948): 451–75.

62. Garrison and Morton, *Medical Bibliography*, no 1102.

63. W. H. Pennell, "Boeck's Sarcoid with Involvement of the Central Nervous System," *Archives of Neurology & Psychiatry* 66 (1951): 728–37; R. F. Gristwood, "Nerve Deafness Associated with Sarcoidosis," *Journal of Laryngology*, 72 (1958): 479–91; W. C. Weiderholt and R. G. Siekert, "Neurological Manifestations of Sarcoidosis," *Neurology* (Minneapolis) 15 (1965): 1147–54; R. Hooper and H. Holden, "Acoustic and Vestibular Problems in Sarcoidosis," *Archives of Otolaryngology* 92 (1970): 386–91.

64. Isselbacher, *Harrison's Principles*, II: 1397; J. C. Seiracki, "Whipple's Disease: Observations on Systemic Involvement," *Archives of Pathology* 66 (1958): 464–67.

65. Om. P. Sharma, "Beethoven's Illness: Whipple's Disease Rather Than Sarcoidosis?" *Journal of the Royal Society of Medicine* 87 (1994): 283–85.

66. Isselbacher, *Harrison's Principles*, II: 1397, 1703.

67. M. Adams, P. A. Rhyer, J. Day, S. de Armond, and E. Smuckler, "Whipple's Disease Confined to the Central Nervous System," *Annals of Neurology* 21 (1987): 104–10; R. A. Weeks, "Cerebral Whipple's Disease," *British Medical Journal* 312 (1996): 371–73.

68. Rolland, *Beethoven the Creator*, 280–81.

69. G. Marage, "Nature de la surdité de Beethoven," *Comptes Rendus Hebdomadaires des Séances de l'Académie des Sciences* 186 (1928): 110–12.

70. G. Marage, "Surdité et composition musicale," *Comptes Rendus Hebdomadaires des Séances de l'Académie des Sciences* 186 (1928): 266–68.

71. G. Marage, "Causes et conséquences de la surdité de Beethoven," *Comptes Rendus Hebdomadaires des Séances de l'Académie des Sciences* 189 (1929): 1036–38, trans. Sheila Krysz.

72. Rolland, *Beethoven the Creator*, 403, n. 291; Ira Frank, "The Deafness of Beethoven," *Annals of Otology and Laryngology* 44 (1935): 327–36.

73. For an overview of intestinal stasis and autointoxication, see J. Lacey Smith, "Sir Arbuthnot Lane, Chronic Intestinal Stasis, and Autointoxication," *Annals of Internal Medicine* 96 (1982): 365–69; and R. P. Hudson, "Theory and Therapy: Ptosis, Stasis and Autointoxication," *Bulletin of the History of Medicine* 63 (1989): 392–413.

74. Baratoux et Natier, "A Propos," 492–96; Neumann, "Beethovens Gehörleiden," 1015–19; M. Sorsby, "Beethoven's Deafness," *Journal of Laryngology and Otology* 45 (1930): 529–44; I. W. Voorhees, "Beethoven from an Otologist's Viewpoint," *Bulletin of New York Academy of Medicine* 12 (1936): 105–18; Schweisheimer, "Beethoven's Physicians," 289–98; Forster, *Beethovens Krankheiten*, 61; L. M. Sellers, "Beethoven the Immortal: His Deafness and His Music," *Laryngoscope* 73 (1963): 1158–83; Neumayr, "Notes," 323.

75. Davies, "Beethoven's Deafness," 648–49.

76. B. F. McCabe, "Autoimmune Sensorineural Hearing Loss," *Annals of Otology* 88 (1979), 585–89.

77. Davies, "Beethoven's Deafness," 648; Y. F. Cuddennec, "Ludwig van Beethoven: Une surdité auto-immune? par Peter J. Davies," *Histoire des Sciences Médicales* 29, no. 3 (1995): 271–76. I am grateful to Parisian otologist Professor Y. F. Cudennec, who translated my article into French and presented it in his lecture to La Société française d'Histoire de la Médecine, in Paris, 30 April 1994.

78. Davies, "The cause of Beethoven's Deafness," 149–50.

79. J. W. Miller, "Beethoven's Deafness," Letter to the Editor, *Journal of the American Medical Association* 213 (1970): 2082.

80. T. von Frimmel, "Beethovens Leiden und Ende," *Die Wiener Presse*, 8 September 1880.

81. Scherf, *Die krankheit Beethovens*, 73.

82. Frank, "Deafness of Beethoven," 334; Gattner, "Zu Beethovens Krankheit," 1009; Davies, "The Cause of Beethoven's Deafness," 150.

83. Ballantyne and Martin, *Deafness*, 210–12.

84. A. Laskiewicz, "Ludwig van Beethovens, Tragödie vom audiologischen Standpunkt," *Zeitschrift für Laryngology, Rhinology, Otology und ihre Grenzgebiete* 43 (1964): 261–70; Neumayr, "Notes," 323; Davies, "The Cause of Beethoven's Deafness," 150.

85. Ballantyne and Martin, *Deafness*, 221–22.

86. Scheidt, "Quecksilbervergiftung," 195–96; R. W. Gutt, "Beethoven's Deafness: An Iatrogenic Disease," *Medizinische Klinik* 65 (1970): 2294–95.

87. Isselbacher, *Harrison's Principles*, II: 2464–65.

88. Ibid., I:895.

89. Neumann, "Beethovens Gehörleiden," 1019.

90. N. Asherton, "The Deafness of Beethoven and the Saga of the Stapes," *Trans. Hunterian Soc.* 24 (1965–66):7–24.

91. V. S. Naiken, "Did Beethoven Have Paget's Disease of Bone?" *Annals of Internal Medicine* 74 (1971): 995–99; V. S. Naiken, "Beethoven's Deafness: Letter to the

Editor," *Journal of the American Medical Association* 215 (1971): 1671; V. S. Naiken, "Paget's Disease and Beethoven's Deafness," *Clinical in Orthopedics and Related Research* 89 (1972), 103–5.

92. Naiken, "Did Beethoven Have," 997.

93. Ibid., 996.

94. Ibid., 997.

95. Ibid., 998. See also D. Davies, "Paget's Disease of the Temporal Bone: A Histopathological Survey," *Acta. Otolaryng.*, (1968): Suppl. 269.

96. Frimmel, *Neue Beethoveniana*, 248.

97. Frimmel, BS, I:165.

98. H. Bankl, "Beethovens Krankheit—Morbus Paget?" *Pathologe* 6 (1985): 46–50; Bankl and Jesserer, *Die Krankheiten*, 119–20.

99. J. D. Clemis, J. Boyles, E. R. Harford, J. P. Petasnick, "The Clinical Diagnosis of Paget's Disease of the Temporal Bone," *Annals of Otology* 76 (1967): 611–23.

100. Klotz-Forest, "La surdité de Beethoven," 331.

101. Bonnier, "La surdité de Beethoven," 521–22.

102. Jacobsohn, "Ludwig van Beethovens Gehörleiden," 1282–85; M. Menier, "La surdité de Ludwig van Beethoven," *Archives Internationales de Laryngologie, d'Otologie, et de Rhinologie* 31 (1911): 179–81.

103. Sorsby, "Beethoven's Deafness," 538.

104. Ballantyne and Martin, *Deafness*, 215.

105. Sorsby, "Beethoven's Deafness," 539.

106. P. H. Beales, *Otosclerosis* (Bristol, England: John Wright and Sons, 1981), 4.

107. Ibid., 12, 51–67.

108. Garrison and Morton, *A Medical Bibliography*, nos. 1537, 1538, 1542.

109. Beales, *Otosclerosis*, 1; Garrison and Morton, *A Medical Bibliography*, no. 3373.

110. Bilancioni, "La sordità di Beethoven," 531–41; Engel, "Views and Reviews," 646–62; Asherton, "Deafness of Beethoven," 7–24; Larkin, "Beethoven's Medical History," 440–41; J. G. O'Shea, "Medical Profile of Ludwig van Beethoven," 44–49.

111. K. M. Stevens and W. G. Hemenway, "Beethoven's Deafness," *Journal of the American Medical Association* 213 (1970): 434–37; M. Landsberger, "Beethoven's Medical History," *New York State Journal of Medicine* 78 (1978): 676–79; N. I. Chalat, "Some Psychologic aspects of Deafness: Beethoven, Goya, and Oscar Wilde," *American Journal of Otology* 1 (1980): 240–46; Bankl and Jesserer, *Die Krankheiten*, 130.

112. Marage, "Nature de la surdité," 110–112.

113. Voorhees, "Beethoven from an Otologist's Viewpoint," 105–18.

114. Schweisheimer, *Beethovens Leiden*, 56–97.

115. Forster, *Beethovens Krankheiten*, 60–61.

116. Laskiewicz, "Beethovens Tragödie," 261–70.

117. Böhme, *Medizinische Porträts*, I:83–86.

118. TF, 644, 967.

119. Beales, *Otosclerosis*, 19.

120. A-51; B-65.

121. TF, 595.

122. American Otological Society, "Symposium on Sensorineural Deafness in Otosclerosis," *Annals of Otology, Rhinology, and Laryngology* 75 (1966): 418–590; A. Larsson, "Otosclerosis: A Genetic and Clinical Study," *Acta Oto Laryngology* (Stockholm), Suppl. 154 (1960): 1–86.

123. Politzer, *History of Otology*, I:288–90.

124. Davies, "Beethoven's Deafness," 648; S. R. Guild, "Histologic Otosclerosis," *Annals of Otology, Rhinology, and Laryngology* 53 (1944): 246–66; T. Cawthorne, "Otosclerosis," *Journal of Laryngology and Otology*, 69 (1955): 437–56; G. T. Nager, "Sensorineural Deafness and Otosclerosis," *Annuals of Otology, Rhinology, and Laryngology* 75 (1966): 481–511; L. Rüedi and H. Spoendlin, "Pathogenesis of Sensorineural Deafness in Otosclerosis," *Annals of Otology, Rhinology, and Laryngology* 75 (1966): 525–52; G. E. Shambaugh, "Sensorineural Deafness due to Cochlear Otospongiosis: Pathogenesis, Clinical Diagnosis and Therapy," *Otolaryngological Clinics of North America* 11 (1978): 135–54.

125. Sorsby, "Beethoven's Deafness," 539.

126. Davies, "Beethoven's Deafness," 648; A. Politzer, "Über primäre Erkrankung der knöchernen Labyrinthkapsel," *Zschr Ohrenheilk* 25 (1894): 309–27; F. R. Nager and F. S. Fraser, "On Bone Formation in the Scala Tympani of Otosclerotics," *Journal of Laryngology and Otology* 53 (1938): 173–80; H. F. Schuknecht and C. W. Gross, "Otosclerosis and the Inner Ear," *Annals of Otology, Rhinology, and Laryngology* 75 (1966): 423–35; J. R. Lindsay and D. D. Beal, "Sensorineural Deafness in Otosclerosis: Observations on Histopathology," *Annals of Otology, Rhinology, and Laryngology* 75 (1966): 436–57; D. Wolff, "Sensorineural Deafness in Otosclerosis," *Annals of Otology, Rhinology, and Laryngology* 75 (1966): 458–68; G. Kelemen and F. H. Linthicum, Jr., "Labyrinthine Otosclerosis," *Acta Oto-Laryngol* 253 Suppl. (1969): 5–68.

127. A. K. Kubba and M. Young, "Ludwig van Beethoven: A Medical Biography," *Lancet* 347 (1996): 167–70.

128. Landon, *Beethoven: A Documentary Study*, 256.

129. Isselbacher, *Harrison's Principles*, II: 2329–32.

130. "Beethoven's Diseases," Editorial, *Lancet* 1 (January 1921): 41.

131. Johann's portrait is illustrated in Landon, *Beethoven: A Documentary Study*, plate 242. I am grateful to Dr. John O'Shea for this information.

132. See Bruce W. Konigsmark, "Hereditary Deafness in Man," in three parts, *New England Journal of Medicine* 281 (1969): 713–20, 774–78, 827–32.

133. K. Aterman, H. M. MacSween, P. E. Perry, H. A. Warner, "Recurrent Infections, Diarrhea, Ascites, and Phonophobia in a 57-Year-Old Man," *Canadian Medical Association Journal* 126 (1982): 623–28.

134. Isselbacher, *Harrison's Principles*, II: 1629.

135. *Goodman and Gilman's the Pharmacological Basis of Therapeutics* 6th ed. (New York: Macmillan, 1980), 1617–18; Isselbacher, *Harrison's Principles*, II: 2463; F. Walshe, *Diseases of the Nervous System*, 9th ed. (Edinburgh: E & S Livingstone, 1958), 283–84.

136. *Goodman and Gilman*, 1618; N. Popoff, S. Weinberg, and I. Feigin, "Pathologic Observations in Lead Encephalopathy," *Neurology* (Minneapolis) 13 (1963): 101–12.

9

Gastrointestinal Disorders

Beethoven suffered his first bouts of abdominal disorder in Bonn. Dr. Gerhard Franz Wegeler stated that when Abbé Georg Joseph Vogler played in Bonn, he was seated at "Beethoven's sickbed."[1] Alexander Wheelock Thayer established that this visit occurred in either 1790 or 1791.[2]

Wegeler also stated that Beethoven was subject to frequent bouts of rather severe, griping abdominal pain (*Kolikschmerzen*), as on the afternoon he was composing the rondo of his first piano concerto, just two days before he performed it.[3] Expert opinion remains divided as to whether it was indeed the First Piano Concerto in C, Op. 15[4] or a much revised and partly rewritten Second Piano Concerto in B-flat Major, Op. 19,[5] which he performed at his first public concert on 29 March 1795, in the Burgtheater, for the benefit of the widows of the Tonkünstlergesellschaft. In any event, Wegeler assisted Beethoven with symptomatic remedies as best he could during those stressful days.

In December 1795 Beethoven wrote in his diary, "Courage. Even with all the frailties of my body, my spirit shall dominate."[6]

THE RECURRENT GASTROINTESTINAL COMPLAINT

In his overview, written barely two months after Beethoven's death, on 20 May 1827, Dr. Andreas Ignaz Wawruch wrote,

After Mozart and Haydn, the last triumphant composer in Austria, has passed away, deeply mourned everywhere. It is my sacred duty as the attending physician of this man who deserves and received the highest respect, and whose enormous talent and celebrated name penetrated the utmost ranges of civilization, to present a few of the peculiarities of the period of his illness. Such rare talents offer rich experiences and interesting moments, and no one is better qualified to relate them than the attending physician. This brief essay is therefore not a formal medical history (for what could it have to offer to the layman that is attractive?), but it is a simple narrative of facts with reference to Beethoven's courageous suffering and devout resignation, with which he faced the end (of his life).

Ludwig van Beethoven could look upon a hardened state of health, based on the hardships of his youth which he courageously encountered, and which the most strenuous work and concentrated studies could not impair. From early on he was most inclined to work at night, when he could give his fantasy free reign. He usually wrote till 3 A.M. He felt fully restored after four to five hours sleep. After breakfast he worked again until 2 o'clock in the afternoon.

But in the beginning of his thirtieth year he began having problems with haemorrhoids (*Hämorrhoidalleiden*) and with annoying whistling and rushing in both ears. . . . At about the same time Beethoven's digestion gave him trouble: impaired appetite resulted in indigestion, annoying belching, soon troublesome constipation, alternating with frequent diarrhoea. Never accustomed to seek medical advice, he began to imbibe in spirits to stimulate his appetite, and to counteract the weakness of his stomach with strong Punsch (punch) and ices, which he partook of in excess. It was this change of his habits which almost brought him to the brink of his grave about seven years ago. He contracted a severe inflammation of the bowels which, although it subsided with treatment, resulted in frequent stomach complaints and colic (pains), which must have been partly responsible for the subsequent development of his fatal illness.

In the late Fall of last year (1826) Beethoven had an irrepressible urge to go to the country to achieve an improvement of his ill health. Since he carefully avoided social contacts because of his complete deafness, he was left to his own resources for days and sometimes for weeks on end. With rare perseverance he often composed his works on a slope of a hill in the woods, and after completion of his work walked around, still sweating from his efforts, in the roughest country areas and in every weather (often in deep snow). His already swollen feet became even more swollen. Since, as he said, he had to forgo all conveniences and comforts of living, he was soon overwhelmed by his intolerable situation.[7]

Not surprisingly, Dr. Wawruch's account of the early history of Beethoven's gastrointestinal complaint was inaccurate. When he obtained the medical history in December 1826, Wawruch's communication with Beethoven was restricted to use of the conversation-books, many of which were subsequently lost or destroyed. No doubt Wawruch would also have obtained some of the history secondhand, through the nephew Carl, or the brother Johann, or Anton Schindler, or Stephan von Breuning, or Carl Holz.

Even so, Dr. Wawruch's report highlighted three important aspects: (1) Beethoven's hemorrhoids; (2) his troublesome constipation alternating with diarrhea, a decisive diagnostic detail which several medical writers have failed to grasp; and (3) a history of excessive consumption of alcohol. The differential diagnosis of Beethoven's abdominal disorders is summarized in Table 9.1.

Table 9.1
Beethoven's Abdominal Disorders

Recurrent Gastrointestinal Complaint	Chronic Pancreatitis
Irritable bowel syndrome	Caused by:
Inflammatory bowel disease	alcohol
Crohn's disease of the ileum	Gallstones
Ulcerative colitis	Hemochromatosis
Post typhus—chronic enteritis	Alpha-1-antitrypsin deficiency
Sarcoidosis	Cystic fibrosis
Intestinal tuberculosis	Congenital syphilis
Chronic brucellosis	Sclerosing cholangitis
Whipple's disease	Hereditary
IgA deficiency	Drugs
Lead poisoning	Idiopathic
Gallstones	Manifest as:
Peptic ulcer	Abdominal pain
Hemorrhoids	Steatorrhea
	Diabetes mellitus

IRRITABLE BOWEL SYNDROME

Following an onset in 1790 or 1791, the long history of intermittent crampy abdominal pain (*Kolikschmerzen*), associated with alternating constipation and diarrhea, flatulence, digestive upsets, weakness, and debility, is typical of one of three clinical variants of the irritable bowel syndrome. This condition, which in the medical literature is also referred to by various other synonyms (irritable colon, irritable gut, spastic colon, spastic colitis, mucous colitis), is associated with alterations of intestinal motility and hypersensitive visceral perception, though without any demonstrable macroscopic or microscopic pathology. Irritable bowel syndrome today is the most common gastrointestinal disorder in clinical practice.

The triggering of symptoms by stress, as for example, in Beethoven's case, the rehearsals for concerts or dramatic stage works, and Napoléon Bonaparte's siege of Vienna, is common in irritable bowel syndrome, as also is an association with depression. Indeed, small doses of antidepressant medication is known often to be of symptomatic benefit in this condition. Furthermore, in Beethoven's case, the prompt response of most of his bouts to bed rest, symptomatic medication, dietary restriction of fatty and spicy foods, and the spa cures add evidence to support this diagnosis.

Three further clinical observations are also deserving of serious consideration: (1) the very long interval of thirty years, between 1790 and 1820, when, despite recurrent bouts of the disorder, there was no physical deterioration; (2) the association with the bout of diarrhea in April 1823 of a burning irritation in his throat, in the face of reassurances from Dr. Carl von Smetana that his throat was not inflamed or ulcerated; and (3) the failure of Dr. Johann Joseph Wagner to detect a segmental abnormality or lesion in either the small intestine or the large bowel, a point which will be further discussed below.

Yet because symptoms of recurrent abdominal pain associated with alternating constipation and diarrhea are nonspecific, and in no way pathognomonic of the irritable bowel syndrome, the consultant gastroenterologist in the 2000s, when faced with such a history, would exclude other causes of such symptoms with a careful physical examination, sigmoidoscopy, and several further tests. In the irritable bowel syndrome, the full blood examination and erythrocyte sedimentation rate are normal. The stools would be examined to exclude parasites and pathogens. Malabsorption would be screened for with a serum folic acid and vitamin B12 assay, a fecal fat estimation, and a lactose tolerance test. An immunoglobulin assay would exclude IgA deficiency. A gastroscopy would exclude the presence of reflux oesophagitis or peptic ulceration, while duodenal biopsies would be examined under the microscope for evidence of celiac sprue, giardiasis, Whipple's disease, amyloidosis, Crohn's disease, or enteropathy. Colonoscopy with multiple biopsies would be performed to exclude inflammatory bowel diseases such as ulcerative colitis and Crohn's disease. The small bowel would be studied by barium x-ray studies or enteroscopy. Negative findings in these tests would confirm the diagnosis of irritable bowel syndrome.[8]

It should be emphasized that Beethoven was obsessional and hypochondriacal about his bowels, with good reason, for he had observed that purgatives, laxatives, and enemas were the mainstay of treatment for inflammations. Consequently, he was anxious that his respiratory and intestinal catarrhs might become transformed into serious inflammations that might cut the thread of his life. He was overly concerned about constipation, and there is no doubt that some of his bouts of diarrhea were iatrogenic.

The diagnosis of irritable bowel syndrome was also proposed and accepted with reservations by S. J. London,[9] F. H. Franken,[10] H. Bankl and H. Jesserer,[11] and T. G. Palferman[12]; this diagnosis was rejected by J. G. O'Shea[13] and by Anton Neumayr.[14] There were two major objections.

Contra Irritable Bowel Syndrome

First, it was argued that Beethoven's more severe bouts, associated with prostration or prolonged illness, were not typical of irritable bowel syndrome, and would be better accounted for by alternative diagnoses such as chronic pancreatitis,[15] renal colic,[16] or Crohn's disease.[17]

Most of Beethoven's bouts of gastrointestinal illness lasted only three or four days, and it would appear that the more prolonged episodes were related to his depression. Prostration, it should be noted, refers to complete physical or mental exhaustion, and Beethoven was readily subject to neurasthenia when depressed. On the other hand, when his mood became more elevated, his strength and well-being increased.[18]

Let us then take another look at three of these more prolonged bouts of illness. In December 1809 he was confined to bed for two weeks with his intestinal disorder, and he was still not fully recovered in February. He was then grumbling about the lack of decent bread to eat, and he was suffering with depression following the French invasion of Austria and the departure of the Archduke Rudolph and many of his friends from Vienna.

He also blamed some indigestible food for his indisposition at Teplitz during the last two weeks of September in 1812, but at that time he was suffering depression in the aftermath of the "Immortal Beloved" affair. Likewise his depression would help to account for his prolonged illness for several months during 1816 and 1817.

Second is the association of the abdominal symptoms with fever, which will be discussed below.

INFLAMMATORY BOWEL DISEASE

Crohn's Disease of the Small Intestine (Regional Enteritis)

Viennese physician Dr. Anton Neumayr argued that a diagnosis of irritable bowel syndrome was contradicted not only by Beethoven's prolonged spells of weakness and infirmity, but especially by the association of his bouts of abdominal pain and diarrhea with fever.[19] "From 1795 on, Beethoven grumbled repeatedly about bouts of sickness with fever that accompanied a worsening of his intestinal complaints."[20]

If this statement were correct, it would warrant significant merit, but it is erroneous. Dr. Neumayr has misread and misinterpreted the accounts of Beethoven's symptoms to suit his own diagnosis. Let us then look again at the accounts of such illnesses.

Beethoven's Illnesses with "Fever"

In his detailed letter of 29 June 1801 to Wegeler, in which he described his deafness and abdominal problems, there was no mention of fever.[21]

With regard to the persistent undulant fever during the latter half of 1804, referred to by Stephan von Breuning, there was no mention of gastrointestinal symptoms.[22] It would appear likely that this fever was due to an infection, and the unusual term undulant fever (*Wechselfieber*) was suggestive of acute brucellosis, as discussed by Horst Scherf,[23] although I dispute that the infection became chronic, for Breuning stated that, on 13 November 1804, Beethoven was completely well again. Alternatively, it could have been some other illness such as malaria, some louse-borne or tick-borne relapsing fever, or some other infection. We will never know for certain for, under such circumstances, the diagnosis can be established only by blood cultures, appropriate serological tests, and response to treatment.

During 1807 or 1808, Beethoven was plagued for a few days with a wretched attack of colic, but he made no mention of fever.[24] In an undated note to Herr Bigot, attributed by Emily Anderson to 1808, but consigned more broadly by Brandenburg to the period between 1807 and 1809, Beethoven told him that he was laid up with a feverish attack caused by a chill. There was no mention of intestinal upset, and it may have been a respiratory infection.[25]

Early in December 1809 he was thoroughly upset by a fever,[26] and hardly had he recovered when he suffered a recurrence of his abdominal complaint in association with depression, as discussed above.[27]

Beethoven's violent attack of colic in May 1810 lasted three days, but there was no mention of fever.[28] Neither of two other bouts of fever was associated with abdominal symptoms. A violent fever in April 1803 kept him in bed for a few days.[29] On this occasion, when he was struck down with such a fever that he fainted when his injured foot gave way under him, once again there was no reference to his abdominal complaint.[30] His fierce attacks during the winter of 1812 could well have been respiratory in nature.[31]

The lingering effects of his dangerous, feverish cold at Baden in October 1816 were discussed above. In an undated note to the Archduke Rudolph, which Anderson attributed to 1816, there was mention of a bout of colic which indisposed him for three days.[32]

During the winter of 1817, Beethoven's pain was so severe that he had to lie down on the couch.[33] Soon after he caught another chill, which caused a violent cold and cough.[34]

Nor was there mention of fever during two other bouts of abdominal illness.[35] Indeed, in all the above episodes, he distinguished his bouts of fever from his usual complaint—his gastrointestinal disorder. However, during his bout of "intestinal inflammation" in the spring of 1825, there was mention of a short bout of fever, but Dr. Anton Braunhofer reassured him on two occasions that it had subsided: "No fever,"[36] and "It is not fever, but a flutter with a tendency towards inflammation."[37]

Even if Beethoven's gastrointestinal symptoms were associated with fever, that would not necessarily support a diagnosis of Crohn's disease, since chronic liver disease, and chronic pancreatitis, and sometimes certain complications of gallstones may also be associated with pyrexia.

Crohn's Disease (Regional Enteritis)

Since inflammatory bowel disease may be associated with chronic disorders of the liver, biliary tract, and pancreas, as well as an enteropathic arthropathy, inflammation of the eyes, and autoimmune sensorineural deafness, the acceptance of a diagnosis of Crohn's disease or ulcerative colitis would also help to account for such other disorders of Beethoven. However, such an argument of recognized association is invalid when satisfactory alternative explanations are more plausible. Admittedly there is also, in inflammatory bowel disease, an increased incidence of gallstones and renal calculi. However, gallstones are common in the general population, and Beethoven's renal lesions will be discussed in a later chapter.

The diagnosis of Crohn's disease in Beethoven's case was first proposed in 1975 by Professor Walter Smith[38] and was again advocated by A. K. Kubba and M. Young.[39] The diagnosis of Crohn's disease has been opposed by Franken,[40] O'Shea,[41] Bankl and Jesserer,[42] and Palferman.[43]

Contra Crohn's Disease

Perianal erosions causing abscesses, sinuses, and fistulae are very common in Crohn's disease. There was no such history in Beethoven's case, but Neumayr proposed that such lesions might have been misdiagnosed as hemorrhoids.[44] While rectal bleeding is not uncommon in colonic Crohn's disease, it is infrequent in regional enteritis. Nor was there a history of intestinal obstruction which is a frequent complication of Crohn's disease.

Another major objection to the diagnosis of regional enteritis is the failure of Dr. Johann Joseph Wagner to note any segmental macroscopic abnormality in the ileum. Dr. Neumayr proposed, as a possible explanation, that in performing the autopsy Dr. Wagner elected to concentrate on the organs of the ear and the liver, giving relatively little attention to the remainder of the gastrointestinal tract.[45] This explanation is unacceptable because Dr. Wagner performed a detailed autopsy, which involved dissection not only of the hearing mechanism, liver, biliary tract, spleen, and pancreas, but also of the brain, heart, lungs, and even the kidneys. Why would he then neglect an examination of the gastrointestinal tract that caused Beethoven so much discomfort and trouble?

Furthermore, Dr. Wagner had a special interest in intestinal perforation and ileus and later wrote a paper on that subject.[46] In order to have stated that "the stomach with the intestines were greatly distended with air," he would need to have dissected the entire gastrointestinal tract. The characteristic thickening and hardening of the segment or segments of regional enteritis in the ileum, together with changes in the mesentery and lymph nodes, associated with narrowing of the lumen and stricture formation, are unlikely to have escaped Dr. Wagner's experienced eye. Nor did he mention such other common features as ulcerations, fistulae, abscesses, or adhesions. Crohn's disease is an unlikely cause of Beethoven's gastrointestinal complaint.

Ulcerative Colitis

Several researchers have proposed a diagnosis of ulcerative colitis, another form of inflammatory bowel disease which may be associated with systemic manifestations similar to Crohn's disease.[47] Physician Dr. Alfred Warner has proposed the clever joint diagnoses of ulcerative colitis associated with IgA deficiency to account also for the frequent respiratory infections, and the possible association with atopic and autoimmune diseases.[48]

Certain types of ulcerative colitis, especially the less extensive cases of distal proctocolitis, may give rise to a long history of diarrhea alternating with constipation, associated with abdominal pain.

Contra Ulcerative Colitis

In patients with ulcerative colitis recurrent bouts of colicky abdominal pain do not usually dominate the clinical picture, as in Beethoven's case. However, the major objection is the absence of rectal bleeding. The most characteristic symptom of ulcerative colitis is the recurrent passage of blood and slime through the rectum. It has been proposed that the diagnosis of hemorrhoids might imply that Beethoven might have been subject to bouts of minor rectal bleeding.[49] However, Beethoven, who was overly concerned about his bowels, liked to mention his symptoms in his correspondence. Among his numerous references to his bowels, there was not one reference to rectal bleeding. Furthermore, he was specifically asked about it in the conversation-books. Nor did Dr. Wagner describe any abnormal changes in the large bowel. Although it is impossible, in the absence of a histological examination, to exclude inflammatory bowel disease with absolute certainty, the balance of all the evidence renders it unlikely.

CHRONIC PANCREATITIS

Dr. Wagner's description of an enlarged pancreas which was firmer than normal, associated with a dilated pancreatic duct, is typical of chronic pancreatitis. Autopsy studies in Germany have established that a goose quill could not be passed into the excretory duct of a normal, nondiseased pancreas, whereas it could be passed readily into the dilated pancreatic duct of subjects with chronic pancreatitis.[50]

It is probable that Beethoven's chronic pancreatitis was caused by his excessive intake of alcohol, although the gallstones could have contributed to its pathogenesis. Autopsy studies have shown that about 30 percent of patients with alcoholic cirrhosis also have an established chronic pancreatitis. Hemochromatosis seems a less likely cause because Dr. Wagner made no mention of brownish, chocolate, or rusty pigmentation of the pancreas.[51]

Sarcoidosis,[52] cystic fibrosis,[53] and alpha-1-antitrypsin deficiency[54] warrant consideration because of Beethoven's concurrent respiratory symptoms, but the other possible causes listed in Table 9.1 are unlikely.

Several authors have favored chronic pancreatitis as the cause of Beethoven's gastrointestinal disorder.[55] However, in the susceptible population it takes a period of from six to twelve years of regular alcohol consumption before the onset of symptoms.[56] Since Beethoven's recurrent gastrointestinal complaint commenced in his early twenties, it is unlikely that the early bouts were due to chronic pancreatitis, although that disorder may have contributed to later attacks. Pari passu with the progress of chronic pancreatitis there is a gradual decline in exocrine glandular function, which when 90 percent of the parenchyma has been destroyed becomes clinically manifest as steatorrhea. The maldigestion and malabsorption associated with chronic pancreatitis may have contributed to Beethoven's weight loss during the last two years of his life. The question of diabetes mellitus, another complication of chronic pancreatitis, will be discussed later.

GALLSTONES

Although an unlikely cause of Beethoven's recurrent gastrointestinal ailment, gallstones may have caused some of his bouts of colicky abdominal pain. In chapter 15 we will return to gallstones in the discussion of the attack of severe pain and jaundice on 10 December 1826.

POST-TYPHUS CHRONIC ENTERITIS

Waldemar Schweisheimer[57] and W. Forster[58] proposed that Beethoven's chronic intestinal catarrh (*chronischen Darmkatarrhes*), following an attack of typhus in his earlier life, caused not only his recurrent gastrointestinal complaint, but also his cirrhosis. However, it is now appreciated that chronic enteritis following a bout of typhus fever, or typhoid fever, is not a recognized entity. Nor does a typhus illness cause cirrhosis. On the other hand, it is well known in clinical practice that a bout of typhus or dysentery might sometimes trigger the onset of irritable bowel syndrome.

INTESTINAL TUBERCULOSIS

Beethoven was at risk of contracting a tuberculous infection because his mother and a brother, Caspar Carl, died of consumption.[59] Involvement of the small intestine and large bowel may occur as a primary infection with the human or bovine strain, or it may be secondary to spread from an active focus in the lung or elsewhere. The most common site of involvement is the ileocaecal region, so that confusion with Crohn's disease poses a problem. The protean symptoms include abdominal pain, fever, night sweats, weight loss, diarrhea, or constipation. Dr. Wagner's failure to identify the characteristic hypertrophic lesions, circumferential transverse ulcers, short strictures, or abundant miliary serosal nodules render a diagnosis of intestinal tuberculosis as unlikely. Nor was there an active focus in the lungs.

SARCOIDOSIS

Sarcoidosis has been advanced as a possible single explanation for all Bee-thoven's illnesses, including the abdominal complaint.[60] Though granulomatous histological involvement of the oesophagus, stomach, small intestine, pancreas, and peritoneum have been reported in patients with sarcoidosis, symptomatic involvement of these organs is rare.[61]

WHIPPLE'S DISEASE

Whipple's disease has been proposed as the cause of Beethoven's recurrent abdominal pain, diarrhea, arthralgia, and weight loss.[62] However, his history of alternating constipation with diarrhea, the usual absence of fever with the ab-dominal symptoms, the long delay in the onset of weight loss, the absence of progression in the severity of the diarrhea, and especially the survival for thirty-five years without antibiotic therapy all render the diagnosis of Whipple's dis-ease unlikely.

LEAD POISONING

The possibility of plumbism as the cause of recurrent abdominal pain and constipation in a man with elevated levels of lead in his hair must be considered. Headache and anemia are common in plumbism, and diarrhea occurs occasion-ally.

An important source of lead poisoning then was the ingestion of fish from the Danube, whose waters were polluted by the dumping of toxic waste. It is interesting to note that Beethoven preferred fish from the ocean.

It might also be argued that Beethoven's abdominal complaints were relieved at the spa resorts because such waters were free of lead contamination.

Contra Lead Poisoning

Beethoven's bouts of diarrhea were frequent, and there is no record of his ever complaining about a metallic taste in his mouth. None of his physicians made note of a blue gum line which results from the periodontal deposition of lead sulfide.[63]

Lead-intoxicated adults with related symptoms of recurrent abdominal pain and headache usually have significantly elevated blood levels of lead.[64] Such subjects commonly develop neurological sequela, to be discussed elsewhere.

It must be emphasized that Beethoven's gastrointestinal disorder commenced in Bonn. It is improbable that symptomatic lead poisoning persisted for thirty-six years without the development of neurological complications.

While it is possible that some of Beethoven's bouts of abdominal pain were related to exacerbations of lead poisoning, the overall picture is more suggestive of irritable bowel syndrome.

PEPTIC ULCER DISEASE

The history of recurrent abdominal pain and indigestion suggests the possibility of peptic ulcer disease. Three quarters of such patients complain of recurrent upper abdominal pain relieved by antacids. In cases with a duodenal ulcer, pain tends to come on when the stomach is empty, and typically the patient is awakened from sleep in the early hours of the morning. When a gastric ulcer is present, the pain is often aggravated by food and may be associated with vomiting. In the less common cases of peptic ulcer without pain, the condition is heralded by a hemorrhage.

Beethoven gave no such history. His indigestion and flatulence were associated by him with his bowels and lower gastrointestinal tract. Furthermore, Dr. Wagner reported no localized lesion in the stomach or duodenum.

SUMMARY AND CONCLUSIONS

The very long history of Beethoven's recurrent gastrointestinal complaint, tracing back to his Bonn period in 1790, or 1791, when viewed against his apparent physical well-being, and the absence of the development of overt serious complications, tends to favor the diagnosis of irritable bowel syndrome.

The history of recurrent abdominal pain associated with indigestion, flatulence, and troublesome constipation alternating with frequent diarrhea, is typical of this disorder.

Such a diagnosis is further supported by the association with stress or depression, and the response to symptomatic medication or spa cures. No doubt the frequent straining at stool, when constipated, aggravated the hemorrhoids.

The absence of a history of rectal bleeding adds considerable weight to arguments against ulcerative colitis. Furthermore, the absence of such intestinal complications as an abscess, a fistula, or an obstruction goes against a diagnosis of Crohn's disease.

Intestinal tuberculosis must be considered against a background of the family history, but Dr. Wagner's findings were negative in this regard.

Although it is possible that gallstones, or lead poisoning, or chronic pancreatitis contributed to or caused some of the later attacks of abdominal pain, the other possible causes listed in Table 9.1 are unlikely.

NOTES

1. Wegeler and Ries, *Remembering Beethoven*, 17.
2. TDR, I: 287.
3. Wegeler and Ries, *Remembering Beethoven*, 38.

4. Ibid., 176, n. 24, by Alfred C. Kalischer; Hans-Werner Küthen, *Klavierkonzerte*, vol. 1, *Kritischer Bericht* (vol. 3, *Beethoven Werke*), (Munich: G. Henle Verlag, 1984), 5; Barry Cooper, *Beethoven and the Creative Process* (Oxford, England: Clarendon Press, 1990, 295.

5. TF, 174; Douglas P. Johnson, *Beethoven's Early Sketches in the 'Fischhof Miscellany': Berlin Autograph, 28*, Ph.D. diss., University of California, Berkeley, 1978 (Ann Arbor, Mich.: University Microfilms, 1979), I: 635.

6. Bankl and Jesserer, *Die Krankheiten*, 10, trans. Erna Schwerin.

7. Alois Fuchs, "Ärztlicher Rückblick auf Ludwig van Beethovens letzte Lebensepoche," *Wiener Zeitschrift für Kunst, Literatur, Theater und Mode*, no. 86, on 30 April 1842; Bankl and Jesserer, *Die Krankheiten*, 46–47, trans. Erna Schwerin.

8. Isselbacher, *Harrison's Principles*, II:1421–22.

9. London, "Beethoven: Case Report," 446.

10. Franken, *Die Krankheiten grosser Komponisten*, I: 102.

11. Bankl and Jesserer, *Die Krankheiten*, 127–29.

12. Palferman, "Beethoven: A Medical Biography," 44.

13. O'Shea, "Medical Profile," *Music and Medicine*, 42.

14. Neumayr, "Notes," *Music and Medicine*, 328.

15. London, "Beethoven: Case Report," 446–48; O'Shea, "Medical Profile," 42.

16. Palferman, "Beethoven: A Medical Biography," 44.

17. Neumayr, "Notes," 328.

18. A-54; B-70.

19. Neumayr, "Notes," 323–31.

20. Ibid., 324.

21. A-51; B-65; Neumayr, "Notes," 324. The letter is misdated 29 July 1801.

22. Neumayr, "Notes," 324; TDR, II: 432; Albrecht, *Letters*, no. 90.

23. Scherf, *Die Krankenheit Beethovens*, 63–65.

24. A-170 (Summer 1808); B-303 (4 December 1807).

25. A-191; B-308.

26. A-230; B-415.

27. A-243–5; B-419, 421, 423.

28. A-260; B-431 (18 April 1810).

29. A-302; B-134 (April 1803).

30. A-330 (December 1811); B-640 (20 April 1813).

31. A-351, 353; B-555, 544.

32. A-729; B-687 (1813–14).

33. A-881; B-1203.

34. A-882; B-1226.

35. A-904, 995; B-1260, 1047.

36. LvBCB, VII: 227–28.

37. Ibid., 232.

38. Critchley and Henson, *Music and the Brain*, 402.

39. Kubba and Young, "Beethoven: A Medical Biography," 170.

40. Franken, *Die Krankheiten grosser Komponisten*, I: 102.

41. O'Shea, "Medical Profiles," 42.

42. Bankl and Jesserer, *Die Krankheiten*, 127–28.

43. Palferman, "Beethoven: A Medical Biography," 42–43.

44. Neumayr, "Notes," 329.

45. Ibid., 330.

46. J. Wagner, "Einige Beobachtungen innerer Brüche," *Medizinische Jahrbücher des K.K. österreichischen Staates, N.S.* 4 (1833): 196–221.

47. Voorhees, "Beethoven from an Otologist's Viewpoint," 106; Sellers, "Beethoven the Immortal," 1169; Larkin, "Beethoven's Medical History," 445; Paul C. Adams, "Historical Hepatology: Ludwig van Beethoven," *Journal of Gastroenterology and Hepatology*, 2 (1987): 377.

48. Aterman et al., "Recurrent Infections," 626.

49. Larkin, "Beethoven's Medical History," 445; Neumayr, "Notes," 324.

50. Franken, *Die Krankheiten grosser Komponisten*, I: 103–4.

51. P. J. Davies, "Was Beethoven's Cirrhosis due to Hemochromatosis?" *Renal Failure* 17 (1995): 82.

52. Palferman, "Beethoven: A Medical Biography," 42.

53. Aterman et al., "Recurrent Infections," 625.

54. Ibid., 625.

55. Piroth, "Beethovens letzte Krankheit," 26, 34; London, "Beethoven: Case Report," 446–47; Y. Cudennec, L. Soubeyrand, and P. Buffe, "Ludwig van Beethoven: L'homme et son enigme médicale," *Les Cahiers d'Otologie, Rhinologie, Laryngologie*, 18 (1983): 49; Franken, I, *Die Krankheiten grosser Komponisten*, 102–8; O'Shea, "Medical Profile," 42.

56. M. H. Sleisinger and J. S. Fordtran, eds., *Gastrointestinal Disease*, 2nd ed. (Philadelphia: W. B. Saunders, 1978), II: 1439.

57. Schweisheimer, *Beethovens Leiden*, 161.

58. Forster, *Beethovens Krankheiten*, 61.

59. Bodros, "La surdité et la maladie," 949–50; Aterman et al., "Recurrent Infections," 625.

60. Palferman, "Beethoven: A Medical Biography," 44.

61. J. G. Scadding, *Sarcoidosis* (London: Eyre and Spottiswoode, 1967), 319–27; Om. P. Sharma, *Sarcoidosis: A Clinical Approach* (Springfield, Ill.: Charles C. Thomas, 1975), 125–26.

62. Sharma, "Beethoven's Illness," 285.

63. Admittedly the blue gum line in lead poisoning was not described by Henry Burton until 1840. See Garrison and Morton, *A Medical Bibliography*, no. 2099.

64. Usually above 4 micromoles/L (80 micrograms/dl).

10

Liver Disease

The first description of a cirrhotic liver was given in 1685 by John Browne.[1] Following another description in 1802 by Matthew Baillie,[2] the term cirrhosis was coined in 1819 by René Laënnec:

The liver [was] reduced to a third of its ordinary size . . . its external surface, lightly mamellated and wrinkled, showed a greyish yellow tint; indented, it seemed entirely composed of a multitude of small grains, round or ovoid in form, the size of which varied from that of a millet seed to that of a hemp seed . . . their colour was fawn or a yellowish russet, bordering on greenish . . . to the touch the sensation of a piece of soft leather.[3]

Dr. Johann Joseph Wagner's description of a liver reduced to half its normal size, hard like leather, slightly bluish-green, with bean-sized nodes throughout its substance was therefore, apart from the color, typical of Laënnec's cirrhosis. The bean in question was the white bean which measures about 15×9 mm.[4] Laënnec's cirrhosis was subsequently classified as atrophic portal cirrhosis[5] and a macronodular or mixed cirrhosis.[6] Dr. Theodore von Frimmel was the first author to diagnose Beethoven's cirrhosis.[7] The differential diagnosis is summarized in Table 10.1. The best evaluations of the pathology are by M. Piroth[8] and William B. Ober.[9]

ALCOHOL-RELATED LIVER DISEASE

The father of modern anatomy, Andreas Vesalius (1514–1564), stated that there was a prevalent opinion among anatomists that the liver was reduced in size by drinking.[10] In his treatise (1858–1861) Professor F. T. Frerichs stated

Table 10.1
Beethoven's Liver Disease

> Hepatic Cirrhosis
>> Alcohol-related
>> Chronic active viral hepatitis
>> Autoimmune chronic active hepatitis
>> Inflammatory bowel disease
>> SLE
>> Sclerosing cholangitis
>> Primary and secondary biliary cirrhosis
>> Sarcoidosis
>> Hereditary liver disease
>>> Alcohol-related liver disease
>>> Genetic hemochromatosis
>>> Alpha 1-Antitrypsin Deficiency
>>> Cystic fibrosis
>> Drugs and toxins
>> Congenital syphilis
>> Cryptogenic
> Acquired syphilis
> Brucellosis
> Amyloidosis

that the leading causes of cirrhosis in Germany were alcohol abuse, congenital syphilis, intermittent fever, and heart failure.[11] It remained unclear why only about one in five heavy drinkers developed cirrhosis of the liver. In the medical literature there was controversy, confusion, and misunderstanding about the pathogenesis of Laënnec's cirrhosis with regard to the precise roles played by alcohol, nutrition, infectious agents, drugs, toxic chemicals, heavy metals, pigments, immunopathic injury, and additive effects.[12]

Klotz-Forest diagnosed a catarrhal jaundice in 1821, complicated by chronic intestinal toxemia and alcohol abuse.[13] In his *Beethoven-Handbuch* Frimmel wrote,

With respect to the prodromal history of Beethoven's liver cirrhosis one has the choice between the cause of the chronic intestinal inflammation, the habitual intake of wine, and the ominous lues, in addition to the complicated common cause of all three factors.[14]

Over the last thirty years, several important advances have shed new light on the pathogenesis of hepatic cirrhosis. It was demonstrated in humans and baboons that alcohol is a direct hepatotoxin which causes a wide range of structural and functional changes. Other major advances were the isolation of the hepatitis viruses A, B, C, D, and E. A progression to cirrhosis was shown in some patients with chronic active hepatitis, whether of the autoimmune type, or in those with chronic viral hepatitis, especially types B and C.

It is now known that the wide spectrum of alcohol-related liver disease extends from a reversible fatty infiltration, through alcoholic hepatitis, to fibrosis and contrasting varieties of cirrhosis. While in the early stages an enlarged fatty liver is often associated with a micronodular cirrhosis, in the later stages the disease may progress to a contracted macronodular or mixed cirrhosis of Laënnec's type.[15] The latter is not widely appreciated and needs to be emphasized. Indeed it is now known that a macronodular, shrunken, fibrotic liver is typical of the end stage of cirrhosis, whatever its cause.[16] During the early phase of the final illness, Beethoven's liver was sufficiently enlarged for Dr. Andreas Ignaz Wawruch to be able to palpate hard nodules on its surface; four months later, the liver had shrunk to half its normal size.

The reasons for the controversy in the literature over Beethoven's alcohol consumption have been discussed in detail elsewhere.[17] Suffice it here to say that he exposed himself to the jeopardy of severe liver disease through his regular consumption of substantial quantities of alcohol.

The first definite evidence of a serious liver disease was the development of jaundice in mid-July 1821. It lasted for six weeks, and unfortunately there are no other details. However, Beethoven informed the Archduke Rudolph that he had been feeling poorly for a long time before the jaundice set in. This might suggest that it was an exacerbation of chronic liver disease, rather than an acute hepatitis. Without the assistance of appropriate serological tests for viral hepatitis and a liver biopsy, it is impossible to be certain what the diagnosis was back in July 1821. Even so, Dr. Wawruch has offered us the important clue that excessive drinking of alcohol brought about a severe inflammation of the bowels which eventually caused his demise.

We know that Anton Schindler often lied or even forged documents to protect Beethoven's reputation, but what would Dr. Wawruch have to gain by lying about Beethoven's alcohol consumption? Several other authors have supported the diagnosis of alcoholic cirrhosis, including Richard Loewe-Cannstatt,[18] Max Grünewald,[19] S. J. London,[20] M. Landsberger,[21] F. H. Franken,[22] J. G. O'Shea,[23] and Anton Neumayr.[24] Several authors have argued erroneously, for reasons discussed above, that the Laënnec's cirrhosis described by Dr. Wagner was inconsistent with alcoholic liver disease.[25]

CHRONIC ACTIVE VIRAL HEPATITIS

It has also been proposed that the bout of jaundice suffered in 1821 was due to viral hepatitis, complicated by the development of chronic active viral hepatitis, which in turn led to the development of cirrhosis, either alone[26] or in conjunction with alcohol.[27] Such a sequence of events is known to occur with hepatitis types B, C, and D. As stated above, it is impossible to substantiate such a diagnosis without appropriate laboratory tests and a liver biopsy. Admittedly prodromal constitutional symptoms may precede the onset of jaundice by a week or two, but Beethoven implied he had been feeling poorly for longer than that. The question of an immune-complex arthritis will be discussed later. There was no evidence of a generalized vasculitis such as polyarteritis nodosa. The autoimmune type is more common in females and is also associated with characteristic autoantibodies.

SYSTEMIC LUPUS ERYTHEMATOSIS

Although E. Larkin diagnosed ulcerative colitis and cirrhosis as a result of chronic active viral hepatitis, he proposed that all of Beethoven's illnesses, other than the deafness, were best accounted for by a multisystem connective tissue disease and immunopathy, such as systemic lupus erythematosis (SLE) or some similar disorder.[28] Though some other medical authors support this diagnosis,[29] the majority oppose it.[30] Such a diagnosis today would be confirmed in the laboratory by the detection of characteristic autoantibodies.

Contra SLE

Although SLE might account for many of Beethoven's symptoms, there are alternative, more plausible explanations for the gastrointestinal, liver, and rheumatic complaints. His history is not suggestive of mesenteric ischemia, and ascites occurs in less than 5 percent of cases of SLE, which is nine times more frequent in females.

Nor is there a history of photosensitivity, one of the eleven important criteria for the classification of SLE; rather the opposite, Beethoven loved a warm sunny day. Though he complained of a sore throat, his doctors found no evidence of oral ulceration.

In the face of his frequent respiratory complaints, if he did suffer with SLE, surely Dr. Wagner would have found some evidence of lupus disease in the lungs, but there was no hint of pleural effusion, or pulmonary fibrosis, or macroscopic anomaly. Nor was there any evidence of heart disease by way of pericarditis, or myocarditis, or endocarditis. Furthermore, there was no history of lymphadenopathy, alopecia, neurological involvement, or suggestion of progressive renal failure. SLE is an unlikely cause of Beethoven's illnesses.[31]

SCLEROSING CHOLANGITIS

Canadian physicians Alfred Warner[32] and Paul Adams[33] have added sclerosing cholangitis to the list. Adams proposed that Dr. Wagner might have mistaken the "greatly narrowed, considerably thickened" hepatic blood vessels for intense inflammatory fibrosis which affects the extrahepatic and intrahepatic bile ducts in primary sclerosing cholangitis.[34] In that event, Beethoven's fevers may have been due to recurrent cholangitis. Liver failure develops about six years after the onset of symptoms, and both postnecrotic and biliary cirrhosis have been documented. Such a diagnosis would also account for the chronic pancreatitis.

Contra Sclerosing Cholangitis

Although it is feasible, the diagnosis of sclerosing cholangitis would be more credible if Beethoven had suffered with ulcerative colitis, with which it has a well-known association. It seems more likely that Dr. Wagner, an experienced pathologist, was in fact describing changes in the hepatic blood vessels, for he would need to have dissected them to have reached the conclusion that they were devoid of blood. In cases of sclerosing cholangitis, it would be unusual for jaundice to remit for six years without treatment. However, it is especially the absence of pruritus that renders a diagnosis of sclerosing cholangitis, or indeed of biliary cirrhosis, improbable.[35]

SARCOIDOSIS

The common granulomatous hepatitis in patients with sarcoidosis is usually asymptomatic, but occasional cases of portal hypertension with ascites are well documented, and postnecrotic scarring or cirrhosis may follow healing of the granulomatous lesions.[36] It would be a more probable diagnosis if Beethoven drank little alcohol. The question of sarcoidosis will be discussed further in chapters concerning the respiratory, rheumatic, eye, and renal disorders.

THE QUESTION OF HEREDITARY LIVER DISEASE

Beethoven's grandmother, Maria-Josepha van Beethoven, née Poll, was confined with alcoholism to a convent in Bonn, where she died at the age of sixty-one in 1775. Her medical condition is unknown, though she is likely to have suffered with liver disease, since females are more susceptible than males to the hepatotoxic effects of alcohol. The alcoholic father, Johann van Beethoven, died at fifty-three with *Brustwasser*, or dropsy of the chest; more accurately, *Brustwassersucht*.[37]

The biblical term dropsy (*Wassersucht*) refers to the abnormal accumulation of serous fluid in cellular tissues, when it is called edema (*Ödem*), or a body cavity. Dropsy of the chest is a pleural effusion (*Brustwassersucht, Hydrothorax*); abdominal dropsy is ascites (*Bauchwassersucht, Aszites*). Abdominal dropsy caused by liver disease is *Ödem od. Aszites bei Leberleiden*. Massive generalized edema, related to the body's retention of water and salt, is called anasarca (*Anasarka, Hautwassersucht*), and it may be due to heart failure, renal failure, nephrotic syndrome, liver failure, or hypoproteinemic states.[38]

In his letter of 29 December 1826, Johann Baptist Jenger informed Marie Pachler-Koschak that Beethoven was suffering from dropsy in the chest (*Brust-wassersucht*).[39] We now know that this term was inaccurate since Beethoven had no evidence of fluid in the pleural cavity. On the other hand, by the same argument, Beethoven's father may also have died with ascites caused by liver failure, which was misdiagnosed as dropsy in the chest.

Beethoven's death certificate and his funeral invitation stated that he died from dropsy (*Wassersucht*), which is a more general term without specific connotation. His nephew Carl van Beethoven (1806–1858) died at the age of fifty-one with liver disease (*Leberkrebs*).[40] He was a drinker, but the precise details of his alcohol consumption are unknown.

The occurrence of alcoholism and liver disease in four generations certainly invites the possibility of a hereditary disorder, and there are four deserving of consideration.

Alcoholic Liver Disease

Since as many as one-third of heavy drinkers have normal liver histology, there must be factors, other than the cumulative amount of alcohol consumed, involved in the pathogenesis of alcoholic liver disease. These include environmental factors, such as nutritional status; coexisting viral hepatitis infection; and especially genetic influences. Genetic research has demonstrated that complex polygenic factors appear to influence the individual susceptibility not only to alcohol addiction as such, but also to alcohol-related diseases such as liver disease, pancreatitis, and cardiomyopathy.[41] In other words, some of the genes inherited by Beethoven influenced not only his proclivity for drinking alcohol, but also his liver disease and pancreatitis.

Hemochromatosis

The association of hepatic cirrhosis with chronic pancreatitis in a fifty-six-year-old man with an arthropathy, pigmented skin, and recurrent abdominal pain, considered against the background of a family history of liver disease, certainly merits serious consideration of hemochromatosis.[42] In this condition, an inappropriate increase in intestinal iron absorption, caused by a genetic mutation, gives rise to the buildup and deposition of iron in such organs as the liver, spleen, pancreas, heart, and pituitary, causing structural and functional impairment. The gene responsible for hereditary hemochromatosis has recently been cloned. The HFE gene on the short arm of chromosome 6 has undergone a C 282 Y mutation.[43]

Abnormal pigmentation of the skin by way of various combinations of slate-grey, brownish-grey, tan, brown, bronze, blue, or grey discoloration may occur in hemochromatosis. Beethoven's blooming red cheeks contrasted with his dark-brown skin, so that his swarthy complexion and coal-black hair earned him the nickname "Spaniard." Despite the inheritance of his dark skin, there is mention from 1823 of a yellowish tan.[44] However, in hyperpigmented racial groups it is often impossible to detect such discolorations. Diabetes mellitus related to chronic pancreatitis occurs in about 65 percent of cases.

The liver is usually the first organ to be affected, and as in the case of alcoholic cirrhosis, the enlarged liver is initially associated with a micronodular cirrhosis, though in the advanced stage a macronodular or mixed cirrhosis may develop. Dr. Wagner's description of a slightly bluish-green cirrhotic liver and enlarged blackish spleen suggest the possibility of hemochromatosis.

Contra Hemochromatosis

The color of a cirrhotic liver depends on such variables as the degree of hyperemia, hemosiderosis, fat content, icterus, and the activity of necrosis or regeneration. The greenish discoloration was probably due to bile stasis. The massive accumulation of iron commonly produces a striking rusty red or ochre color. We do not have any information about Dr. Wagner's color vision or the intensity of brightness in Beethoven's apartment in the Schwarzspanierhaus on the morning of the autopsy—both factors might have influenced his capacity for color discrimination. Also, the autopsy was performed about sixteen hours after death, and there might have been some degree of postmortem change.[45]

Dr. Wagner described narrowing and considerable thickening of the hepatic vessels. An endarteritis of the branches of the hepatic artery, associated with hemosiderin deposition in the vessel walls is described in hemochromatosis, but in the absence of a histological examination, it remains unknown whether this was arteriosclerosis, or arteritis, or a combination of the two.[46]

An enlarged, firm spleen is common in hemochromatosis, though the color is usually a normal dark red. While the spleen in this condition usually contains only four to five times the normal amount of iron, in occasional cases considerable amounts may be accumulated, and a black color might develop. Alternative explanations have been proposed, such as an acquired hemolytic anemia[47] and oxygen desaturation of the blood in the congested spleen after death.[48]

Chronic pancreatitis is common in hemochromatosis, though the hundredfold increase in iron pigments is usually associated, as in the liver, with visible pigmentation, by way of a brownish or chocolate or rusty tint. Even so, there was no mention of calcification which is common in alcoholic pancreatitis. Nor did Dr. Wagner note pigmentation or enlargement of Beethoven's heart.

While hemochromatosis cannot be excluded with certainty without a chemical analysis and measurement of hepatic iron concentration in necropsy tissue, it would appear to be a less probable cause than alcohol for Beethoven's liver disease. If, however, he was a heterozygote carrier of the hemochromatosis gene, his liver disease might have been aggravated by his habitual intake of wines rich in iron.[49]

Alpha 1-Antitrypsin Deficiency

This hereditary disorder, associated with reduced serum levels of this anti-protease, warrants consideration because it may be associated with the development of emphysema, micronodular or macronodular cirrhosis, and chronic pancreatitis. However, Beethoven is unlikely to have suffered with severe emphysema for he never complained of shortness of breath while out walking.

Cystic Fibrosis

This monogenetic disorder, though commonly manifesting in childhood, may be first diagnosed in adult life.[50] It warrants consideration because of its multisystem features by way of chronic respiratory infections, chronic pancreatitis, biliary cirrhosis, gallstones, and infertility. It is an unlikely cause of Beethoven's illnesses because of the absence of a history of progressive lung disease and the negative autopsy findings in the lungs.

INFLAMMATORY BOWEL DISEASE

Beethoven and his physicians believed that his gastrointestinal disorder was linked in some way to his liver disease. Dr. Wawruch was of the opinion that an excessive intake of alcohol was responsible. It was later proposed that his cirrhosis was caused by an autointoxication associated with a chronic enteritis.[51]

Because inflammatory bowel disorders, such as ulcerative colitis and Crohn's disease, may be associated with liver disease, they therefore warrant consideration as a cause of Beethoven's cirrhosis. In chapter 9 I argued that inflammatory bowel disease was a less likely cause of Beethoven's gastrointestinal complaint.

MISCELLANY

In the absence of photosensitivity, skin lesions, or neuropathy, one of the porphyrias is unlikely. Nor were Beethoven's attacks of abdominal pain directly precipitated by alcohol. There was no evidence of Wilson's disease, glycogen storage disease, or lysosomal storage disorder, such as Fabry's disease.[52]

Drugs and Toxins

Drugs and toxins always need to be considered in patients with liver disease. Arsenicals are hepatotoxic, and they were formerly used for a wide variety of complaints including all forms of neuroses, malaria, intermittent fevers, malignant lymphoma, and all manner of cutaneous afflictions.[53] Oxyphenisatin, formerly used in laxatives, causes chronic active hepatitis and cirrhosis.[54]

Cryptogenic Cirrhosis

Some authors maintain that the cause of Beethoven's liver disease is unknown.[55] Even today there are patients with cirrhosis the cause of which cannot be discerned.

Syphilis

Although congenital syphilis was a common cause of cirrhosis in eighteenth-century Europe, that diagnosis has been discredited. Nor is Dr. Wagner's description of Beethoven's liver suggestive of multiple gummata or the *hepar lobatum* of acquired late lues.[56]

Brucellosis

Horst Scherf proposed that Beethoven contracted brucellosis in his seventeenth year, and this became chronic with recurrent relapses, causing his fevers, recurrent abdominal pain and diarrhea, cirrhosis, deafness, rheumatic complaints, eye disorder, respiratory symptoms, and melancholic depressive state.[57] As discussed above, Beethoven's persistent undulant fever during the latter half of 1804 might have been due to acute brucellosis, but by November he was well again. Though brucellosis causes a granulomatous hepatitis, it is not a recognized cause of cirrhosis.

Amyloidosis

Systemic amyloidosis, whether primary, familial, or secondary to chronic inflammatory disease, warrants consideration because of its multisystem effects.[58] The characteristic amyloid fibril proteins are deposited in the liver, kidneys, gastrointestinal tract, skin, brain, or other tissues. The liver is frequently involved, and ascites occurs in 20 percent of cases. The diagnosis is established by the demonstration in sections from the liver of the characteristic Congo red-staining deposits by polarizing microscopy.[59] In the amyloid liver there are diffuse waxy deposits of the fibril proteins throughout the organ, but amyloidosis is not a cause of cirrhosis. The liver described by Dr. Wagner is not suggestive of amyloidosis.

SUMMARY AND CONCLUSIONS

The controversies in the music and medical literature about Beethoven's liver disease were related to several errors. Schindler wickedly sullied the reputations of Dr. Wawruch and Carl Holz, attempting to undermine the veracity of their accounts of Beethoven's decided inclination to imbibe alcoholic beverages.

After a careful study of Beethoven's daily housekeeping records, Alexander

Wheelock Thayer concluded that the cost of his purchases of alcohol was far from moderate, and yet he failed to point this out in his biography.

Some medical writers have argued erroneously that Dr. Wagner's description of Beethoven's liver disease was inconsistent with an alcohol-related disorder.

It is clear that he exposed himself to the risk of developing serious liver disease by regularly consuming substantial quantities of alcohol.

It would appear that his genetic constitution predisposed him not only to alcohol dependency, but also to the consequent development of hepatic cirrhosis and chronic pancreatitis.

Dr. Wagner's description of his liver disease was typical of the end stage of alcohol-related cirrhosis, which diagnosis is most probable.

It is impossible to exclude a contributing chronic viral hepatitis without appropriate blood tests for serological markers and a microscopic study of liver sections.

Hemochromatosis is a less likely cause of the cirrhosis because of the absence of visible pigmentation in the liver and pancreas.

An association with inflammatory bowel diseases is worthy of consideration, but the other possible causes, listed in Table 10.1, are much less likely.

NOTES

1. J. Browne, "A Remarkable Account of a Liver, Appearing Glandulous to the Eye," *Philosophical Transactions* 15 (1685): 1266–68; Garrison and Morton, *A Medical Bibliography*, no. 3613.

2. H. D. Attwood, "Some Specimens from William Clift's Copy of Matthew Baillie's *The Morbid Anatomy of the Human Body (1799–1802)*," *Aust. N.Z.J. Surg* 58 (1988): 665–70.

3. R. H. Major, *Classic Descriptions of Disease*, 3rd ed. (Springfield, Ill.: C. C. Thomas, 1945), 635.

4. I am grateful to Dr. Karl Portele and Dr. Beatrix Patzak of the Federal Anatomical Pathology Museum in Vienna for this information about the weisse Bohne.

5. O. D. Ratnoff and A. J. Patek, Jr., "The Natural History of Laënnec's Cirrhosis of the Liver," *Medicine* (Baltimore) 21 (1942): 207–67; H. T. Karsner, "Morphology and Pathogenesis of Hepatic Cirrhosis," *American Journal of Clinical Pathology* 13 (1943): 569–605.

6. Peter J. Scheuer, *Liver Biopsy Interpretation*, 3rd ed. (London: Baillière and Tindall 1980), 117.

7. Frimmel, "Beethovens Leiden und Ende."

8. M. Piroth, "Beethovens letzte Krankheit," 7–35.

9. William B. Ober, "Beethoven: A Medical View," *The Practitioner* 205 (1970): 819–24.

10. A. Vesalius, *De humani corporis fabrica libri septem* (Basileae: J. Oporinus, 1543), V: 507.

11. F. T. Frerichs, *A Clinical Treatise on Diseases of the Liver* (London: New Sydenham Society, 1861), II: 30–35.

12. Ratnoff and Patek, "Natural History," 207–67; Karsner, "Morphology and Path-

ogenesis," 569–606; R. A. MacDonald and G. K. Mallory, "The Natural History of Post-necrotic Cirrhosis," *American Journal of Medicine* 25 (1958): 334–57; Edward A. Gall, "Posthepatitic, Postnecrotic, and Nutritional Cirrhosis: A Pathologic Analysis," *American Journal of Pathology* 36 (1960): 241–71.

13. Klotz-Forest, "La dernière maladie," 248.

14. FRHB, I: 300, trans. Erna Schwerin.

15. E. Rubin, S. Krus, and H. Popper, "Pathogenesis of Postnecrotic Cirrhosis in Alcoholics," *Archives of Pathology* 73 (1973): 40–51; Pauline Hall, ed., *Alcoholic Liver Disease* (London: Edward Arnold, 1985), 41–68; Isselbacher, *Harrison's Principles*, II: 1483–86.

16. Peter J. Scheuer, *Liver Biopsy Interpretation*, 3rd ed. (London: Baillière and Tindall, 1980), 117.

17. P. J. Davies, *Beethoven in Person: The Character of a Genius*, chap. 4 (forthcoming).

18. Richard Loewe-Cannstatt, "Beethovens Krankheit und Ende: Eine medizinische Studie," *Die Musik* 19 (1927): 418–24.

19. Max Grünewald, "Beethovens Leiden und Sterben," *Signale für die musikalische Welt* 85 (1927): 514–16; MacArdle, *Beethoven Abstracts*, 274, E.

20. London, "Beethoven: Case Report," 447–48.

21. Landsberger, "Beethoven's Medical History," 679.

22. Franken, *Die Krankheiten grosser Komponisten*, I: 98–101, 104–8.

23. O'Shea, "Medical Profiles," 49–55.

24. Neumayr, "Notes," 333–35.

25. Piroth, "Beethovens letzte Krankheit," 22–23; Scherf, *"Die Krankheit Beethovens"* 24–26; Larkin, "Beethoven's Medical History," 447; Palferman, "Beethoven: A Medical Biography," 42.

26. Piroth, "Beethovens letzte Krankheit," 22–24; Larkin, "Beethoven's Medical History," 447–48.

27. Cudennec, Soubeyrand, and Buffe, "Ludwig van Beethoven," 49; Bankl and Jesserer, *Die Krankheiten* 125–26; Ivan Teply, "Ludwig van Beethoven in the Mirror of Medicine," *Bratisl. lek.listy* 89 (1988): 858–59.

28. Larkin, "Beethoven's Medical History," 448–49.

29. Beryl D. Corner, "Beethoven: Muss es sein? Es muss sein" (The difficult question—Must it be? It must be!), *Bristol-Medico-Chirurgical Journal* 86 (1971): 50; I. E. Willetts, "Beethoven's demise," Letter to the editor, *Journal of the Royal Society of Medicine* 86 (1993): 677–78; Milo Keynes, "Beethoven's Medical History," Letter to the editor, *Journal of Medical Biography* 2 (1994): 59.

30. Ober, *"Beethoven: A Medical View,"* 822–24; Landsberger, "Beethoven's Medical History," 679; Aterman et al., "Recurrent Infections," 626; O'Shea, "Medical Profiles," 53; Palferman, "Beethoven: A Medical Biography," 43–44; Kubba and Young, "Beethoven: A Medical Biography," 169.

31. Isselbacher, *Harrison's Principles*, II: 1643–48.

32. Aterman et al., "Recurrent Infections," 625.

33. Adams, "Historical Hepatology," 375–79.

34. Ibid., 378.

35. Davies, "Was Beethoven's Cirrhosis," 83.

36. Palferman, "Beethoven: A Medical Biography," 44; Isselbacher, *Harrison's Principles*, II: 1500.

37. Solomon, *Beethoven*, 43.

38. Werner E. Bunjes, *Medical and Pharmaceutical Dictionary: English-German* (Stuttgart: G. Thieme Verlag, 1981), 32, 159.

39. TDR, V: 435; Albrecht, *Letters*, no. 451.

40. FRHB, I: 459. I am grateful to Dr. Hans-Werner Küthen for this information.

41. C. P. Day and M. F. Bassendine, "Genetic Predisposition to Alcoholic Liver Disease," *Gut* 33 (1992): 1444–47; P. Hall, "Genetic and Acquired Factors That Influence Individual Susceptibility to Alcohol-associated Liver Disease," *Journal of Gastroenterology and Hepatology* 7 (1992): 417–26.

42. Piroth, "Beethovens letzte Krankheit," 24–25; Adams, "Historical Hepatology," 378; Davies, "Was Beethoven's Cirrhosis," 77–86.

43. J. N. Feder, A. Gnirke, W. Thomas et al., "A Novel MHC Class-1 Like Gene Is Mutated in Patients with Hereditary Haemochromatosis," *Nature Genetics* 13 (1996): 399–408.

44. Sonneck, *Beethoven: Impressions*, 166, 180; H. Zeraschi, "Das Beethoven Porträt von Waldmüller," *Musik und Gesellschaft* 21 (1971): 630–35.

45. Davies, "Was Beethoven's Cirrhosis," 81.

46. Ibid., 82.

47. London, "Beethoven: Case Report," 446.

48. Davies, "Was Beethoven's Cirrhosis," 82.

49. Ibid., 82.

50. Aterman et al., "Recurrent Infections," 625.

51. Schweisheimer, *Beethovens Leiden*, 161; Forster, *Beethovens Krankheiten*, 61.

52. Aterman et al., "Recurrent Infections," 625.

53. Binz, *Lectures on Pharmacology*, II: 88.

54. Sheila Sherlock, *Diseases of the Liver and Biliary System*, 5th ed. (Oxford: Blackwell, 1975), 368.

55. M. Schachter, "Beethoven devant ses maladies et ses médecins," *Journal de Médecine de Lyon* 55 (1974): 1319–27; Böhme, *Medizinische Porträts*, I: 83.

56. R. D. Hahn, "Syphilis of the Liver," *American Journal of Syphilis, Gonorrhea, and Venereal Disease* 27 (1943): 529–62; P. J. Davies, "Hepatic Syphilis: An Historical Review," *Journal of Gastroenterology and Hepatology* 3 (1988): 287–94.

57. Scherf, *Die Krankheit Beethovens*, 64–82.

58. Aterman et al., "Recurrent Infections," 625; Anthony J. Richards, "Beethoven's Illness," Letter to the Editor, *Journal of the Royal Society of Medicine* 87 (1994): 722.

59. Isselbacher, *Harrison's Principles*, II: 1500.

11

Respiratory Catarrhs

Soon after his return to Bonn from Vienna in May 1787, during his mother's final illness, the sixteen-year-old Beethoven suffered his first recorded sickness. The details were included in his letter, dated 15 September, to Dr. Joseph Wilhelm von Schaden,

Since my return to Bonn I have as yet enjoyed very few happy hours. For the whole time I have been plagued with asthma [*engbrustigkeit*]; and I am inclined to fear that this malady may even turn to consumption. Furthermore, I have been suffering from melancholia [*melankolie*], which in my case is almost as great a torture as my illness.[1]

In the facsimile of the autograph of this letter, reproduced by Ludwig Schiedermair, the composer signed his name, "I. v. beethowen."[2]

At that time, Beethoven was under the impression that he was fifteen years old, for he later informed Fanny Giannatasio del Rio, "It is a poor man who does not know how to die! I knew it already as a fifteen-year-old boy."[3]

A variety of diagnoses have been proposed in the literature: typhoid fever, [4] consumption,[5] bronchitis,[6] "a feverish attack with asthma,"[7] pulmonary sarcoidosis,[8] asthma,[9] "fever and a chest illness,"[10] and "a persistent bronchitis."[11]

There are insufficient details to diagnose typhoid fever.[12] Beethoven was then at high risk of contracting tuberculosis since his mother was dying of consumption. He might have then contracted a primary tuberculous infection of the lung, which commonly presented as a subapical pneumonia. The associated hilar lymph node enlargement sometimes caused difficulty in breathing owing to bronchial obstruction.

However, if he did suffer a tuberculous infection at that time, his recovery was complete, and he did not appear to have suffered any reactivation later.

Though Beethoven remained fearful of developing consumption, he never showed any evidence of it.

It might have been an early manifestation of pulmonary sarcoidosis. Although the associated hilar lymph node enlargement in that condition is usually asymptomatic (and today discovered incidentally on a chest x-ray), it may sometimes cause difficulty in breathing.

Beethoven used the term *engbrüstigkeit*,[13] which was translated as "asthma" by Lady Wallace,[14] J. S. Shedlock,[15] and Emily Anderson.[16] However, this German word conveys a broader meaning, such as "tightness in the chest."[17]

Lung involvement occurs in over 90 percent of subjects with sarcoidosis. While asthma is unusual, tightness in the chest or breathlessness is common.

Yet Beethoven continued with frequent respiratory complaints throughout his life. Admittedly, the earliest change of bilateral hilar node enlargement is completely reversible and may resolve after further dissemination.

However, when the background of Beethoven's further frequent respiratory complaints is considered, if he did suffer with pulmonary sarcoidosis, his lungs would surely have shown evidence of sarcoid infiltration or fibrosis at the autopsy.

Dr. Johann Joseph Wagner's finding of normal lungs weighs heavily against the diagnosis of sarcoidosis, yet it is compatible with chronic bronchitis. Furthermore, a diagnosis of chronic bronchitis is consistent with the recurrent respiratory infections that ensued.

When bronchitis is associated with wheezing, it is called asthmatic bronchitis. I favor a diagnosis of asthmatic bronchitis, aggravated by emotional stress and depression, to account for Beethoven's serious illness in May 1787.

Admittedly his bronchitis then might have been complicated by the contraction of viral or bacterial pneumonia, which resolved completely. But forever after this illness he regarded all his respiratory infections as serious, and he remained fearful that such fierce or dangerous attacks would turn to consumption or severe inflammation, which would in turn cut the thread of his survival.

Little wonder that Beethoven dreaded the misery of dreary, freezing cold winters in Vienna, without the comfort of adequate heating. Many of the frequent complaints about his health were directed to his respiratory catarrhs and coughs.

Other researchers too have concluded that the most likely cause of his recurrent cough was chronic bronchitis, a common disorder which afflicts one in five of the adult males in the current population.[18]

The bouts of bronchitis usually followed a common cold, or influenza, or some other upper respiratory infection, whether of viral or bacterial origin.

In association with his hypochondriasis, he tended to exaggerate the severity of his condition to gain sympathy.[19] Furthermore, especially when he was weary with depression, he was readily prone to take to his bed for a rest.[20]

The prolonged bout following the feverish cold on 15 October 1816 was diagnosed by Dr. Jakob Staudenheim as *Lungenkrankheit*.[21] This was probably a persistent bronchitis in association with his depression at that time. Persistent bronchitis was difficult to eradicate in the pre-antibiotic era.

Following "a violent cold and cough" in January 1818, he was indisposed for a few months.[22]

An upper respiratory tract infection in January 1822 was complicated not only by an earache on 11 February, but also a recurrence of his chest ailment, which continued to trouble him for four months. Dr. Staudenheim diagnosed "gout on my chest," advised rest, and treated him with medicines.[23] The ailment lingered on so that in May he moved to Oberdöbling, lodging at no. 135 Alleegasse. While there he took the baths, gave two lessons a week to the Cardinal Archduke Rudolph, and became reconciled with his brother Johann. By 26 July he was feeling better: "For the last few days I have had to drink [Johannes mineral] water and take the powders four times a day."[24]

Dr. Staudenheim then directed Beethoven to the spa at Baden for six weeks to take thirty baths. He arrived on 1 September, lodging initially at the Golden Swan inn, with instructions to spend an hour and a half in each bath. While in Baden he suffered a cough which kept him in bed for two days.[25]

These further respiratory ailments were most probably due to persistent bronchitis. A lack of information about his sputum production prevents comment about the likelihood of bronchiectasis.

The arguments against the diagnoses of systemic lupus erythematosus (SLE), cystic fibrosis, and alpha 1-antitrypsin deficiency have been presented in previous chapters.

Chronic bronchitis may often be associated with emphysema, although of variable severity. Since Beethoven never complained of shortness of breath while out walking, it is unlikely that he suffered with significant emphysema. His bronchitis would have been aggravated by pipe smoking.

NOTES

1. A-1; B-3.
2. Schiedermair, *Der junge Beethoven*, 184–85.
3. Dana Steichen, *Beethoven's Beloved* (New York: Doubleday, 1959), 292. Diary entry on 11 April 1816.
4. Schweisheimer, *Beethovens Leiden*, 131.
5. Bodros, "La surdité et la maladie," 949–50.
6. Forster, *Beethovens Krankheiten*, 11, 60.
7. Larkin, "Beethoven's Medical History," 441–42.
8. Palferman, "Beethoven's Medical History," 644.
9. O'Shea, "Medical Profiles," *Music and Medicine*, 41.
10. Sharma, "Beethoven's Illness," 283.
11. Neumayr, "Notes," *Music and Medicine*, 233.
12. For an account of Mozart's typhoid fever in the Hague in November 1765, see Davies, *Mozart in Person*, 22–23.
13. B-3.

14. Nohl, *Beethoven's Letters*, no. 2.

15. Kalischer, *Beethoven's Letters*, no. 2.

16. A-1.

17. W. E. Bunjes, *Medical and Pharmaceutical Dictionary* (German-English edition) (Stuttgart, New York: Georg Thieme Verlag, 1981), 145.

18. Forster, *Beethovens Krankheiten*, 60; Neumayr, *Music and Medicine*, 265.

19. For a discussion of Beethoven's hypochondriasis, see P. J. Davies, *Beethoven in Person: The Character of a Genius*, chap. 5 (forthcoming).

20. For a discussion of Beethoven's depression, and its effects on his music, see ibid., chap. 7.

21. B-1137; A-785.

22. A-882; B-1226; A-898; B-1258 (19 May 1818).

23. A-1076, 1078; B-1466, 1461.

24. A-1086; B-1483.

25. A-1097; B-1493.

12

Rheumatic Complaints

In the middle of November 1810 Beethoven's sore foot prevented him from walking very far, but he made light of it in his letter to Johann Andreas Streicher, "On account of my foot I cannot yet walk so far. But if you keep me waiting any longer I will invade your premises with a horrible modulation."[1] Three weeks later there was no mention of it.[2]

The following year in October he was troubled with his feet for eight days.[3] As noted above, in April 1813 he fainted during a fever and made mention of an injured foot. There is insufficient evidence in these episodes to clinch a diagnosis of gout.

For the next six years he was free of rheumatic complaints until the autumn of 1817 when he suffered "a frightful attack of rheumatism" [einen fürchterlichen rheumatischen Anfall], which kept him indoors for three days.[4] Dr. Jakob Staudenheim sent him back to the spa at Nussdorf, and there was no further mention of it in his correspondence in November. Following another chill in December, he took to his bed again, scarcely able to move a limb. It seems like a viral infection.

It was a much more serious ailment in January 1821, when in the AMZ he was reported to be ill with a rheumatic fever [ein rheumatisches Fieber].[5] However previous commentators appear to have missed a vital clue in Beethoven's letter of 14 March to Nikolaus Simrock: his translator and all the people he knew in his neighborhood were similarly afflicted.[6] This violent attack of rheumatism [einem starken Rheumatischen Anfall] laid him up for six weeks.[7] He was treated with various medicines and not permitted to work.

Self-limited polyarthritis or synovitis are well-recognized complications of certain viral infections, such as the adenoviral, coxsackieviral, and parvoviral varieties. There was no hint of rubella, mumps, or varicella. It was probably not type B hepatitis as there was no history of a rash, and the interval between the arthritis and the jaundice was six months. Nor was it a genuine rheumatic fever since that affliction becomes manifest earlier in life.

Before turning to Beethoven's last rheumatic complaint, it should be noted that he suffered an eye disorder in 1823 since there might be a connection.[8] The significance of Dr. Staudenheim's diagnosis of gout on his chest [*Gicht auf der Brust*] in May 1822 has already been discussed.

In his undated letter to Dr. Anton Braunhofer, assigned by Sieghard Brandenburg to 20 or 21 February 1826, Beethoven complained that he had been plagued for some time with rheumatism or gout [*einem rheumatisch oder Gichtis*].[9] In stating this, he was indicating that he was uncertain whether it was gout or some other rheumatic complaint, which had accompanied a flare-up of his bowel trouble. We learn, in his next letter of 23 February to Dr. Braunhofer, that the complaint is a pain in his back, which though not severe is persistent.[10] Four or five days later, in his last letter to Dr. Braunhofer, he stated that his back was not yet fully restored, and with a republican quip he grumbled that he hoped he would not have to bow.[11]

From his conversation-book entry, we know that Dr. Braunhofer diagnosed a gouty affliction [*der gichtischen Affecktion*] and treated him with a strict diet, moderation of alcohol, and powders. The bowel trouble cleared up in about five days, but the back pain persisted a little longer. There was no further mention of it.

It was almost certainly not gout, which rarely involves the sacroiliac joints or the spine. At no stage was there a history of acute monarticular arthritis so characteristic of gouty arthritis, and nor was there evidence of tophi.

It was a genuine back pain, rather than referred pain from pancreatitis, because of aggravation by bending. Of course one needs to consider a common disorder such as low back derangement or strain, but there was no history of heavy lifting, fall, or accident. Protrusion of a lumbar intervertebral disc is high on the list of possibilities.

One other clue might provide the answer. At the first exhumation in 1863, it was noted that the spine was complete from the neck to the coccyx, and all of the individual vertebrae were intact, except one which had disintegrated into two parts. This might suggest that a vertebral compression fracture was responsible for his back pain. Admittedly vertebral collapse with minimal trauma, or when occurring spontaneously, would happen only with pathological bone disease. But in hepatic cirrhosis, metabolic bone diseases, such as osteoporosis and osteomalacia are well-recognized complications.

Beethoven was not afflicted with ankylosing spondylitis since an onset after forty is unusual, while the pain and stiffness are worse after prolonged inactivity. Nor was any evidence of pathology, such as erosions or obliteration, noted in the sacroiliac joints at the time of the first exhumation.

Could Beethoven's bowel complaint have caused his rheumatic problems? An enteropathic arthritis and spondylitis, sometimes associated with uveitis, is common in inflammatory bowel disease, especially in patients with expression of the HLA-B27 gene product. But the arguments against ankylosing spondylitis also apply here, and the case for inflammatory bowel disease has been discredited.

A post-dysenteric spondyloarthropathy is a possibility that warrants consideration.[12] If Beethoven was positive for the histocompatibility antigen HLA-B27, and if he had contracted a bowel infection within a few weeks of the onset of his back pain, then such a reactive spondyloarthropathy, within the spectrum of Reiter's syndrome, would need to be considered. While there was no history of urethritis it is possible that Beethoven contracted an enteric infection with any of several *Shigella, Salmonella, Yersinia,* or Campylobacter species. However, the joint symptoms usually persist in this condition, and there was no history of the characteristic skin lesions.

Any consideration of more exotic diagnoses seems unnecessary, and Beethoven's rheumatic complaints are not well accounted for by the systemic multisystem disorders that have been proposed, such as systemic lupus erythematosus (SLE), hemochromatosis, Whipple's disease, syphilis, or amyloidosis. While a diagnosis of sarcoidosis might account for some of the rheumatic complaints, and also the uveitis, the absence of erythema nodosum weighs against it, and the above explanations seem more plausible.

NOTES

1. A-283; B-478.
2. A-284; B-480.
3. A-328; B-529.
4. A-830; B-1179.
5. TDR, IV: 219, n. 4.
6. A-1051; B-1429.
7. A-1050; B-1428.
8. A-1180; B-1650.
9. B-2119; A-1471.
10. A-1469; B-2122.
11. Albrecht, *Letters*, no. 427; B-2123.
12. Palferman, "Beethoven: A Medical Biography," 44.

13

Headaches

Had Beethoven complained of headaches during 1796–1797, then they could have been attributed to his bout of basal meningitis. However, there is no record of the details of that illness. Nor did Dr. Johann Joseph Wagner describe changes suggestive of hydrocephalus, which might sometimes be a sequela of meningitis.

In his letter of 13 June 1807 to Baron Ignaz von Gleichenstein, Beethoven wrote, "Yesterday and today I have been very ill, and I still have a terrible headache—Heaven help me to get rid of it—I have quite enough with one complaint."[1] Three days later he informed the baron that he was still not well.[2]

He consulted Dr. Johann Adam Schmidt who performed a bloodletting and arranged a tooth extraction; however, his headache persisted and delayed the completion of his Mass in C, Op. 86, which Prince Nikolaus Esterházy had commissioned for his wife.[3]

On 22 July, Dr. Schmidt wrote to Beethoven to inform him that in his opinion his headache was caused by gout. Schmidt, advising him to leave Baden, since his ailment was being aggravated by the north wind (Boreas), recommended him to take the baths at Rodaun or Heiligenstadt. Dr. Schmidt also prescribed the application of a poultice to his arm, less working, more rest, wholesome food, and moderation of alcohol intake.[4]

By 20 September Beethoven's headache had begun to abate, as he stated in his letter to his beloved Countess Josephine Deym, "This condition persisted for almost that whole month. . . . My health is daily improving."[5]

Such a sequence of events, though too vague to permit an accurate diagnosis, is compatible with septic complications of a dental abscess.[6]

Little wonder then that his creative outflow was in this year restricted to the completion of the *Coriolan* Overture, the Mass in C, the transcription for piano

of the violin concerto, and the Overture to *Leonore* no. 1, though he did commence work on the Fifth Symphony and the Opus 69 Cello Sonata.

During the early days of December 1810, he complained of headache.[7] During
the spring of 1811, Beethoven was troubled with a recurrence of headache and
fever. Toward the end of March, he sent to be copied the manuscript of his
glorious Piano Trio in B-flat, Op. 97 to the Archduke Rudolph: "For over a
fortnight now I have been afflicted with a headache which is plaguing me. I
have kept on hoping that the pain would subside, but in vain. Now that the
weather is improving, however, my doctor has promised me an early recovery."[8]
The association of this headache with fever suggests the probability of sinusitis.

Nanette Streicher and her family supported Beethoven during the miserable
months of autumn in 1817. She acted as courier, brought him medicines and
emetic powders, mended his clothing, and provided such necessities as bed
linen, nightshirts, and a pewter spoon. Dr. Jakob Staudenheim forbade him to
be out of doors later than six o'clock in the evening. For a time in December
his condition improved, until Boxing Day when

My splendid servants took three hours, from seven until ten in the evening, to get a fire
going in the stove. The bitter cold, particularly in this house, gave me a bad chill; and
almost the whole day yesterday I could scarcely move a limb. Coughing and the most
terrible headaches I have ever had plagued me the whole day. As early as six o'clock in
the evening I had to go to bed, where I still am.[9]

Beethoven was also troubled by a host of other worries and depression. Little
wonder that his creative outflow was restricted in this most dismal year. However he commenced work on the massive *Hammerklavier* Sonata, and he composed several songs.[10] He also revised and amended Herr Kaufmann's
transcription of the C Minor Piano Trio, Op. 1, no. 3, for the Op. 104 String
Quintet.[11]

In an undated letter to the Archduke Rudolph, assigned by Emily Anderson
to 1814, though by Sieghard Brandenburg to 1816–1817, he wrote, "All this
long while I have been ill and suffering pain, especially in my head; and I am
still unwell. . . . Since yesterday evening I have had to apply vesicatories, with
the help of which the physician hopes to cure me not merely for a time, but
permanently."[12]

During the winter Beethoven sat for engraver Joseph Daniel Böhm's medal-
lion. In late February 1820 the following entry appeared in a conversation-book,
"Yesterday I had a bad headache, I get it often but don't know why. [Carl von]
Smetana is only a surgeon."[13]

In March Beethoven jotted down in a conversation-book, "Braunhofer im
Gundel Hof."[14] Dr. Anton Braunhofer lived at Gundelhofe no. 627.[15] On 4
March Beethoven composed the song "Evening Song under the Starred Sky" to
a text by H. Goeble, WoO 150. It was published in the Wiener *Modenzeitung*

Supplement on 28 March, with a dedication to Dr. Anton Braunhofer.[16] Fanny Giannatasio and her family visited Beethoven on the evening of 19 April. Fanny recorded in her diary that his hearing had declined a little over the previous year, and that the composer gave her a copy of this beautiful song.[17] It seems likely that Beethoven consulted Dr. Braunhofer about his headaches at this time.

The Archduke Rudolph was consecrated Archbishop of Olmütz on 20 March, but the *Missa solemnis*, intended to honor this occasion, was not ready.

Early in May Beethoven went again to Mödling to take the baths. However, in view of his noisy disturbances the previous year, the landlord of the Hafner House had served notice on him, and he rented lodgings in the Christof House at Babenbergerstrasse no. 116. He paid an extra twelve florins for a balcony view, and he even considered purchasing this house, though he decided against it. While in Mödling Beethoven sat for sculptor Anton Dietrich.[18]

On Saturday 2 September, at Mödling, he informed the Archduke Rudolph that he had not been feeling well since Tuesday evening. He ascribed his indisposition to having caught a chill when he was drenched with rain in an open post chaise on a cold day, and he went on to say, "Nature seems indeed to have taken umbrage at my foolishness or audacity and to have punished me for my stupidity."[19]

On 20 September he informed Berlin publisher Adolf Martin Schlesinger that persistent ill health had delayed his proofreading of the songs (Op. 108), but that now his health was completely restored. He also emphasized that the first of the three sonatas (Op. 109) was only awaiting his correction of the proof.[20]

Klotz-Forest proposed a diagnosis of migraine,[21] but this cannot be substantiated because Beethoven left us no description of his headaches. Nor did he complain of suggestive accompanying symptoms such as nausea, vomiting, photophobia, visual disturbances, or scalp tenderness.

Recurrent headaches are common in plumbism; however, headaches symptomatic of chronic lead poisoning are usually associated with one of three neurological sequela: (1) cramps and shooting pains in the limbs, (2) lead palsy, and (3) lead encephalopathy, which is uncommon in adults.[22]

Lead palsy gives rise to the characteristic disorder of wrist drop resulting from paralysis of the extensor muscles of the fingers and the wrists. Beethoven showed no evidence of this. Though some of his headaches, for example those in the winter of 1819–1820, may have been related to plumbism, it seems more probable that Beethoven's lead poisoning was subclinical, as is usual with slightly elevated blood levels.[23]

Tension headaches, related to stress, anxiety, or depression, are common. Dr. Wagner found no evidence of an intracranial space-occupying lesion such as a tumor or an abscess, a cyst, or a hematoma.

NOTES

1. A-144; B-283.
2. A-145; B-285.
3. A-150; B-291.
4. TDR, III: 33; Landon, *Beethoven: A Documentary Study*, 217–18; Albrecht, *Letters*, no. 122. Albrecht concluded that the bleeding was performed by the application of leeches.
5. A-151; B-294.
6. Edward Larkin diagnosed an abscess of the jaw. See Larkin, "Beethoven's Medical History," 443.
7. A-284; B-480.
8. A-300; B-489.
9. A-839; B-1206.
10. Op. 108; WoO 156, 157, 158, 171; Hess 168.
11. Alan Tyson, "The Authors of the Op. 104 String Quintet," in BS, I (New York: W. W. Norton, 1973), 158–73.
12. A-511; B-1051 (1816–1817).
13. Schünemann, *Beethovens Konversationshefte*, I: 278, trans. Erna Schwerin; LvBCB, I: 283.
14. LvBCB, I: 372.
15. FRHB, I: 60; LvBCB; I: 502, n. 857.
16. TF, 772; KHV, 621–22.
17. TDR, IV: 200; TF, 761.
18. A-1031; B-1377.
19. A-1032; B-1409.
20. A-1033; B-1410.
21. Klotz-Forest, "La dernière maladie," 247.
22. F. Walshe, *Diseases of the Nervous System*, 9th ed. (Edinburgh: E. & S. Livingstone, 1958), 283–85; Isselbacher, *Harrison's Principles*, II: 2463; P. B. Beeson and W. McDermott, eds., *Cecil-Loeb Textbook of Medicine*, 12th ed. (Philadelphia: W. B. Saunders, 1967), II: 1689–91.
23. Adults with blood levels in the range between 40 and 60 micrograms/dl (2–3 micromoles/L) are often asymptomatic.

14

Eye Disorder

During his youth Beethoven was shortsighted, although Ignaz von Seyfried in-correctly attributed this myopia to a sequela of his smallpox in childhood.[1] A shortsighted, or nearsighted, or myopic person can see near objects more clearly than distant ones.

According to Ferdinand Ries, Beethoven liked to look at lovely young women, and if he passed a pretty girl on the street he would turn to study her through his eyeglass.[2] Franz Grillparzer referred to his wearing glasses in 1804–1805 for shortsightedness.[3] In the unsigned portrait of the Brunswick House, attributed to Isidor Neugass in 1806, Beethoven is wearing a double chain around his neck for attachment to a double lorgnette.[4] Gerhard von Breuning made note of how Beethoven's shortsightedness troubled him when he was stumbling across a plowed field at dusk.[5]

Designed about 1780 by an English optician, George Adams, the lorgnette, after its introduction at a Leipzig fair in 1800, became very popular in the Germanic countries. Often worn on a string or chain around the neck, the single or double lorgnette was held by a lateral handle attached to the frame. The spring lorgnette allowed both lenses to be apposed, one behind the other, till released by a catch. Lorgnettes became popular with women and were often adorned with precious gems.[6]

With the development of presbyopia, Beethoven required reading glasses for fine print. During 1816–1817 Carl Hirsch noted that Beethoven sometimes used spectacles for reading.[7] In the conversation-books during March and August in 1820, there is mention of an oculist, Dr. Wilhelm Schmidt, and two opticians, Gottlieb Schönstadt and Johann Burghardt.[8]

After completing the Ninth Symphony in February 1824, his Viennese friends and acquaintances were delighted to greet him on the street, as he gazed into shopwindows through his eyeglasses, which hung on a black ribbon around his neck.[9] A cord around his neck for his lorgnette was included in Anton Dietrich's pencil drawing done in 1826.[10]

Three of Beethoven's eyeglasses, preserved in the Beethoven House in Bonn, have been subjected to optometric study.[11] One pair of spectacles, with concave lenses of -4.0 diopters and straight temple pieces, would have been used for distant vision. On the cardboard case Beethoven wrote, "Alt" (old). A glued-on note bears the following printed legend, "To be found at the court turner Jos. Respini at no. 628 Stephansplatz." There is also preserved a pair of reading glasses, with concave lenses of -1.75 diopters and double sidebars. On the case Beethoven wrote, "Vor de O Stu" (presumably for near vision).[12] His framed monocle, with a concave lens of -3.0 diopters, would have been useful for surveying music scores.[13]

A PAINFUL EYE DISORDER

During the first week or early May 1823, Beethoven suffered the onset of a painful eye ailment. He informed Anton Schindler,

I have to bandage my eyes at night and must spare them a good deal, for, if I don't, as [Carl von] Smetana writes, I shall write very few more notes. . . . My eyes allow me to see to everything only very slowly . . . I can no longer stand this accursed flannel which I am wearing at present.[14]

In his letter to Antonio Diabelli, in late May, he stated,

Quite recently for a whole three weeks I had in addition sore eyes, and by the doctor's orders I was forbidden to write or to read. Today at last is the first day I have been using my eyes again, and even so very carefully and very sparingly.[15]

Toward the end of April Beethoven began sitting for an oil portrait by Ferdinand Georg Waldmüller. During the latter part of May, angry about being seated with his face toward the window, he refused a further sitting. No doubt his painful eye complaint was aggravated by glare. In this portrait Waldmüller has captured the annoyed, angry Beethoven in a bluster of commotion.

Throughout the month of June he continued to use his eyes sparingly, and in his letter of 1 July, he informed the Cardinal Archduke, "Latterly I have been having bad pain in my eyes. This has subsided, however, but only to the extent that during the last week I have been able to use my eyes again, though sparingly."[16]

A fortnight later, his eyes were slowly improving, but he complained, "If only I did not have to wear glasses, the trouble would clear up more quickly."[17]

In the conversation-books at this time, there is mention of two oculists that Beethoven may have attended: Professor Georg Joseph Beer (1763–1821), the professor of ophthalmology at Vienna University, and his pupil, Dr. Friedrich Jäger (1784–1871).[18]

During a very hot summer day in July, or August, Beethoven informed Schindler, "I am feeling very ill and have violent diarrhoea today. Anything may happen to me amongst these veritable Hottentots. I am taking medicine to help my poor stomach which is completely ruined."[19]

Beethoven went into Vienna twice to consult his doctors (Smetana and Jakob Staudenheim), but, noting that the town air aggravated his eye complaint, he was happy to move out to Baden on 13 August. Three days later he told his nephew,

I came here with catarrh and a cold in my head, both serious complaints for me, seeing that, as it is, the fundamental condition is still catarrh; and I fear that this trouble will soon cut the thread of my life or, worse still, will gradually gnaw it through—Moreover my abdomen, which is thoroughly upset, must still be restored to health by medicines and dieting; and for this we have to thank our loyal servants![20]

On 19 August Beethoven informed his brother Johann,

My eyes are not yet quite cured; and I came here with a ruined stomach and a horrible cold, the former thanks to that arch-swine, my housekeeper, the latter handed onto me by a beast of a kitchen-maid whom I had already chucked out once and then taken on again.[21]

However, this complete undermining of his constitution seemed gradually to respond to the baths and mineral waters at Baden. On 17 September he informed Louis Spohr, "I now feel better than I did. My eye complaint too is rapidly clearing up."[22]

Despite this eventful year of illness Beethoven completed the *Missa solemnis* and the *Diabelli Variations*. He also composed a cantata for the birthday of Prince Ferdinand Lobkowitz, WoO 106, on 12 April, and a few trifles.[23]

In October he moved into an apartment at Landstrasse no. 323 (corner of Bockgasse and Ungargasse), where he became preoccupied with composing the choral finale of the Ninth Symphony.

During the first three months of this year, his eye complaint was gradually resolved, and after his completion of the Ninth Symphony in February, he was again to be seen peering into shopwindows through glasses which dangled on a black ribbon necklace. Beethoven was cautioned not to rub his eyes when they were itchy, and his nephew Carl advised wearing a shade to counteract glare. There is no further mention of the eye complaint after the end of March.[24]

BEETHOVEN'S EYE DISORDER

A. C. Kalischer concluded it was impossible to diagnose the cause of Beethoven's eye trouble,[25] although Klotz-Forest suggested conjunctivitis,[26] and Dieter Kerner asserted it was an iritis caused by congenital syphilis.[27] More recent authors have diagnosed an ophthalmia resulting from an immunopathy,[28] an iridocyclitis,[29] or uveitis.[30]

Beethoven's bilateral, painful eye complaint commenced in early May 1823, and it was aggravated by glare so that he spent his day in a darkened room, and his eyes were bandaged at night. His vision was blurred so that his eyes allowed him to see fine details only very slowly. Complete rest was advised, and he was forbidden to read or write for three weeks. During the latter part of May he was troubled by glare while seated facing the window for Waldmüller's portrait. In June his eyes were still painful so that he had to spare them, and in July he complained of having to wear glasses.

While at Hetzendorf in July he also suffered a relapse of diarrhea, so that he returned to Vienna to visit his doctors (Smetana and Staudenheim). However, his eyes were upset by the town air, and he went to the spa at Baden. In September his eye complaint was rapidly clearing up, and there was no further mention of it after the end of March 1824.

In January 1826, when troubled with his bowels and backache, he again suffered with his eyes until his brother dispensed eyedrops. Then there was no further mention of it.

UVEITIS

The triad of photophobia, ocular discomfort, and blurred vision suggest a diagnosis of uveitis, which is any combination of inflammation of the iris, ciliary body, or choroid. The diagnosis would today be confirmed by the detection under the slit lamp of haziness from *keratitis punctata* in the anterior chamber. In conjunctivitis there is no photophobia; the complaint is of a discomfort, burning, or itching; impairment of vision is absent or slight; and there is secretion of a mucoid or purulent discharge. There is no description of Beethoven's eyes during this illness, but they would have been red, with a muddy iris. The pupil might have been contracted and irregular. The lachrymation caused by the secretion of clear watery tears would have hindered the use of glasses. An outline of the differential diagnosis is given in Table 14.1.

SARCOIDOSIS

One third of patients with sarcoidosis suffer with a granular uveitis, which runs either a subacute or chronic course. The cases of acute uveitis are usually associated with erythema nodosum and bilateral hilar adenopathy.[31]

ENTERIC CAUSES

Iritis, uveitis, and episcleritis are well-recognized extraintestinal manifestations of inflammatory bowel diseases such as ulcerative colitis and Crohn's

Table 14.1
Beethoven's Uveitis

Diabetes mellitus

Idiopathic

Inflammatory bowel disease

HLA-B27 associated

Sarcoidosis

Congenital syphilis

Rheumatoid arthritis

Relapsing polychondritis

Lyme borreliosis

Toxoplasmosis

disease, which are discussed above. The association of uveitis with the HLA-B27 histocompatibility antigen has also been considered.

Beethoven had no evidence of rheumatoid arthritis. Nor was there a history of the characteristic expanding skin lesion of erythema migrans to suggest the tick-transmitted spirochetal illness, Lyme borreliosis. Nor did he suffer with relapsing polychondritis.

Toxoplasmosis is a common cause of chorioretinitis, especially the congenital type, acquired in utero. The acquired infection is more common in the immunocompromised host. Although Beethoven's resistance to infection was impaired by his cirrhosis, toxoplasmosis is an unlikely cause of his eye disorder.

CONGENITAL SYPHILIS

Interstitial keratitis is the most common late lesion in congenital syphilis, and it may begin at any age from two to seventy. It is generally associated with iridocyclitis, and it is complicated by varying degrees of corneal scarring. Sixteen percent of luetic subjects with interstitial keratitis develop deafness, but the hearing impairment usually becomes manifest after the eye complaint.[32] Interstitial keratitis usually starts in one eye, with affliction of the other eye following after weeks, or months, or even years. Congenital syphilis is an unlikely cause of Beethoven's eye trouble.

IDIOPATHIC

The majority of patients with bilateral uveitis are of idiopathic cause, and Beethoven's case also appeared to be in this category until the recent discovery of an association with diabetes.

DIABETES MELLITUS

Iritis was first reported in 1984 as a feature of severe symptomatic diabetic autonomic neuropathy.[33] Since then Dr. P. J. Watkins has seen several cases of iritis in diabetics, up to five years in advance of autonomic neuropathy, and occasionally in association with it. These cases of iritis are usually, though not invariably, nonrecurring, and nondeforming.[34] Such a natural history is in keeping with Beethoven's eye disorder.

Beethoven's diabetes mellitus, which was secondary to his chronic pancreatitis, will be discussed in the next chapter. It should also be noted, with regard to Johann van Beethoven's eye disorder, that an isolated oculomotor nerve palsy may be a sequela of diabetes mellitus.

Although lead encephalopathy may cause blindness owing to optic neuritis or optic atrophy, Beethoven showed no evidence of it.

NOTES

1. TF, 371. For an early review of Beethoven's eyesight, see Alfred C. Kalischer, "Beethovens Augen und Augenleiden" (first of two parts), *Die Musik* 1 (1902): 1062–71; "La myopie de Beethoven," *La Chronique Médicale* 9 (1902): 197.

2. Wegeler and Ries, *Remembering Beethoven*, 104.

3. Sonneck, *Beethoven: Impressions*, 154.

4. This portrait was probably commissioned by Franz von Brunswick for his sister Josephine Deym. See FRHB, I: 43; Landon, *Beethoven: A Documentary Study*, 11. The Brunswick portrait is illustrated in Frimmel, *Beethoven im zeitgenössischen Bildnis*, no. 4; and in Landon, no. 157. A signed oil portrait in 1806 by Neugass, commissioned by Prince Carl Lichnowsky, formerly hung in Grätz Castle. It was inherited by his heirs, now in South America. See Frimmel, no. 5.

5. Breuning, *Memories of Beethoven*, 81.

6. H. W. Holtmann, "A Short History of Spectacles," in *Atlas on the History of Spectacles*, ed., W. Poulet, trans. Frederick C. Blodi, 3 vols. (Bonn: Verlag J. P. Wayenborgh, 1978), I: vii–xxi.

7. TF, 665.

8. Schünemann, *Beethovens Konversationshefte*, I: 377; II: 247.

9. TF, 887.

10. Faust Herr's lithograph, c. 1840, of Dietrich's drawing is illustrated in Bory, *Beethoven: His Life and Work in Pictures*, 176; Hans Conrad Fischer and Erich Kock, *Ludwig van Beethoven: A Study in Text and Pictures* (New York: Macmillan, 1970), 144; Alessandra Comini, *The Changing Image of Beethoven: A Study in Mythmaking* (New York: Rizzoli, 1987), no. 25.

11. H. Cohn, "Beethovens Brillen," *Wschr. für Therapie und Hygiene des Auges* 5 (1901): 5–6; K. Müller, "Beethovens Brillen," *Klin.Monatsbl. Augenklinik* 138 (1961): 412–14.

12. Bankl and Jesserer, *Die Krankheiten*, 140, trans. Erna Schwerin.

13. Beethoven's spectacles are illustrated in Schmidt-Görg and Schmidt, *Beethoven*, 247, Fischer and Kock, *Beethoven: A Study in Text and Pictures*, 154.

14. A-1180, 1181 (after 17 May 1823); B-1650, 1635 (23 April 1823).

15. A-1182 (late May 1823); B-1661 (end May/early June 1823).

16. A-1203; B-1686.

17. A-1208; B-1701.

18. LvBCB, III: 383, 493 n. 905, n. 906.

19. A-1219; B-1725.

20. A-1230; B-1729.

21. A-1231; B-1731.

22. A-1240; B-1742.

23. WoO151, 183, 184, 185, 202.

24. A-1260, 1268; B-1773, 1776; TDR, V:5; TF, 880, 887.

25. Kalischer, "Beethovens Augen," part 2; 1 (1902): 1160.

26. Klotz-Forest, "La dernière maladie," 247.

27. Kerner, *Krankheiten grosser Musiker*, I: 121.

28. Larkin, "Beethoven's Medical History," 439.

29. Neumayr, "Notes," 274.

30. Palferman, "Beethoven: A Medical Biography," 44.

31. Om. P. Sharma, *Sarcoidosis* (Springfield, Ill.: Charles C. Thomas, 1975), 81.

32. Dalsgaard-Nielsen, "Correlation between Syphilitic Interstitial Keratitis and Deafness," *Acta Ophthalmologica* 16 (1938): 635–47.

33. R.J.C. Guy, F. Richards, M. E. Edmonds, and P. J. Watkins, "Diabetic Autonomic Neuropathy and Iritis: An Association Suggesting an Immunological Cause," *British Medical Journal* 189 (1984): 343–45.

34. P. J. Watkins, "The Enigma of Autonomic Failure in Diabetes," *Journal of the Royal College of Physicians in London* 32 (1998): 360–65.

15

The Cause of Beethoven's Death

Following the ominous winter nose bleeds in 1824, there was further evidence of the progression of serious liver disease during the spring of 1825, when there was a general breakdown of Beethoven's health. It was not functional or depressive in origin this time. There was a fever and he was so weak and debilitated that he could not walk properly—a severe hindrance for him. But even more distressing was his inability to compose properly, or to sleep soundly.

Beethoven felt dizzy and heavy in the head. There was malaise and belching, and the nosebleeds recurred. He felt weak and faint, suffered from excessive thirst, and was concerned over his loss of weight.

Then there was recurrence of his usual complaints of abdominal pain and intermittent diarrhea, and Dr. Anton Braunhofer diagnosed intestinal inflammation. Beethoven, however, knew it was something new. His urine had darkened, and Ludwig Rellstab noted a sickly yellowish complexion.

THE STRING QUARTET IN A MINOR OP. 132

The vague symptoms of Beethoven's breakdown of health at this time were the vague symptoms of liver disease. Unexplained pyrexia is one of the nebulous presentations of liver disease. Today the diagnosis would have been confirmed with the demonstration of bile salts in his urine and other laboratory tests. However, it was not possible to test his urine for bile salts then, for it was not until 1844 that Max Josef von Pettenkofer first described a chemical test for bile salts.[1]

Although the symptoms were vague, it was fortunate for us that Beethoven acted out a cathexis of his suffering at this time in the first movement *Assai sostenuto-Allegro* of the Opus 132 Quartet. This is yet another example of his extraordinary perception of his own destiny. He knew that this was a serious illness. He sensed the approach of Death with his scythe. In fact, he then had less than two years to live. Following his recovery, albeit temporary, he thanked God in the *Molto adagio* of the third movement, and then described his return of strength in the *Andante* of this sublime movement.

The reprieve lasted till the autumn of 1826 at Gneixendorf. He knew Op. 135 would be his last quartet. At Gniexendorf he developed for the first time definite evidence of hepatic decompensation, by way of ascites and edema of his feet.

Why the deterioration of his hepatic cirrhosis? Was it the arrival of the end stage liver disease, or had some new disorder added further insult to his liver? Why did he suffer from excessive thirst and a disturbing weight loss?

PROGRESSION OF LIVER DISEASE—DIABETES MELLITUS

Admittedly, pancreatic malabsorption and the cirrhosis per se would have contributed to the weight loss. Liver failure is associated with defective albumin synthesis, which is reflected as a low blood albumin concentration, which when associated with portal hypertension gives rise to ascites and peripheral edema, which is associated with a compensatory breakdown of the body's muscle mass.

However, Beethoven was concerned about his weight loss in the spring of 1825, and his appetite remained fairly good until December 1826. The insidious development of diabetes mellitus accounts nicely for the weight loss, increased thirst, and deterioration of the liver disease.[2] The subacute onset of diabetes mellitus is associated with fatty infiltration of the liver which further impairs hepatic function.

With regard to its pathogenesis, diabetes mellitus is a common complication of chronic pancreatitis; patients with cirrhosis are twice as likely to develop diabetes. There are three other clinical observations that lend support to the diagnosis of diabetes mellitus. Subjects with uncontrolled diabetes are susceptible to wound infections, and we have noted that Beethoven suffered this complication after the abdominal paracenteses.

The vermin infestation of the straw under Beethoven's bed may have been related to the sweet glucose taste of the ascitic fluid, although admittedly infection of the fluid may also have contributed. The strongest evidence of all is the specific nature of the renal papillary lesions. Even so, his physicians did not suspect diabetes, and at that time there was no simple chemical test available to detect sugar in the urine.

Early Hindu physicians described honey-like urine which attracted ants in certain cases of carbuncles and skin afflictions, but it was the Cappadocian physician Aretaeus (81–138?) who gave the first accurate description of diabetes, emphasizing the importance of the symptom of thirst.[3] In 1674 Thomas Willis described the sweetness of diabetics' urine, but physicians remained reluctant to taste their patient's urine.[4] It is fascinating to recall that Francis Home, in 1780 in England, and Johann Peter Frank, in 1791 in Pavia, both employed the yeast test to detect sugar in diabetic urine, but this time-consuming fermentation test was not in clinical use in 1827 in Vienna. Carl August Trommer in 1841 introduced his test for the detection of grape sugar in urine, and in 1848 Herman von Fehling described his quantitative method. Stanley Benedict's test was reported in 1915.[5]

RENAL PAPILLARY NECROSIS

Both of Beethoven's septic kidneys were oozing a dark turbid fluid. Dr. Johann Joseph Wagner described unusual lesions which are pathognomonic of renal papillary necrosis, "Every single calyx was filled with a calcareous concretion like a pea which had been cut across the middle."

Dr. Wagner's description of symmetrical, soft calyceal concretions, like a pea cut across the middle, is so typical of papillary necrosis concretions that the diagnosis is as near to certain as is possible, in the absence of a histological examination. Renal papillary necrosis is the only condition that would explain the findings of "calcareous concretions" filling every calyx of both kidneys.

The use of the words "calcareous concretions" suggests that Dr. Wagner recognized these lesions as being quite different from the stones usually found in the kidney, for which the word "calculus," in use since the time of Celsus, would have served. Renal papillary necrosis is the only disease process that can affect, at least in some cases, especially those associated with diabetes mellitus, all the papillae of both kidneys in this way. Indeed, Beethoven's case appears to be the first report in the medical literature of an autopsy-proven case of renal papillary necrosis.[6]

It is an uncommon condition which is difficult to diagnose. In one large series, acute necrosis of the renal papillae was observed in 29 of 859 diabetic patients in a series of 32,000 necropsies. It was noted that the papillary lesions in diabetic patients "usually stand alone as gross pillars of pathologic change."[7]

The cause of renal papillary necrosis is a combination of impaired blood supply and infection. The condition was first described in 1877 in a man with a urinary tract obstruction caused by an enlarged prostate gland.[8] The association with diabetes was first emphasized in 1937; other susceptible groups include chronic alcoholism, sickle-cell disease, and vascular disorders.[9] Those cases related to compound analgesic abuse are usually asymptomatic in the early stages, and they present late with chronic renal failure.

Were Beethoven's symptoms consistent with renal papillary necrosis? Yes.

BEETHOVEN'S FINAL ILLNESS: RENAL PAPILLARY
NECROSIS AND LIVER FAILURE

The common presenting symptoms of renal papillary necrosis are pain in the flank, febrile chills, and abdominal pain of variable site and severity. Less commonly the sloughing of the renal papillae is associated with blood in the urine, frequency and scolding, or even the voiding of tissue fragments or concretions, accompanied by renal or ureteric colic.[10]

The question of error in Dr. Andreas Ignaz Wawruch's diagnosis of pneumonia, first raised by Gerhard von Breuning, has already been discussed. In the early morning hours of 2 December 1826, Beethoven's final illness was ushered in with fever, chills, thirst, and pain in his sides. Such symptoms are compatible with diabetic renal papillary necrosis. His condition improved for a few days until the severe exacerbation on the eighth day of the illness.

THE SECOND ATTACK ON 10 DECEMBER 1826

Beethoven awakened during the early morning with a second febrile chill associated with violent abdominal pain (in his liver and bowels), vomiting, and diarrhea. But that was not all, for there was also a worsening of his jaundice and fluid retention (ascites and peripheral edema) and oliguria (he urinated less). Once again, these symptoms are consistent with renal papillary necrosis causing aggravation of the liver failure. In the differential diagnosis one would need to consider (1) gallstones causing biliary colic and the passage of calculi into the common bile duct with cholangitis, (2) relapse of pancreatitis, and (3) an exacerbation of inflammatory bowel disease, which is less likely.

The subacute course of his illness over a period of four months is also characteristic of renal papillary necrosis. In one large series 50 percent exhibited a short fulminating course to succumb with acute renal failure; 34 percent ran a subacute course over several months; and the remainder were chronic. The lethal nature of the condition, with a survival of less than 10 percent, was emphasized. Death occurred within fourteen hours to ten months (mean 43 days) of admission to the hospital.[11]

THE DIFFERENTIAL DIAGNOSIS OF RENAL PAPILLARY NECROSIS

Although M. Piroth mentioned the possibility of renal papillary necrosis, the majority of authors have proposed that the kidney lesions were renal calculi.[12] J. G. O'Shea diagnosed "renal stones, parenchymal oedema and chronic pyelonephritis."[13] T. G. Palferman proposed that the renal calculi might have been a sequela of sarcoidosis, hypercalcemia, and hypercalciuria.[14]

The diagnosis of stony hard renal calculi is impossible. Not only did Dr. Wagner avoid the use of the ancient term "calculus," but also, in order for him to have stated that the calcareous concretions were like a pea cut across the middle, they must have been soft enough to have been bisected by his knife, when he sectioned the kidneys.[15]

In the presence of hypercalcemia, calcification in the kidneys is deposited in the tubules, especially of the pyramids, in the parenchyma, or in cases of the milk-alkali syndrome, in the cortex. While at times small calculi may be extruded into the renal pelvis and be passed after renal colic, the lesions found in Beethoven's kidneys are quite dissimilar to those of hypercalcemia.

Furthermore, the only circumstance in which calculi appear to form casts of the calyces is when these are part of a "stag-horn" calculus. In that event, the major pelvic portion of the calculus would not have escaped Dr. Wagner's notice. Nor was there any evidence of other conditions that might sometimes be confused with papillary necrosis: medullary sponge kidney, tuberculosis, calyceal cysts or diverticula, renal hypoplasia, or tumors of the renal pelvis.[16]

The nephropathy of lead poisoning also needs to be discussed. Plumbism, especially in adults, may become manifest as progressive renal failure associated with hypertension and gout. Though Beethoven's blood pressure was never recorded, Dr. Wagner's finding of a normal-sized heart is evidence against hypertension, which commonly causes cardiomegaly.[17] The case against gout was presented in a previous chapter.

Furthermore, the nephropathy of plumbism is characterized by atrophic small kidneys, sometimes with focal areas of cortical scarring.[18] Lead poisoning would not account for the pealike concretions described by Dr. Wagner.

BEETHOVEN'S ASCITES

Cirrhotic ascites is a serious disorder with a poor prognosis, insofar as only about 50 percent survive two years. Though two authors have proposed a cardiac cause, by way of coronary artery disease,[19] or high output cardiac failure from Paget's disease,[20] such proposals are nullified by Dr. Wagner's findings of a normal heart and lungs.

Today, at the initial diagnostic paracentesis, 50 milliliters of ascitic fluid would be aspirated for analysis. Beethoven showed no evidence of blood-stained fluid, which would suggest malignant disease. The protein concentration would be estimated, for if it is high this would suggest the possibility of tuberculous ascites or Budd-Chiari syndrome (thrombosis of the hepatic veins).[21] The ascitic fluid would also be examined in the microbiology laboratory to exclude spontaneous bacterial peritonitis, or other infections, especially if there was pyrexia or abdominal tenderness.[22] Dr. Wagner removed 5.6 liters of rust-colored fluid, suggesting contamination from infection, altered blood, and bile. Little wonder that there was some infection, since Dr. Johann Seibert was then unaware of the importance of a strict aseptic technique in performing an abdominal paracentesis.

THE FOUR ABDOMINAL PUNCTURE OPERATIONS

Prior to 1950, abdominal paracentesis was the mainstay of treatment for symptomatic ascites.[23] However, it was only a palliative or temporary solution, as Beethoven soon realized. Following the drainage of 7.7 liters at the first paracentesis on 20 December 1826, from 10.25 to 14 liters were removed at subsequent punctures at intervals of nineteen, twenty-six, and twenty-four days. On 14 March Beethoven informed Ignace Moscheles that there was already a further buildup of fluid so that a fifth operation would soon be necessary.[24]

An excessively rapid removal of fluid may cause syncope, shock, or acute renal failure. The impairment of renal function that is associated with a large-volume paracentesis can now be prevented by an intravenous albumin infusion.[25] The long-term complications of repeated paracentesis include infection; depletion of electrolytes and liver proteins, such as complement, clotting factors, and opsonins; and the hepato-renal syndrome.

Following a visit to the Vienna Pathology Museum, physician Dr. Johann Lucas Schönlein (1793–1864) made an undated entry in his diary that Beethoven's kidney lesions would have prevented a satisfactory diuresis.[26] He was right up to a point, but effective diuretics were not then available. Beethoven was treated with herbal teas and a hayseed vapor bath!

The first effective drugs, the mercurial diuretics, given by injection, were tried in cases of ascites in the 1940s. Despite a dramatic initial diuresis, the buildup of a metabolic alkalosis restricted their long-term effectiveness. The low salt diet was introduced in the early 1950s, when it became appreciated that ascites was associated with avid sodium retention. The use of appropriate oral diuretics is now an effective treatment for the majority of cases of ascites.[27] For the 5 to 10 percent of patients with ascites who fail to respond to salt restriction and diuretics, surgical treatment may be considered.[28]

LIVER FAILURE: HEPATIC ENCEPHALOPATHY

Beethoven's hepatocellular failure and portal hypertension became manifested as jaundice, ascites, peripheral edema, anemia, splenomegaly, and coagulopathy. The splenomegaly may have been associated with hypersplenism, which would have aggravated his anemia and could have caused a reduction of his platelet count (thrombocytopenia), which together with the coagulopathy might account for the black petechiae described by Dr. Wagner. Although there was no specific mention of jaundice in the autopsy report, Dr. Wawruch stated that the jaundice increased from the eighth day of the illness.

PORTAL-SYSTEMIC ENCEPHALOPATHY

The indolent form of hepatic encephalopathy that complicates cirrhosis is referred to as portal-systemic encephalopathy (PSE). It is due to an abnormality in nitrogen metabolism with a buildup of ammonia and other amines in the systemic circulation, which impairs cerebral metabolism. Normally, the ammonia and amines that are formed in the bowel by the action of urease-containing microorganisms on dietary protein are detoxified in the liver. In cirrhosis the buildup of nitrogenous end products may result from either hepatocellular failure or portal-systemic shunting.

The duration and severity of PSE is variable. In the early prodromal phase, the disturbances of awareness and mentation are slight, manifest as forgetfulness, slight confusion, and drowsiness. Constructional apraxia and writing difficulty are common, while asterixis or a flapping tremor of the extremities, head, and trunk is a characteristic feature.

Beethoven only signed his letters written from Gneixendorf in the autumn of 1826, and those from the Schwarzspanierhaus in December, which were written by his nephew Carl. Most of his letters from Vienna in 1827 were written by Anton Schindler, but it is possible to follow the evolution of PSE in the script of his letters to Baron Johann Pasqualati. For example, in his letter to the kind baron, assigned by Sieghard Brandenburg to 7 March 1827, Beethoven confusedly wrote *Seine* in lieu of the intended *Weine*.[29] Note also the variability of emphasis and the unsteadiness of his hand in his letter of 14 March to the baron.[30] A more obvious contrast is a comparison of the script of his will, written to Dr. Johann Baptist Bach on 3 January, to that of the codicil on 23 March.[31] Gerhard von Breuning claimed that, if he was not mistaken, Beethoven also signed the testamentary letter to Bach on 23 March.[32] A comparison of the two signatures renders that unlikely.

Another characteristic of PSE is *foetor hepaticus*, a sickly, musty odor of the breath and urine, resulting from the presence of mercaptans, but there is no record of this.

The earlier stages of PSE are associated with loss of affect, euphoria, depression, apathy, or inappropriate behavior. Following Dr. Johann Malfatti's prescription of iced punch, the good cheer was evident in Beethoven's already quoted letter to Schindler, "Truly a miracle," recently assigned by Sieghard Brandenburg to 11 January 1827.[33] After a few days, it was necessary to withdraw the delicious treat because he became intoxicated. The inflammatory sore throat, hoarseness, and voicelessness described by Dr. Wawruch was presumably a laryngitis.

With progression of PSE, there is an associated gradual clouding of the sensorium through the stages of drowsiness, stupor, and coma. At the time of Hummel's first visit on 8 March, Beethoven was able to stand, recognize, and embrace him. During his second visit on 13 March, Beethoven's apathy and fluctuations of mood were again evident.

On 23 March he was in a state of stupor, and it was with great difficulty that he was aroused to copy and sign the codicil to his will which had been drafted by Stephan von Breuning. He ceased passing urine on 23 March, and he remained in a state of stupor the next morning when he was anointed. He lapsed into a coma on the evening of 24 March, and he remained unconscious until his death at 5:45 P.M. on 26 March.

At the autopsy, Dr. Wagner found that "the sulci of the brain were much softer and more watery, twice as deep as usual and (much more) more numerous than is usually seen." Such a report is consistent with cerebral edema which is a common finding in patients dying in hepatic coma.[34]

Table 15.1
The Precipitants of Beethoven's Liver Failure

Malnutrition and dehydration

Azotemia and renal failure

Constipation

Electrolyte imbalance especially hypokalemia (?)

Acid base disturbance (?)

Hypovolemia

Infection

Surgery

Drugs (?)

Lead poisoning (?)

THE CAUSES OF BEETHOVEN'S HEPATIC COMA

The precipitants of Beethoven's hepatic encephalopathy are summarized in Table 15.1. The renal failure associated with the severe assault of the renal papillary necrosis was aggravated by dehydration and hypovolemia. His urine was retained in a measuring glass, for observation each day by Dr. Wawruch, who stated that he urinated less from the eighth day of the illness. Gerhard von Breuning noted in a conversation-book that Beethoven usually passed only a small glass full of urine each day.[35] On 27 February, after the fourth paracentesis, he passed a little more than a glass full of urine.

On 16 March H. Rau found Beethoven more cheerful and relieved following the spontaneous gush of ascitic fluid through his abdominal wound during the night. This helps to account for the measurement, by Dr. Wagner, of only 5.6 liters of fluid, twenty-seven days after the fourth paracentesis.

The buildup of nitrogenous products in the blood resulting from renal failure was aggravated by constipation, which in turn was related not only to the immobility and inadequate intake of fluids and fiber, but especially to the severe hypokalemia that is usually associated with cirrhotic ascites treated by repeated paracentesis.

The severe infection in Beethoven's kidneys was evident at the autopsy. Care must be taken with the administration of drugs such as narcotics, tranquilizers, sedatives, and diuretics, which may precipitate encephalopathy. Perhaps some of the numerous drugs prescribed by Dr. Wawruch and Dr. Malfatti caused adverse effects and contributed to Beethoven's encephalopathy. As discussed earlier, plumbism is an unlikely cause of Beethoven's terminal coma.

ADYNAMIC ILEUS

The French aptly described ascites as *"le vent avant la pluie"* to emphasize the accompanying flatulent abdominal distention. At the autopsy, Dr. Wagner found that "the stomach together with the intestines were greatly distended with air." In the absence of evidence of a mechanical intestinal obstruction, this suggests the diagnosis of adynamic ileus, which is common in such patients. The adynamic ileus was presumably related to the combination of the peritoneal insult of the infected ascites, the four abdominal operations, the renal sepsis, the hypokalemia, and possibly the diabetes.

Gallstone ileus is unlikely. Although poor Beethoven appeared to be groaning in pain at the time of Hummel's second visit on 13 March, suggesting the possibility of biliary colic, with subsequent passage of a gallstone, there was no subsequent history of obstructive jaundice, vomiting, or increasing abdominal distention. Furthermore, Dr. Wagner found no evidence of a large gallstone obstructing the intestinal lumen. Nor did Beethoven show evidence of primary intestinal pseudoobstruction. A diabetic autonomic neuropathy may also have contributed to the ileus.

NOTES

1. Garrison and Morton, *A Medical Bibliography*, no. 679.

2. Davies, "Beethoven's Nephropathy," *Journal of the Royal Society of Medicine* 86 (1993): 161.

3. Garrison and Morton, *A Medical Bibliography*, no. 3925.

4. Ibid., no. 3926.

5. L. Gershenfeld, *Urine and Urinalysis*, 2nd ed. (Philadelphia: Lea and Febinger, 1943), 19–21.

6. Davies, "Beethoven's Nephropathy," 159. I am grateful to the late Melbourne urologist and medical historian Leonard Murphy, MD, MS, FRACS, FACS, who after a detailed study of Beethoven's case history and the autopsy report, concurred that the diagnosis of renal papillary necrosis was nearly certain.

7. H. A. Edmondson, H. E. Martin, and N. Evans, "Necrosis of Renal Papillae and Acute Pyelonephritis in Diabetes Mellitus," *Archives of Internal Medicine* 78 (1947): 169.

8. N. von Friedreich, "Ueber Necrose der Niefenpapillen bei Hydronephrose," *Archives of Pathological Anatomy* 69 (1877): 308–12.

9. Isselbacher, *Harrison's Principles*, I:553.

10. Edmondson, Martin, and Evans, "Necrosis," 153–69; D. F. Richfield, "Chronic Interstitial Pancreatitis with Diabetes Mellitus and Terminal Necrotizing Renal Papillitis," *Ohio State Medical Journal* 44 (1948): 59–60; E. E. Mandel, "Renal Medullary Necrosis," *American Journal of Medicine* 13 (1952): 322–27; D. P. Lauler, G. E. Schreiner, and A. David, "Renal Medullary Necrosis," *American Journal of Medicine* 29 (1960): 132–56; N. Hultengren, "Renal Papillary Necrosis: A Clinical Study of 103 Patients," Acta Chir Scandinavica Suppl. 277 (1961): 1–84.

11. Lauler, Schreiner, and David, "Renal Medullary Necrosis," 146–49.

12. Piroth, "Beethoven letzte Krankheit," 26; London, "Beethoven: Case Report," 448; Böhme, *Medizinishe Porträts*, I:80; Franken, *Die Krankheiten grosser Komponisten*, I:95; Bankl and Jesserer, *Die Krankheiten*, 115; Neumayr, "Notes," 330.

13. O'Shea, "Medical Profile," 53.

14. Palferman, "Beethoven: A Medical Biography," 44; T. G. Palferman, "Beethoven's Nephropathy and Death," Letters to the editor, *Journal of the Royal Society of Medicine* 87 (1994): 247; Palferman, Letter to the editor, *Journal of the Royal Society of Medicine* 88 (1995): 303.

15. P. J. Davies, "Beethoven's Nephropathy and Death," *Journal of the Royal Society of Medicine* 87 (1994): 772.

16. Davies, "Beethoven's Nephropathy," 160.

17. In 1834 Jules Hérisson invented a device for recording blood pressure. See Garrison and Morton, *A Medical Bibliography*, no. 2748–2.

18. Isselbacher, *Harrison's Principles*, II:1315.

19. J. Niemack-Charles, "Herzschlag und Rhythmus," *Die Musik* 7 (1908): 20–25.

20. D. Golding, "Beethoven's Deafness," Letter to the editor, *Journal of the American Medical Association* 215 (1971): 119.

21. Aterman et al., "Recurrent Infections," 625.

22. Ibid., 625.

23. For reviews see T. B. Reynolds, "Renaissance of Paracentesis in the Treatment of Ascites," *Advances in Internal Medicine* 35 (1990): 365–73; B. H. Lerner, "Abdominal paracentesis: A Casualty of Reductionist Medical Therapeutics," *Bulletin of the History of Medicine* 67 (1993): 439–62; R. Bataller, V. Arroyo, and P. Ginès, "Management of Ascites in Cirrhosis," *Journal of Gastroenterology and Hepatology* 12 (1997): 723–33.

24. A-1563; B-2281.

25. Reynolds, "Renaissance of Paracentesis," 368–71; Bataller, Arroyo, and Ginès, "Management of Ascites," 727–28.

26. Schweisheimer, *Beethovens Leiden*, 207.

27. Chlorothiazide was introduced in 1958; the aldosterone antagonists were available in the early 1960s.

28. The insertion of a LeVeen shunt, or TIPS (transjugular intrahepatic portosystemic shunt), or liver transplantation. Periodic paracentesis was reintroduced in 1987.

29. B-2275.

30. A facsimile of this letter is reproduced in R. Bory, *Beethoven: His Life and Works in Pictures*, 212.

31. Ibid., 212–13.

32. Breuning, *Memories of Beethoven*, 102–3.

33. B-2249.

34. Isselbacher, *Harrison's Principles*, II:2336.

35. Between 10:00 A.M. and evening. Presumably Beethoven's urinal was emptied twice a day at these times.

Appendix 1

Beethoven's Conversation with Herr Sandra

In April 1823 Beethoven struck up an interesting conversation with a deaf man named Sandra.[1] Some of the details were recorded in one of Beethoven's conversation-books.[2] Little is known about Herr Sandra other than that he was a deaf fellow countryman who had formerly been a traveling salesman.

Sandra showed Beethoven a book written by a famous sixteenth-century physician, which he had purchased for twenty Kreuzer at the flea market. Sandra wrote that the account of deafness in the book squared exactly with his ailment.

He wrote that he had already spent more than 800 Ducats in seeking a cure. He offered to give Beethoven a recipe for a remedy using the young tips of the fir tree.

However, Beethoven's own comments about his ailment are of the greatest interest. He wrote that his was "an unhappy malady, [about which] the doctors know so little, and it makes you so weary, especially when you must constantly be busy."[3]

With regard to the treatments he had experienced, Beethoven wrote that he had tried Galvanism (*Galvanisiren*) earlier, but he could not endure it.[4]

While he felt better after taking the country air and the spa, he warned Sandra to avoid using an ear-trumpet, and to use writing for communication:

The waters, the country air can improve many things, only don't make use of an ear-trumpet too soon; by not doing so I have rather preserved my left ear.[5]

When possible, writing is better, that protects the hearing, which is worsened with the ear-trumpet.[6]

Sandra advised Beethoven to go to London where his great genius would be better appreciated, especially in the aftermath of the huge popularity of his "Battle of Vittoria."[7] Beethoven responded that he had been "constantly in poor health for 3 years, otherwise I would already be in London."[8]

Much of the remainder of the conversation was devoted to a scathing attack by Beethoven on his brother. He criticized Johann as an immoral, avaricious, stupid commoner, who had been corrupted by the French. Despite his apparent exterior success as a landlord with his own carriage, he was a barbarian whose life was dominated by the pursuit of wealth.

NOTES

1. Bruce Cooper Clarke has suggested that the name "Sandra" might be a Germanized version of the Hungarian "Sandor."

2. Conversation-book No. 28. The editors, Karl-Heinz Köhler, Dagmar Beck, and Günter Brosche, have attempted to reconstruct the chronological sequence of the conversation. See LvBCB, III: 172–74.

3. LvBCB, III: 173, 44 r, trans. Bruce Cooper Clarke.

4. LvBCB, III: 172, 43 r.

5. LvBCB, III: 41 v, trans. Bruce Cooper Clarke.

6. LvBCB, III: 172, 42 v, trans. Bruce Cooper Clarke.

7. *Wellingtons Sieq oder Schlacht bei Vittoria* ("Battle Symphony"), Op. 91.

8. LvBCB, III: 173, 36 v, trans. Bruce Cooper Clarke.

Appendix 2

Beethoven's Compositions

Year	Op. No.	Work
1782	WoO 63	Variations in C Minor for Piano on Dressler's March
1782–1783	WoO 47	Three Piano Sonatas in E-flat, F Minor, and D
1783	WoO 31	Fugue in D for Organ
	WoO 48	Rondo in C for Piano
	WoO 107	Song: "Schilderung eines Mädchens"
1784	WoO 108	Song: "An einen Säugling"
	WoO 4	Piano Concerto in E-flat
	WoO 49	Rondo in A for Piano
1785	WoO 36	Three Piano Quartets in E-flat, D, and C
	WoO 82	Minuet in E-flat for Piano
1787–1790(?)	WoO 110	Song: "Elegie auf den Tod eines Pudels"
1789(?)	Op. 39	Two Preludes through the Twelve Major Keys for Piano or Organ
1786–1790	WoO 37	Trio in G for Piano, Flute, and Bassoon
1790	WoO 64	Six Variations on a Swiss Air in F for Piano or Harp
	WoO 65	Twenty-four Variations in D for Piano on Righini's Aria: "Venni amore"
(March–June)	WoO 87	Cantata: "On the Death of Emperor Joseph II"
	WoO 113	Song: "Klage"
(September–October)	WoO 88	Cantata: "On the Elevation of Leopold II"

1790–1791(?)	WoO 38	Piano Trio in E-flat
	WoO 1	Music for a Ritterballet
1791	WoO 111	Song: "Punschlied"
1790–1792(?)	Op. 52	Eight Songs
	WoO 92	Concert Aria: "Primo Amore"
	WoO 50	Two Movements of a Piano Sonata in F
	WoO 89	Aria for Bass and Orchestra: "Prüfung des Küssens"
1791–1792	WoO 67	Eight Variations in C for Piano Four Hands on a Theme by Count Waldstein
	WoO 51	Sonata for Piano in C (fragment)
	WoO 90	Aria for Bass and Orchestra: "Mit Mädeln sich vertagen"
1792	WoO 117	Song: "Der freie Mann" (rev. 1794)
	Op. 3	String Trio in E-flat for Violin, Viola, and Cello
	Op. 103	Octet for Winds in E-flat
	WoO 26	Duo in G for Two Flutes
	WoO 66	Thirteen Variations in A for Piano
	WoO 114	Song: "Selbstgespräch"
	WoO 109	Drinking Song: "Erhebt das Glas mit froher Hand"
	WoO 112	Song: "An Laura"
1792–1793	WoO 40	Twelve Variations in F for Piano and Violin on "Se vuol ballare" from Mozart's *Le Nozze di Figaro*
	WoO 115	Song: "An Minna"
1793	Op. 52, no. 2	Song: "Feuerfarb"
	WoO 6	Rondo for Piano and Orchestra in B-flat
	WoO 25	Rondino for Wind Octet in E-flat
1792–1794	WoO 99	Italian Songs
1793–1794	WoO 41	Rondo in G for Piano and Violin
1794	WoO 116	Song: "Que le temps me dure"
	WoO 119	Song: "O care selve"
1793–1795	Op. 1	Three Trios for Piano, Violin, and Cello in E-flat, G, and C Minor
	Op. 2	Piano Sonatas no. 1 in F-minor, no. 2 in A, no. 3 in C
1794–1795	Op. 81b	Sextet in E-flat for String Quartet and Two Horns
	WoO 118	Song: "Seufzer eines Ungeliebten und Gegenliebe"
1795	WoO 7	Twelve Minuets for Orchestra

	WoO 8	Twelve German Dances for Orchestra
	WoO 9	Six Minuets for Two Violins and Bass
	WoO 10	Six Minuets for Orchestra
	WoO 68	Twelve Variations in C for Piano
	WoO 69	Nine Variations in A for Piano
	WoO 70	Six Variations in G for Piano
	WoO 159	Canon: "Im Arm der Liebe ruht sich's wohl"
	Op. 87	Trio in C for Two Oboes and English Horn
	Op. 129	Rondo a Cappriccio for Piano in G ("The Rage over the Lost Penny")
	WoO 52	Presto for Piano in C Minor
	WoO 123	Song: "Zärtliche Liebe"
	Op. 15	Piano Concerto no. 1 in C (rev. 1800)
1794–1796	WoO 126	Song: "Opferlied" (first version)
	WoO 131	Song: "Erlkönig" (unfinished)
1795 or 1796	WoO 42	Six German Dances for Piano and Violin
1795–1796	Op. 4	String Quintet in E-flat (arr. of Op. 103)
	WoO 99	Italian Songs
	Op. 46	Song: "Adelaide"
	Op. 49, no. 2	Piano Sonata in G
	WoO 124	Song: "La Partenza"
1796	WoO 43	Sonatina in C Minor and Adagio in E-flat for Mandolin and Cembalo
	WoO 44	Sonatina in C and Variations on a Theme in D for Mandolin and Cembalo
	WoO 45	Twelve Variations in G for Piano and Cello on a Theme from *Judas Maccabeus*
	Op. 65	Concert Aria: "Ah Perfido"
	Op. 71	Sextet for Winds in E-flat
	Op. 16	Quintet for Piano and Winds in E-flat
	Op. 5	Two Sonatas for Piano and Cello in F and G Minor
	WoO 91	Two Arias for the Singspiel: "Die schöne Schusterin"
(November)	WoO 121	Song: "Abschiedsgesang an Wiens Bürger"
	Op. 66	Twelve Variations for Piano and Cello in F on "Ein Mädchen oder Weibchen" from Mozart's *Die Zauberflöte*
1792–1797	WoO 13	Twelve German Dances for Orchestra

1795–1797	WoO 72	Eight Variations for Piano in C
1796–1797	WoO 71	Twelve Variations for Piano in A on a Russian Dance
	Op. 6	Sonata in D for Piano, Four Hands
	Op. 7	Piano Sonata no. 4 in E-flat
	Op. 8	Serenade in D for String Trio
	Op. 51, no. 1	Rondo in C for Piano
	WoO 28	Variations in C for Two Oboes and English Horn on "La ci darem la mano" from Mozart's *Don Giovanni*
	WoO 32	Duo for Viola and Cello in E-flat
	WoO 53	Allegretto for Piano in C Minor
1797 (April)	WoO 122	Song: "Kriegslied der Österreicher"
	WoO 99	Italian Songs
	Op. 11	Trio in B-flat for Piano, Clarinet, and Cello
1797(?)	Op. 49, no. 1	Piano Sonata no. 19 in G Minor
1795–1798	Op. 10	Piano Sonatas no. 5 in C Minor, no. 6 in F, and no. 7 in D
	Op. 50	Romance in F for Violin and Orchestra
1797–1798	Op. 9	Three Trios for Violin, Viola, and Cello in G, D, and C Minor
	Op. 13	Piano Sonata no. 8 in C Minor ("Pathétique")
	WoO 29	March in B-flat for Winds
	Op. 12	Three Violin Sonatas in D, A, and E-flat
1798	Op. 51, no. 2	Rondo for Piano in G
1798–1799	WoO 125	Song: "La Tiranna"
	Op. 14	Piano Sonatas no. 9 in E and no. 10 in G
	WoO 127	Song: "Neue Liebe, neues Leben"
1799 (January)	WoO 73	Ten Variations in B for Piano on "La stessa, la stessissima" from Salieri's opera *Falstaff*
	WoO 99	Italian Song (no. 2)
	WoO 33	Five Pieces for Mechanical Instrument
(May)	WoO 74	Song: "Ich denke dein" in D (Goethe), with Four of Six Variations for Piano Four Hands (nos. 1, 2, 5, and 6)
	WoO 75	Seven Variations in F for Piano
	WoO 76	Six Variations in F for Piano
(November)	WoO 12	Twelve Minuets for Orchestra
	WoO 11	Seven Ländler for Piano in D

1798–1800	Op. 18	Six String Quartets in F, G, D, C Minor, A, and B-flat ("La Malinconia")
1799–1800	Op. 21	Symphony no. 1 in C
	Op. 20	Septet in E-flat for Violin, Viola, Clarinet, Horn, Oboe, Cello, and Contrabass
1800	Op. 22	Piano Sonata no. 11 in B-flat
(April)	Op. 17	Sonata in F for Piano and Horn
	WoO 77	Six Variations for Piano in G on an Original Theme
	Op. 23	Violin Sonata no. 4 in A Minor
1788–1801	Op. 19	Piano Concerto no. 2 in B-flat
1791–1801	WoO 14	Twelve Contredanses for Orchestra
1800–1801	Op. 43	Music for Vigano's Ballet *The Creatures of Prometheus* (first perf. on 28 March 1801)
	Op. 24	Violin Sonata no. 5 in F (*Spring*)
	Op. 26	Piano Sonata no. 12 in A-flat
1801	Op. 25	Serenade for Flute, Violin, and Viola in D
	Op. 27, no. 1	Piano Sonata no. 13 in E-flat ("Quasi una Fantasia")
	Op. 27, no. 2	Piano Sonata no. 14 in C-sharp Minor ("Quasi una Fantasia": *Moonlight*)
	Op. 28	Piano Sonata no. 15 in D (*Pastoral*)
	Op. 29	String Quintet in C
	WoO 46	Variations for Piano and Cello in E-flat on "Bei Männern, welche Liebe pühlen" from Mozart's *Die Zauberflöte*
	WoO 100	Musical Joke: "Lob auf den Dicken" for Three Voices and Chorus
1800–1802	Op. 40	Romance for Violin and Orchestra in G
	WoO 99, no. 5	Italian Song: "Giura il nocchier"
1801–1802	Op. 36	Symphony no. 2 in D
	Op. 30, no. 1	Violin Sonata no. 6 in A
	Op. 30, no. 2	Violin Sonata no. 7 in C Minor
	Op. 30, no. 3	Violin Sonata no. 8 in G
	Op. 33	Seven Bagatelles for Piano
	Op. 48	Six Songs to Poems by C. F. Gellert
	Op. 14, no. 1	String Quartet in F: transcription of Piano Sonata no. 9 in E
1802	Op. 31, no. 1	Piano Sonata no. 16 in G

	Op. 31, no. 2	Piano Sonata no. 17 in D Minor (*Tempest*)
	Op. 31, no. 3	Piano Sonata no. 18 in E-flat
	Op. 34	Six Variations for Piano in F
	Op. 35	Fifteen Variations and a Fugue for Piano in E-flat on an Original Theme "Prometheus" Variations)
	WoO 92a	Scene and Aria for Soprano and String Quartet: "No, non turbati"
	WoO 15	Six Ländler for Two Violins and Bass
	WoO 120	Song: "Man strebt die Flamme zu verhehlen"
	WoO 93	Duet for Soprano and Tenor with Orchestra: "Nei giorni tuoi felici"
	WoO 101	Musical Joke: "Graf, Graf, liebster Graf"
1800–1803	Op. 37	Piano Concerto no. 3 in C Minor
1802–1803	Op. 47	Violin Sonata no. 9 in A (*Kreutzer*)
	Op. 38	Trio for Piano, Clarinet, or Violin, and Cello in E-flat, from the Septet, Op. 20
	WoO 78	Seven Variations for Piano in C on "God Save the King"
1803	Op. 85	Oratorio: *Christus am Ölberge* (first perf. on 5 April 1803, rev. 1804)
	Op. 55	Symphony no. 3 in E-flat (*Eroica*)
	Op. 45, no. 1	March for Piano Four Hands in C
	Op. 45, no. 2	March for Piano Four Hands in E-flat
	Op. 45, no. 3	March for Piano Four Hands in D
	Op. 88	Song: "Das Glück der Freundschaft"
	WoO 55	Prelude for Piano in F Minor
	WoO 56	Allegretto for Piano in C (rev. 1822)
	WoO 57	Andante for Piano in F ("Andante favori")
	WoO 74	Variations nos. 3 and 4 for Piano Four Hands in D on Goethe's Song: "Ich denke dein"
	WoO 79	Five Variations for Piano in D on "Rule Britannia"
	WoO 129	Song: "Der Wachtelschlag"
1792–1804(?)	Op. 44	Fourteen Variations for Piano, Violin, and Cello in E-flat
1803–1804	Op. 53	Piano Sonata no. 21 in C (*Waldstein*)
1804	Op. 54	Piano Sonata no. 22 in F
1804–1805	Op. 32	Song: "An die Hoffnung"
	Op. 56	Concerto for Piano, Violin, and Cello in C (*Triple Concerto*)
	Op. 57	Piano Sonata no. 23 in F Minor (*Appassionata*)

	Op. 72	Opera: *Leonore I* (with Overture: Leonore no. 2, first perf. on 20 November 1805)
1805	Op. 36	Arrangement of the Second Symphony in D for Piano—Trio
1805–1806	Op. 72	Opera: *Leonore II* (with Overture: Leonore no. 3, first perf. on 29 March 1806)
	Op. 58	Piano Concerto no. 4 in G
	Op. 59, no. 1	String Quartet in F (*Razumovsky*)
	Op. 59, no. 2	String Quartet in E Minor (*Razumovsky*)
	Op. 59, no. 3	String Quartet in C (*Razumovsky*)
1806	Op. 60	Symphony no. 4 in B-flat
	Op. 61	Violin Concerto in D
	WoO 80	Thirty-two Variations for Piano in C Minor on an Original Theme
	WoO 83	Six Ecossaises in E-flat for Piano or Orchestra
	WoO 132	Song: "Als die Geliebte sich trennen wollte"
1806–1807	WoO 133	Arietta: "In questa tomba oscura"
1807	Op. 61	Piano Concerto in D: arrangement of the violin concerto
	Op. 62	*Coriolan*: Overture in C Minor
	Op. 86	Mass in C
	Op. 138	*Leonore* Overture no. 1 in C
	WoO 16	Twelve Ecossaises for Orchestra(?) spurious
1807–1808	Op. 67	Symphony no. 5 in C Minor
	Op. 69	Cello Sonata in A
	WoO 134	Song: "Sehnsucht" (four settings)
1808	Op. 68	Symphony no. 6 in F (*Pastoral*)
	Op. 70, no. 1	Piano Trio in D (*Ghost*)
	Op. 70, no. 2	Piano Trio in E-flat
	Op. 80	Fantasia in C Minor for Piano, Chorus, and Orchestra (first perf. on 22 December 1808, rev. 1809)
1809	Op. 73	Piano Concerto no. 5 in E-flat (*Emperor*)
	Op. 74	String Quartet in E-flat (*Harp*)
	Op. 76	Six Variations for Piano in D on an Original Theme
	Op. 77	Fantasia for Piano in G Minor
	Op. 78	Piano Sonata no. 24 in F-sharp (*À Thérèse*)
	Op. 79	Piano Sonata no. 25 in G (*Cuckoo*)
	Op. 82	Four Ariettas and a Duet
	Op. 75	Six Songs to Poems by Goethe and Matthisson

	WoO 18	March for Military Band no. 1 in F
	WoO 136	Song: "Andenken"
	WoO 137	Song: "Lied aus der Ferne"
	WoO 138	Song: "Der Jüngling in der Fremde"
	WoO 139	Song: "Der Liebende"
1809–1810	Op. 81a	Piano Sonata no. 26 in E-flat (*Das Lebewohl; Les Adieux*)
	Op. 84	Overture and Incidental Music for Goethe's *Egmont* (first perf. on 15 June 1810)
1810	Op. 83	Three Songs to Poems by Goethe
	WoO 19	March for Military Band no. 2 in F
	WoO 20	March for Military Band no. 3 in C
	WoO 21	Polonaise for Military Band in D
	WoO 22	Ecossaise for Military Band in D
	WoO 23	Ecossaise for Military Band in G
	WoO 59	Bagatelle in A Minor ("Für Elise")
	WoO 152	Twenty-five Irish Songs: nos. 1–9, 12, 14–18, 20, 23
	WoO 153	Twenty Irish Songs: nos. 1–4, 10, 14
	WoO 155	Twenty-six Welsh Songs: nos. 1–14, 16–19, 21–24, 26
	WoO 158/2	Seven British Folksongs: no. 7
	WoO 158/3	Six Assorted Folksongs: no. 6
	Hess 194	Song: "I Dreamed I Lay"
	Hess 196	Song: "I'll Praise the Saints"
	Hess 197	Song: " 'Tis but in Vain"
	Hess 203	Song: "Faithfu' Johnie"
	Hess 206	Song: "To the Blackbird"
1810–1811	Op. 95	String Quartet in F Minor (*Serioso*)
	Op. 97	Trio for Piano, Violin, and Cello in B-flat (*Archduke*)
1811	Op. 113	Incidental Music to "Die Rulnen von Athen" (first perf. on 10 February 1812)
	Op. 117	Incidental Music to "König Stephan" (first perf. on 10 February 1812)
	WoO 140	Song: "An die Geliebte" (rev. 1814)
	WoO 161	Canon: "Ewig dein"
1811–1812	Op. 92	Symphony no. 7 in A
1812	Op. 93	Symphony no. 8 in F

	Op. 96	Violin Sonata no. 10 in G
(June)	WoO 39	Allegretto for Piano Trio in B-flat
(November)	WoO 30	Three Equali for Four Trombones in D Minor, D, and B-flat
	WoO 162	Canon: "Ta ta ta" (spurious)
	Hess 198	Song: "Oh Would I Were"
1813	Op. 91	"Wellingtons Sieg oder die Schlacht bei Vittoria für Orchester" (first perf. on 3 December 1813)
	WoO 2	March and Entr'acte for Kuffner's Tarpeja (first perf. on 26 March 1813)
	WoO 141	Song: "Der Gesang der Nachtigall"
(November)	WoO 142	Song: "Der Bardengeist"
(November)	WoO 163	Canon: "Kurz ist der Schmerz" (first version)
	WoO 153	Twenty Irish Songs: nos. 5, 7–9, 11–12, 15–20
	WoO 154	Twelve Irish Songs: nos. 1–12
	WoO 155	Twenty-six Welsh Songs: nos. 15, 20
	WoO 158/2	Seven British Folksongs: nos. 1?, 2
	Hess 192	Scottish Song: "On the Massacre of Glencoe"
	Hess 195	Song: "When Far from the Home"
	Op. 108	Scottish Songs: no. 20
1814	Op. 116	Vocal Trio: "Tremate, empi, tremate" (c. 1802, rev. 1814)
	WoO 94	Aria for Bass: Germania in B-flat for Treitschke's Singspiel: "Die gute Nachricht" (first perf. on 11 April 1814)
	Op. 72	Opera: *Fidelio*, with Overture in E (first perf. on 23 May 1814)
(May)	WoO 102	Song: "Abschiedsgesang" (for the retirement of Dr. Leopold Weiss)
(June)	WoO 103	"Un lieto brindisi": Cantata campestre (for Giovanni Malfatti, first perf. on 24 June 1814)
(July)	Op. 118	"Elegischer Gesang" for Four Voices and String Quartet (for Baron Pasqualati, first perf. on 5 August 1814)
	Op. 90	Piano Sonata no. 27 in E Minor
(September)	WoO 95	Chor auf die verbündeten Fürsten
(September)	WoO 164	Canon: "Freundschaft ist die Quelle wahrer Glückseligkeit"
	WoO 199	Musical Joke: "Ich bin der Herr von zu, Du bist der Herr von von"

	Op. 136	Cantata: "Der glorreiche Augenblick" (first perf. on 29 November 1814)
	WoO 143	Des Kreigers Abschied
	WoO 144	Song: "Merkenstein"
	WoO 140	Song: "An die Geliebte" (second version)
	Op. 100	Song: "Merkenstein" (for two voices)
	Op. 89	Polonaise for Piano in C
1813–1815	Op. 94	Song: "An die Höffnung" (second version)
1814–1815	Op. 115	Overture in C: *Zur Namensfeier* (first perf. on 25 December 1815)
	Op. 112	Goethe: *Meeresstille und glückliche Fahrt* for Chorus and Orchestra
1815	WoO 165	Canon: "Glück zum neuen Jahr"
	WoO 166	Canon: "Kurz ist der Schmerz"
	WoO 96	Incidental Music for Leonore Prohaska
	WoO 97	Arla for Bass in D: "Es ist vollbracht" for Treitschke's Singspiel: "Die Ehrenpforten" (first perf. on 15 July)
	Op. 102, no. 1	Cello and Piano Sonata in C
	Op. 102, no. 2	Cello and Piano Sonata in D
(?)	WoO 135	Song: Die laute Klage"
	WoO 145	Song: "Das Geheimnis"
	Op. 108	Twenty-five Scottish Songs: nos. 5–7, 10–11, 19
	WoO 153	Twenty Irish Songs: nos. 6, 13
	WoO 155	Twenty-six Welsh Songs: no. 25
	WoO 156	Twelve Scottish Songs: no. 6
	WoO 157	Twelve Folksongs: nos. 6–8, 11
	WoO 158/2	Seven British Folksongs: nos. 5, 6
	WoO 167	Canon: "Brauchle, Linke"
1816	WoO 146	Song: "Sehnsucht"
	Op. 121a	Variations for Piano, Viola, and Cello on "Ich bin der Schneider Kakadu" (c. 1803 (?), rev. 1816)
	Op. 98	Song Cycle: "An die ferne Geliebte"
	Op. 99	Song: "Der Mann von Wort"
	WoO 24	March in D for Military Band
	Op. 101	Piano Sonata no. 28 in A
	WoO 147	Song: "Ruf vom Berge"
	Op. 108	Twenty-five Scottish Songs: nos. 8, 12, 14, 15–16
	WoO 157	Twelve Folksongs: no. 12

	WoO 158/1	Twenty-three Continental Folksongs: nos. 2–6, 9–16, 18–21, 23
	WoO 168	Two Canons: "Das Schweigen" and "Das Reden"
	WoO 169	Canon: "Ich Küsse Sie"
	WoO 170	Canon: "Ars longa, vita brevis"
1817	WoO 148	Song: "So oder so"
	WoO 149	Song: "Resignation"
(May)	WoO 104	"Gesang der Mönche" for Unaccompanied Chorus
	Op. 104	String Quintet in C Minor (initially arr. from Piano Trio, op. 1, no. 3 by Kaufmann)
	Op. 137	Fugue for String Quintet in D
	Op. 108	Twenty-five Scottish Songs: nos. 1, 3–4, 9, 13, 17, 21–22, 25
	WoO 156	Scottish Songs: no. 5
	WoO 157	Assorted Folksongs: nos. 1, 4, 10
	WoO 158/1	Twenty-three Continental Folksongs: nos. 1, 7–8(?), 17(?); 22(?)
	WoO 158/2	Seven British Folksongs: nos. 3–4
	WoO 158/3	Six Assorted Folksongs: nos. 1–2
	Hess 168	Folksong without title
	WoO 171	Canon: "Glück fehl' dir vor allem"
1817–1818	Op. 106	Piano Sonata no. 29 in B-flat (*Hammerklavier*)
1818	WoO 200	Theme: "O Hoffnung" (for Archduke Rudolph who composed forty variations on it)
	WoO 60	Bagatelle for Piano in B-flat
	Op. 105	Six National Airs with Variations: nos. 1–2, 4–6
	Op. 107	Ten National Airs with Variations: nos. 1–2, 4–5, 8–10
	Op. 108	Scottish Songs: nos. 2, 18, 23
	WoO 156	Scottish Songs: nos. 2, 4, 7–9, 11–12
	WoO 158/3	Folksongs: no. 5
	WoO 201	Musical Joke: "Ich bin bereit! Amen"
	WoO 172	Canon: "Ich bitt' dich, schreib' mir die Es-scala auf"
1819	WoO 105	Song with Chorus: "Hochzeitslied"
1819, 1823	Op. 120	Thirty-three Variations for Piano on a Waltz in C by Antonio Diabelli
1819	Op. 105	Six National Airs with Variations: no. 3
	Op. 107	Ten National Airs with Variations: nos. 3, 6–7

	WoO 157	Assorted Folksongs: no. 3
	WoO 173	Canon: "Hol'euch der Teufel!"
	WoO 174	Canon: "Glaube und hoffe"
	WoO 176	Canon: "Glück zum neuen Jahr"
	WoO 17	Eleven "Mödling" Dances (spurious)
	WoO 179	Canon: "Alles Gute, alles Schöne"
1819–1820	WoO 130	Song: "Gedenke mein"
1820	Op. 109	Piano Sonata no. 30 in E
	WoO 150	Song: "Abendlied unterm gestirnten Himmel"
	WoO 157	Folksongs: no. 9
	WoO 158/3	Folksongs: nos. 3, 4(?)
	Hess 133	Austrian Song: "Das liebe Kätzchen"
	Hess 134	Austrian Song: "Der Knabe auf dem Berge"
	WoO 177	Canon: "Bester Magistrat"
	WoO 178	Canon: "Signor Abate"
	WoO 180	Canon: "Hoffmann, sei ja kein Hofmann"
	WoO 181	Three Canons: "Gedenket heute an Baden," Gehabt euch wohl," and "Tugend ist kein leerer Name"
1821	WoO 61	Allegretto in B Minor for Piano
	WoO 182	Canon: "O Tobias!"
1820–1822	Op. 119	Eleven Bagatelles for Piano
1821–1822	Op. 110	Piano Sonata no. 31 in A-flat
	Op. 111	Piano Sonata no. 32 in C Minor
1822	WoO 34	Duet for Two Violins in A
	WoO 81	Allemande for Piano in A (c. 1793, rev. 1822)
	Op. 124	Overture in C: *Die Weihe des Hauses* (first perf. on 3 October 1822)
	Op. 114	March with Chorus: "Die Weihe des Hauses" (adaptation of *Die Ruinen von Athen*, no. 6, first perf. on 3 October 1822)
	WoO 98	Chorus: "Wo sich die Pulse: Die Weihe des Haus" (first perf. on 3 October 1822)
	WoO 3	"Gratulations-Menuett" in E-flat (first perf. on 3 November 1822)
	Op. 121b	*Opferlied* for Three Soloists, Chorus, and Orchestra (first perf. on 23 December 1822, rev. 1824)
	Op. 128	Arietta: "Der Kuss"
1819–1823	Op. 123	*Missa solemnis* in D

1823	WoO 151	Song: "Der edle Mensch sei hülfreich und gut"
	WoO 106	Birthday Cantata for Prince Lobkowitz
	WoO 183	Canon: "Bester Herr Graf"
	WoO 184	Canon: "Falstafferel, lass'dich sehen!"
	WoO 185	Canon: "Edel sei der Mensch" (two versions)
	WoO 202	Musical Motto: "Das Schöne zu dem Guten" for Marie Pachler-Koschak
1823–1824	Op. 122	*Bundeslied* for Voices, Chorus, and Winds
	Op. 125	Ninth Symphony in D Minor (*Choral*)
	—	Mass in C-sharp Minor (unfinished)
1824	Op. 126	Six Bagatelles for Piano
	WoO 84	Waltz in E-flat for Piano
	Op. 121b	*Opferlied* for Soprano, Choir, and Orchestra
	WoO 186	Canon: "Te solo adoro"
	WoO 187	Canon: "Schwenke dich ohne Schwänke!"
1822–1825	—	Tenth Symphony in E-flat (unfinished)
	—	Overture on B-A-C-H (unfinished)
1823–1825	Op. 127	String Quartet in E-flat (first perf. on 6 March 1825)
1825	Op. 132	String Quartet in A Minor (first perf. on 6 November)
	WoO 61a	Allegretto quasi andante for Piano in G Minor
	WoO 85	Waltz for Piano in D
	WoO 86	Ecossaise for Piano in E-flat
	WoO 188	Canon: "Gott ist eine feste Burg"
	WoO 189	Canon: "Doktor, sperrt das Tor dem Tod"
	WoO 190	Canon: "Ich war hier, Doktor"
	WoO 35	Instrumental Canon for Two Violins in A
	WoO 191	Canon: "Kühl, nicht lau"
	WoO 192	Canon: "Ars longa, vita brevis"
	WoO 193	Canon: "Ars longa, vita brevis"
	WoO 194	Canon: "Si non per portas, per muros"
	WoO 195	Canon: "Freu'dich des Lebens"
	WoO 203	Puzzle Canon: "Das Schöne zu dem Guten"
	WoO 204	Musical Joke: "Holz, Holz geigt die Quartette so"
1825–1826	Op. 130	String Quartet in B-flat (first perf. with *Grosse Fuge* as finale on 21 March 1826; with new finale on 22 April 1827)

	Op. 133	*Grosse Fuge* for String Quartet in B-flat
	Op. 131	String Quartet in C-sharp Minor
1826	Op. 134	*Grosse Fuge* in B-flat arr. for Piano Four Hands
	Op. 130	String Quartet in B-flat: New finale: *Allegro* (completed by 22 November 1826)
	Op. 135	String Quartet in F
1826	WoO 196	Canon: "Es muss sein"
	Hess 299	Canon: "Bester Magistrat"
	WoO 197	Canon: "Da ist das Werk"
	Hess 277	Canon: "Esel aller Esel"
	WoO 198	Canon: "Wir irren allesamt"
1826–1827	WoO 62	String Quintet in C (unfinished)

Glossary of Medical Terms

Acoustic nerves: Of, or related to, the sense or organs of hearing, to sound, or to the science of sounds.

Adynamic: Lacking in movement.

Alopecia: Absence of hair from skin areas where it is normally present.

Amyloidosis: A condition characterized by the deposition of amyloid in organs or tissues of the animal body.

Ankylosis: Stiffness or fixation of a joint by disease or surgery.

Aperient: A gentle laxative.

Apoplectic: Relating to, or causing stroke.

Apothecary: One who prepares and sells drugs or compounds for medicinal purposes.

Arteritis: Arterial inflammation.

Arthralgia: Pain in one or more joints.

Arthropathy: A disease of a joint.

Ascites: Accumulation of serous fluid in the spaces between tissues and organs in the cavity of the abdomen.

Ataxia: An inability to coordinate voluntary muscular movements that is symptomatic of some nervous disorders.

Atrophy: Decrease in size or wasting away of a body part or tissue.

Balneology: The science of the therapeutic use of baths.

Bipolar disorder: An affective disorder characterized by the alternation of manic and depressive states.

Blood letting: The opening of a vein.

Botany: A branch of biology dealing with plant life.

Brucellosis: A disease caused by bacteria of the genus *Brucella*.

Calculus: A hard concretion, usually of mineral salts, around organic material, found especially in hollow organs or ducts.

Cardiomegaly: Enlargement of the heart.

Catarrh: Inflammation of a mucous membrane in humans or animals.

Catharsis: 1. Purgation. 2. Elimination of a complex by bringing it to consciousness and affording it expression.

Celiac disease: A chronic nutritional disturbance associated with malabsorption, related to gluten sensitivity.

Cerebellum: A large dorsally projecting part of the brain concerned especially with the coordination of muscles and the maintenance of bodily equilibrium.

Cerebral: Of, or relating to, the brain or the intellect.

Cholangitis: Inflammation of one or more bile ducts.

Cholesteatoma: A tumor in the middle ear or mastoid constituting a sequel to chronic otitis media.

Chorioretinitis: Inflammation of the retina and choroid of the eye.

Cirrhosis: Fibrosis of the liver with hardening caused by excessive formation of connective tissue followed by contraction.

Coagulopathy: A disease affecting blood coagulation.

Coccyx: The lower end of the spine, beyond the sacrum.

Cochlea: A division of the labyrinth of the ear coiled into the form of a snail shell and consisting of a spiral canal in the petrous part of the temporal bone in which lies a smaller membranous spiral passage that communicates with the sacculus at the base of the spiral, ends blindly near its apex, and contains the organ of corti.

Colitis: Inflammation of the colon or large bowel.

Comatose: Of, resembling, or affected with coma.

Concha: The largest and deepest concavity of the external ear.

Cortex: The outer or superficial part of an organ or body structure.

Coryza: Common cold.

Cranial nerve: Any of the twelve paired nerves that arise from the lower surface of the brain.

Cupping: A technique formally employed for drawing blood to the surface of the body by application of a glass vessel from which air had been evacuated by heat, forming a partial vacuum.

Cystic fibrosis: A common hereditary disease that usually appears in childhood involving generalized disorder of exocrine glands.

Diabetes: Any of various abnormal conditions characterized by secretion and excretion of excessive amounts of urine, especially diabetes mellitus.

Diaphoresis: Artificially induced profuse perspiration.

Digitalis: The dried leaf of the foxglove, serving as a powerful cardiac stimulant and diuretic.

Diploe: Cancellous bony tissue between the external and internal layers of the skull.

Diuretic: An agent that increases the flow of urine.

Dropsy: Edema.

Dystonia: A state of disordered tonicity of tissues.

Eczema: An inflammatory condition of the skin characterized by redness, itching, and oozing vesicular lesions, which become scaly, crusted, or hardened.

Edema: Swelling due to an accumulation of tissue fluid.

Emesis: Vomiting.

Empyema: The presence of pus in the pleural cavity.

Encephalitis: Inflammation of the brain.

Endarteritis: Inflammation of the intima of one or more arteries.

Endocarditis: Inflammation of the lining of the heart and its valves.

Enteritis: Inflammation of the small intestine.

Enteropathy: A disease of the intestinal tract.

Enteroscopy: The viewing of the lining of the small intestine through a special endoscope.

Epistaxis: Nose bleed.

Erysipelas: An acute febrile disease that is associated with intense, often vesicular and edematous, local inflammation of the skin and subcutaneous tissues and that is caused by a hemolytic streptococcus.

Erythema nodosum: A skin condition characterized by small tender reddened nodules under the skin, often accompanied by fever and transitory arthritic pains and commonly considered a manifestation of hypersensitivity.

Eustachian tube: A bony and cartilaginous tube connecting the middle ear with the nasopharynx and equalizing air pressure on both sides of the tympanic membrane.

Facial nerve: The seventh cranial nerve.

Faradic: Related to an alternating current of electricity produced by an induction coil.

Febrile: Feverish.

Femur: The thighbone.

Fistula: An abnormal passage leading from an abscess or hollow organ to the body surface or from one hollow organ to another, and permitting passage of fluids or secretions.

Galvanism: A direct current of electricity.

Gangrene: Local death of soft tissues due to loss of blood supply.

Giardiasis: Infestation with or disease caused by a flagellate protozoan of the genus *Giardia*.

Gout: A metabolic disease marked by a painful inflammation of the joints, deposits of urates in and around the joints, and usually an excessive amount of uric acid in the blood.

Granulomatous: Of, relating to, or characterized by granuloma (chronic inflammation).

Gummata: A tumor of gummy or rubbery consistency that is characteristic of the tertiary stage of syphilis.

Hemochromatosis: A disorder of iron metabolism that occurs more often in males and is characterized by a bronze color of the skin due to deposition of iron-containing pigments in the tissues and frequently by diabetic symptoms.

Hemosiderosis: Excessive deposition of hemosiderin in bodily tissues as a result of the breakdown of red blood cells.

Hepato-renal syndrome: Functional kidney failure associated with cirrhosis of the liver and characterized typically by jaundice, ascites, hypoalbuminemia, hypoprothrombinemia, and encephalopathy.

Histology: A branch of anatomy that deals with the minute structure of animal and plant tissues as discernible with the microscope.

Homeopathy: A system of medical practice that treats a disease especially by the administration of minute doses of a remedy that would in healthy persons produce symptoms of the disease treated.

Humerus: The longest bone of the upper arm extending from the shoulder to the elbow.

Humors: One of the four fluids that were believed to enter into the constitution of the body and to determine by their relative proportions a person's health and temperament (black bile, blood, phlegm, and yellow bile).

Hydrocephalus: An abnormal increase in the amount of cerebrospinal fluid within the cranial cavity that is accompanied by expansion of the cerebral ventricles, enlargement of the skull and especially the forehead, and atrophy of the brain.

Hyoid bone: A bone or complex of bones situated at the base of the tongue and supporting the tongue and its muscles.

Hypercalcemia: Excess calcium in the blood.

Hypercalciuria: Excess calcium in the urine.

Hyperemia: Excess of blood in a body part.

Hypersplenism: A condition marked by excessive destruction of one or more kinds of blood cells in the spleen.

Hypertrophic: Of, relating to, or affected with hypertrophy (excessive development of an organ or part).

Hypokalemia: A deficiency of potassium in the blood.

Hypovolemia: Decrease in the volume of the circulating blood.

Iatrogenic: Induced inadvertently by the medical treatment or procedure of a physician.

Ileocecal: Of, relating to, or connecting the ileum and the cecum.

Ileum: The last division of the small intestine that constitutes the part between the jejunum and large intestine.

Ileus: A condition of distention of the intestine due to defective peristalsis.

Immunopathy: A condition associated with disturbance of the immune system.

Inflammation: A local response to cellular injury that is marked by capillary dilatation, leukocytic infiltration, redness, heat, pain, swelling, and often loss of function, and that serves as a mechanism initiating the elimination of noxious agents and of damaged tissue.

Inoculation: The introduction of a pathogen or antigen into a living organism to stimulate the production of antibodies to confer immunity.

Interstitial keratitis: A chronic progressive keratitis of the corneal stroma often resulting in blindness and frequently associated with congenital syphilis.

Iridocyclitis: Inflammation of the iris and the ciliary body.

Iritis: Inflammation of the iris of the eye.

Jaundice: A yellowish discoloration of the skin, sclerae, and certain body fluids, caused by the deposition of bile pigments that follows interference with normal production and discharge of bile, as in certain liver diseases, excessive hemolysis of red blood cells, or obstruction of the bile ducts.

Labyrinth: A tortuous anatomical structure.

Labyrinthitis: Inflammation of the labyrinth of the internal ear.

Lacrimal gland: An acinous gland, about the size and shape of an almond, that secretes tears and is situated laterally and superiorly to the bulb of the eye in a shallow depression on the inner surface of the frontal bone (tear gland).

Laudanum: Any of various formerly used preparations of opium.

Lues: Syphilis.

Luetic: A person affected with syphilis.

Lymphadenopathy: Abnormal enlargement of the lymph nodes.

Lymphoma: Malignant tumor of lymphoid tissue.

Mastoid process: The process of the temporal bone behind the ear that is well developed and of somewhat conical form in adults but inconspicuous in children.

Materia medica: Substances used in the composition of medical remedies.

Ménière's disease: A disorder of the membranous labyrinth of the inner ear marked by recurrent attacks of dizziness, tinnitus, and deafness.

Meningitis: Inflammation of the meninges and especially of the pia mater and the arachnoid.

Meningo-neuro-labyrinthitis: Inflammation of the meninges, adjacent auditory nerves, and the labyrinth of the inner ear.

Middle ear ossicle: Any of three small bones in the middle ear, including the malleus, incus, and stapes.

Mucous: Secreting or containing mucus.

Myalgia: Pain in one or more muscles.

Myocarditis: Inflammation of the myocardium.

Myopia: A condition in which visual images come to a focus in front of the retina of the eye because of defects in the refractive media of the eye or of abnormal length of the eyeball, resulting especially in defective vision of distant objects (nearsightedness).

Necrosis: Death of living tissue.

Neurasthenia: An emotional and psychic disorder characterized especially by easy fatigability and often by lack of motivation, feelings of inadequacy, and psychosomatic symptoms.

Neuritis: An inflammatory or degenerative lesion of a nerve, marked especially by pain, sensory disturbances, and impaired or lost reflexes.

Neurosyphilis: Syphilis of the central nervous system.

Nystagmus: A rapid involuntary oscillation of the eyeballs occurring normally with dizziness during and after bodily rotation or abnormally after injuries (as to the cerebellum or the vestibule of the ear).

Oculomotor nerve: The third cranial nerve which supplies motor and autonomic fibers to certain muscles of the eye and the ciliary body.

Oliguria: Reduced excretion of urine.

Ophthalmia: Inflammation of the conjunctiva or the eyeball.

Osteitis: Inflammation of bone.

Osteomyelitis: An infectious inflammatory disease of bone marked by local death and separation of tissue.

Otology: A science that deals with the ear and its diseases.

Otosclerosis: Growth of spongy bone in the inner ear where it gradually obstructs the oval window or round window or both and causes progressively increasing deafness.

Paget's disease of bone: A chronic bone disease characterized by their great enlargement and rarefaction with bowing of the long bones and deformation of the flat bones; also called *osteitis deformans*.

Pancreatitis: Inflammation of the pancreas.

Paracentesis: A surgical puncture of a cavity of the body, to draw off a collection of fluid.

Paracousis: A disorder in the sense of hearing.

Parenchyma: The essential and distinctive tissue of an organ or an abnormal growth as distinguished from its supportive framework.

Parietal bone: Either of a pair of membrane bones of the roof of the skull between the frontal and occipital bones that are large and quadrilateral in outline, meet in the sagittal suture, and form much of the top and sides of the cranium.

Patella: Kneecap.

Pathognomonic: Distinctively characteristic of a particular disease or condition.

Pathology: The study of the essential nature of diseases and especially of the structural and functional changes produced by them.

Pellagra: A disease marked by dermatitis, gastrointestinal disorders, and central nervous symptoms, associated with a diet deficient in niacin and protein.

Pericarditis: Inflammation of the pericardium, the conical sac of serous membrane that encloses the heart and the roots of the great vessels.

Periostitis: Inflammation of the periosteum.

Petechiae: Minute reddish or purplish spots containing blood that appear in the skin or mucous membranes especially in some infectious diseases, for example, typhus fever.

Petrous part of temporal bone: Of, relating to, or constituting the exceptionally hard and dense portion of the human temporal bone that contains the internal auditory organs and is a pyramidal process wedged in at the base of the skull between the sphenoid and occipital bones, with its lower half exposed on the surface of the skull and pierced by the external auditory meatus.

Photophobia: Painful sensitiveness to strong light.

Phrenology: The study of the conformation of the skull based on the belief that it is indicative of mental faculties and character.

Phthisis: A wasting of the body due to tuberculosis.

Physiology: A branch of biology that deals with the functions and activities of life or of living matter.

Plumbism: Chronic lead poisoning.

Pneumococcus: A bacterium of the genus *Streptococcus pneumoniae* that causes an acute pneumonia involving one or more lobes of the lung.

Polyarteritis nodosa: An acute inflammatory disease that involves all layers of the arterial wall, characterized by degeneration, necrosis, exudation, and the formation of inflammatory nodules along the outer layer; also called periarteritis nodosa.

Polyarthritis: Arthritis involving two or more joints.

Polyarticular: Having or affecting many joints.

Polydipsia: Excessive or abnormal thirst.

Polyuria: Excessive secretion of urine.

Porphyria: Any of several usually hereditary abnormalities of porphyrin metabolism characterized by excretion of excess porphyrins in the urine and by extreme sensitivity to light.

Portal hypertension: Hypertension in the hepatic portal system caused by venous obstruction or occlusion that produces splenomegaly and ascites in its later stages.

Presbycusis: A lessening of hearing acuteness resulting from degenerative changes in the ear that occur especially in old age.

Presbyopia: A visual condition apparent especially in middle age in which loss of elasticity of the lens of the eye causes defective accommodation and inability to focus sharply for near vision.

Ptosis: A drooping of the upper eyelid (as from paralysis of the oculomotor nerve).

Pyramidal tract: Any of four columns of motor fibers of which two run on each side of the spinal cord and which are continuations of the pyramids of the medulla oblongata; also called corticospinal tract.

Pyrexia: Abnormal elevation of body temperature (fever).

Quinine: Bitter crystalline alkaloid from cinchona bark used in medicine as an antipyretic, antimalarial, antiperiodic, and bitter tonic.

Recruitment: An abnormally rapid increase in the sensation of loudness with increasing sound intensity that occurs in deafness of neural origin and especially in neural deafness of the aged in which soft sounds may be completely inaudible while louder sounds are distressingly loud.

Renal papilla: The apex of a renal pyramid which projects into the lumen of a calyx of the kidney and through which collecting tubules discharge urine.

Rhagades: Linear cracks or fissures in the skin, occurring especially at the angles of the mouth or about the anus.

Rheumatism: Any of various conditions characterized by inflammation or pain in muscles, joints, or fibrous tissue.

Rickets: A deficiency disease that affects the young during the period of skeletal growth, is characterized especially by soft and deformed bones, and is caused by failure to assimilate and use calcium and phosphorus normally due to inadequate sunlight or vitamin D.

Sacrum: The part of the spinal column that is directly connected with or forms a part of the pelvis by articulation with the ilia and that in man forms the dorsal wall of the pelvis and consists of five united vertebrae diminishing in size to the apex at the lower end which bears the coccyx.

Sarcoidosis: A chronic disease of unknown cause that is characterized by the formation of nodules resembling true tubercles especially in the lymph nodes, lungs, bones, and skin.

Scala tympani: The lymph-filled spirally arranged canal in the bony canal of the cochlea that is separated from the scala media by the basilar membrane, communicates at its upper end with the scala vestibuli, and abuts at its lower end upon the membrane that separates the round window from the middle ear.

Scurvy: A disease characterized by spongy gums, loosening of the teeth, and a bleeding into the skin and mucous membranes, caused by a lack of ascorbic acid.

Sigmoidoscopy: The process of using a sigmoidoscope for the inspection, diagnosis, treatment, and photography of the last 25–30 centimeters of the rectum and lower sigmoid colon.

Splenomegaly: Abnormal enlargement of the spleen.

Spondylitis: Inflammation of the vertebrae.

Sprue: A chronic deficiency disease characterized by digestive disturbances, fatty diarrhea, a sore mouth and tongue; a macrocytic anemia that chiefly attacks adults in tropical form and that affects children and adults due to a gluten sensitivity in nontropical form.

Squamous: Covered with or consisting of scales.

Steatorrhea: Excess of fat in the stools.

Sudorific: An agent or medicine which induces sweating.

Sulci: Shallow furrows on the surface of the brain separating adjacent convolutions.

Syncope: A faint or temporary loss of consciousness due to generalized cerebral ischemia.

Synovitis: Inflammation of the synovial membrane, usually with pain and swelling of the joint.

Syphilis: A chronic, contagious, usually venereal and often congenital disease caused by a spirochete of the genus *Treponema pallidum*; if left untreated it is characterized by a clinical course in three stages—primary, secondary, and tertiary.

Temporal bone: A compound bone on the side of the skull that has four principal parts, including the squamous, petrous, and tympanic portions and the mastoid process.

Therapeutic: Of, or relating to, the treatment of disease or disorders by remedial agents or methods.

Thrombocytopenic: A condition associated with a reduction in circulating blood platelets and prolonged bleeding time.

Tibia: The inner and usually larger of the two leg bones between the knee and the ankle that articulates above with the femur and below with the talus; also called shinbone.

Tincture: A solution of a medicinal substance in an alcoholic or hydroalcoholic menstruum.

Tinnitus: A sensation of noise (as a ringing or roaring) that is caused by a bodily condition and can usually be heard only by the one affected.

Tophi: Deposits of urates in tissues characteristic of gout.

Toxoplasmosis: Infection with or disease caused by microorganisms of the genus *Toxoplasma* that invade the tissues and may seriously damage the central nervous system, especially in infants.

Tympanic membrane: A thin membrane that separates the middle ear from the inner part of the external auditory meatus and functions in the mechanical reception of sound waves and their transmission to the site of sensory reception; also called eardrum.

Typhus: A severe human febrile disease marked by high fever, stupor alternating with delirium, intense headache, and a dark red rash, caused by rickettsia, and transmitted especially by body lice.

Ulna: The bone on the little finger side of the human forearm that forms with the humerus the elbow joint and serves as a pivot in rotation of the hand.

Undulant fever: Brucellosis.

Urethritis: Inflammation of the urethra.

Urticaria: An allergic disorder marked by raised edematous patches of skin or mucous membrane and usually intense itching, caused by contact with a specific precipitating factor, either externally or internally; also called hives.

Uveitis: Inflammation of the uvea, that is, the middle layer of the eye consisting of the iris and ciliary body together with the choroid coat.

Varices: Abnormally dilated and lengthened veins or blood vessels.

Venesection: Bloodletting (phlebotomy).

Vertigo: Disordered state associated with various disorders (as of the inner ear) in which the individual or his surroundings seem to whirl dizzily.

Vesicatories: Substances which cause the process of blistering.

Volatile ointment: An ointment that vaporizes readily.

Zygomatic bone: A bone on the side of the face below the eye that in mammals forms part of the zygomatic arch and part of the orbit and articulates with the temporal, sphenoid, and frontal bones and with the maxilla of the upper jaw; called also cheek bone, zygoma, malar bone.

Select Bibliography

Adams, L. Ashby. "Beethoven's Deafness." Personal communication to Elliot Forbes. Cited in 1964.

Adams, P. C. "Historical Hepatology: Ludwig van Beethoven." *Journal of Gastroenterology and Hepatology* 2 (1987): 375–79.

Albrecht, T., ed. *Letters to Beethoven and Other Correspondence*. 3 vols. Lincoln: University of Nebraska Press, 1996.

Anderson, E., ed. *The Letters of Beethoven*. 3 vols. London: Macmillan, 1961.

Antonini, I. "Sordità e personalità di Beethoven." *Minerva Medicina* 56 (1965): 133–37.

Archimbaud, J. "Beethoven: Souffrances et surdité." In two parts. *Lyon Médit. Medical* 6 (1970): 59–62; 7 (1971): 65–74.

Arnold, D., and N. Fortune, eds. *The Beethoven Reader*. New York: W. W. Norton, 1971.

Asherton, N. "The Deafness of Beethoven and the Saga of the Stapes." *Transactions Hunterian Society* 24 (1965–66): 7–24.

Aterman, K., H. M. MacSween, P. E. Perry, and H. A. Warner. "Recurrent Infections, Diarrhea, Ascites, and Phonophobia in a 57-Year-Old Man." *Canadian Medical Association Journal* 126 (1982): 623–28.

Baker, D. "The Deafness of Beethoven." *History of Medicine* 5 (1973): 10–13.

Ballantyne, J., and J.A.M. Martin. *Deafness*. 4th ed. Edinburgh: Churchill Livingstone, 1984.

Bankl, H. "Beethovens Krankheit—Morbus Paget?" *Pathologe* 6 (1985): 46–50.

Bankl, H., and H. Jesserer. *Die Krankheiten Ludwig van Beethovens*. Vienna: W. Maudrich, 1987.

Beales, P. H. *Noise Hearing and Deafness*. London: Michael Joseph, 1965.

———. *Otosclerosis*. Bristol, England: John Wright and Sons, 1981.

Becker, W. H. "Wie sie endeten." *Die Thorraduran-Therapie* 21 (1950): 49–50.

Beethoven, L. v. *Ninth Symphony in D Minor, Op. 125*. Facsimile. Leipzig: Kistner and Siegal, 1924.

————. *Piano Sonata in C Minor, Op. 111.* Facsimile. Munich: Drei Masken Verlages, 1922.

————. *Piano Sonata in F Minor, Op. 57.* Facsimile. Leipzig: Edition Peters, undated.

————. *Violin Sonata in G, Op. 30, no. 3.* Facsimile. London: B.L., 1980.

————. "Beethoven's Deafness." *New England Journal of Medicine* 217 (1971): 1697.

"Beethoven's Diseases." *Lancet* 1 (1921): 41.

Behrend, W. *Ludwig van Beethoven's Pianoforte Sonatas.* Translated by I. Lund. London: J. M. Dent, 1927.

Bekker, P., *Beethoven.* Translated by M. M. Bozman. London: J. M. Dent, 1925.

Berberich, J. "Beethovens Krankheit." *Berliner Tageblatt*, 7 February 1928.

Bergfors, P. H. "Hade Beethoven syfilis?" *Lakartidningen* 63 (1966): 3842–44.

Bertein, P., and M. R. Apperce. "Le cas Beethoven." *Oto-rhinolaryng. Internat.* 14 (1930): 113–17.

Biechteler, W. "Krankheiten und Todesursachen berühmter Männer." *Med. Inaug. Diss.*, Munich, 1938.

Bilancioni, G. "La sordità di Beethoven." *Giornale di medicina militare* 69 (1921): 531–41.

————. "*La sordità di Beethoven: Considerazioni di un otologo.*" Rome: A. F. Formiggini, 1921.

Binz, C. *Lectures on Pharmacology.* Translated by Peter W. Latham. 2 vols. London: New Sydenham Society, 1897.

Blondel, R. "The Deafness of Beethoven." Translated by F. Rothwell. *London Quarterly Review* 155 (1931): 52–60.

Bodros, P. "La Surdité et la Maladie de Beethoven." *Presse Médicale* 48 (1938): 949–50.

Böhme, G. *Medizinische Porträts berühmter Komponisten: Ludwig von Beethoven.* 2 vols. Stuttgart: Gustav Fischer Verlag, 1981. I: 41–90.

Bokay, J. "The Deafness, Last Illness and Death of Beethoven." Diss., University of Budapest, 1927.

Bory, R. *Ludwig van Beethoven: His Life and Work in Pictures.* London: Thames and Hudson, 1966.

Boyle, Henry L.F.A. *Beethoven vu par les medicins.* Paris, 1928.

Brandenburg, S. *Ludwig van Beethoven: Briefwechsel Gesamtausgabe.* 7 vols. Munich: G. Henle, 1996–1998.

Breuning, G. von. *Memories of Beethoven.* Edited by M. Solomon and translated by H. Mins and M. Solomon. Cambridge: Cambridge University Press, 1992.

Brünger, E. "Betrachtungen über van Beethovens Krankheit, insbesondere seine Schwerhörigkeit." Med. inaug. diss., University of Cologne, 1942.

Brunton, T. Lauder. *Lectures on the Action of Medicines.* London: Macmillan, 1897.

Bynum, W. F., and R. Porter, eds. *Brunonianism in Britain and Europe.* London: Wellcome Institute for the History of Medicine, 1988.

Caldwell, A. E. "La Malinconia: Final Movement of Beethoven's Quartet, Op. 18, No. 6—A Musical Account of Manic-Depressive States." *Journal of American Medical Women's Association*, 27 (1972): 241–48.

Canuyt, J. G. "La surdité de Beethoven." *Le Médecine Internationale Illustrée* (Paris), March 1934.

Carpenter, C. K. "Disease or Deformation?" *Annals of Otology, Rhinology and Laryngology* 45 (1936): 1069–81.

Cawthorne, T. "The Influence of Deafness on the Creative Instinct." *Laryngoscope* (St. Louis) 70 (1960): 1110–18.

Chalat, N. J. "Some Psychologic Aspects of Deafness: Beethoven, Goya, and Oscar Wilde." *American Journal of Otology* 1 (1980): 240–46.

Comini, A. *The Changing Image of Beethoven: A Study in Mythmaking.* New York: Rizzoli, 1987.

Coon, E. H. "The Deafness of Beethoven: Tragedy and Triumph." *Nassau Medical News* 24 (1951): 1–7.

Cooper, B. *Beethoven and the Creative Process.* Oxford, England: Clarendon Press, 1990.

Cooper, B., ed. *The Beethoven Compendium.* London: Thames and Hudson, 1991.

Cooper, M. *Beethoven: The Last Decade 1817–1827.* Oxford: Oxford University Press, 1985.

Corner, B. D. "Beethoven: Muss es sein? Es muss sein!" *Bristol Medico-Chirurgical Journal* 86 (1971): 43–50.

Critchley, M., and R. A. Henson. *Music and the Brain.* London: William Heinemann, 1977.

Cudennec, Y. F., L. Soubeyrand, and P. Buffe. "Ludwig van Beethoven: L'homme et son enigme médicale." *Les Cahiers d'otologie-Rhinologie-Laryngologie,* 18 (1983): 41–55.

Czeizel, A. "Murdering Beethoven." Letter to the editor. *Lancet* 2 (1977): 1127.

Davies, P. J. "Alexander Porfir'yevich Borodin (1833–1887): Composer, Chemist, Physician, and Social Reformer." *Journal of Medical Biography* 3 (1995): 207–17.

———. "Beethoven's Deafness: A New Theory." *Medical Journal of Australia* 149 (1988): 644–49.

———. "Beethoven's Nephropathy and Death: A Discussion Paper." *Journal of the Royal Society of Medicine* 86 (1993): 159–61.

———. "The Cause of Beethoven's Deafness." In *Aflame with Music: 100 Years of Music at the University of Melbourne.* Edited by Brenton Broadstock et al. Parkville: University of Melbourne, Center for Studies in Australian Music, 1996. 143–51.

———. "Ludwig van Beethoven: Une surdité autoimmune?" Translated by Y. F. Cudennec. *Histoire des Sciences Médicales* 29 (1995): 271–76.

———. *Mozart in Person: His Character and Health.* Westport, Conn.: Greenwood Press, 1989.

———. "Was Beethoven's Cirrhosis due to Hemochromatosis?" *Renal Failure* 17 (1995): 77–86.

De Hevesy, A. *Beethoven the Man.* Translated by F. S. Flint. London: Faber and Gwyer, 1927.

Ealy, G. T. "Of Ear Trumpets and a Resonance Plate: Early Hearing Aids and Beethoven's Hearing Perception." *NCM* 17 (1994): 262–73.

Engel, C. *Discords Mingled.* New York: Alfred Knopf, 1931.

———. "Views and Reviews." *Musical Quarterly* 13 (1927): 646–62.

Ermoloff, J. "The Influence of Beethoven's Malady upon His Spiritual Nature." *The Musician* (Boston) 12 (1907): 373–75.

Ernest, G. "Der Kranke Beethoven." *Med. Welt.* 13 (1927); 491–95.

Forbes, E., ed. *Thayer's Life of Beethoven.* Princeton, N.J.: University Press Princeton 1967.

Forster, W. *Beethovens Krankheiten und ihre Beurteilung.* Wiesbaden, Germany: Breit-
  kopf and Härtel, 1956.
Foster, M. G. *Baths and Medicinal Waters of Britain and Europe.* Bristol, England: John
  Wright, 1933.
Frank, I. "The Deafness of Beethoven." *Annals of Otology and Laryngology* 44 (1935):
  327–36.
Franken, F. H. *Die Krankheiten grosser Komponisten:* 2 vols. Wilhelmshaven, Germany:
  Florian Noetzel Verlag, Heinrichshoffen-Bücher, 1986, 1: 61–110.
Frimmel, T. von. *Beethoven Handbuch.* 2 vols. Leipzig: Breitkopf and Härtel, 1926.
———. *Beethoven im zeitgenössischen Bildnis.* Vienna: Karl König, 1923.
———. "Beethovens Taubheit." *Beethoven-Forschung* 1 (1912): 82–89.
———. "Beethovens Leiden und Ende." *Die Wiener Presse,* 8 September 1880.
———. BS. 2 vols. Munich: Georg Müller, 1905–1906.
———. *Neue Beethoveniana.* Vienna: Carl Gerold's Sohn, 1890.
Garrison, F., and L. Morton. *A Medical Bibliography.* 4th ed. Edited by Leslie T. Morton.
  Aldershot; England: Gower, 1983.
Gattner, H. "Zu Beethovens Krankheit und sein Tod." *Münchener medizinische Wöch-
  enschrift* 100 (1958): 1009–10.
Geiser, S., and R. Steblin. "The Unknown Portrait of Beethoven As a Thirteen-year old."
  BN 6 (1991): 57, 64–67.
Goldschmidt, H. *Zu Beethoven.* vol. 1, *Aufsätze und Annotationen.* Berlin: Verlag Neue
  Musik, 1979.
Gradenigo, G. "La sordità di Beethoven." *Archives of Italian Otology* 32 (1921): 221–
  26.
Grove, G. *Beethoven and His Nine Symphonies.* 2nd ed. London: Novello, Ewer, 1896.
———. *Beethoven Schubert Mendelssohn.* London: Macmillan, 1951.
Grünewald, M. "Beethovens Leiden und Sterben." *Signale für die musikalische Welt* 85
  (1927): 514.
Gully, J. M. *The Water Cure in Chronic Diseases.* 4th ed. London: John Churchill, 1851.
Gutt, R. W. "Beethoven's Deafness: An Iatrogenic Disease." *Medizinische Kliniks* 65
  (1970): 2294–95.
Hahnemann, S. *Organon of Medicine.* London: Victor Gollancz, 1986.
Hamburger, M., ed. *Beethoven Letters, Journals, and Conversations.* New York: Thames
  and Hudson, 1984.
Hanson, A. M. *Musical Life in Biedermeier Vienna.* Cambridge: Cambridge University
  Press, 1985.
Harris, T. J. "Beethoven's Deafness." Diss., New York Academy of Medicine, 1936.
"The Health of Beethoven." *Medical Journal of Australia* 97 (1936): 435–37.
Hoffmann, E. "Die Bedeutung der Syphilis für unser Fach und darüber hinaus." *Arch.
  F. Dermatol. und Syphilis* 189 (1949): 285–94.
Hood, J. D. "Deafness and Musical Appreciation." In *Music and the Brain,* ed. M. Critch-
  ley and R. A. Henson. London: W. Heinemann, 1977, 323–43.
Isselbacher, K. J., et al., eds. *Harrison's Principles of Internal Medicine.* 13th ed. 2 vols.
  New York: McGraw-Hill, 1994.
Jacobsohn, L. "Beethovens Gehörleiden und letzte Krankheit." *Deutsche Medizinische
  Wöchenschrift* 53 (1927): 1610–12.
———. "Ludwig van Beethovens Gehörleiden." *Deutsche Medizinische Wöchenschrift*
  36 (1910): 1282–85.

Johnson, D. P. *Beethoven's Early Sketches in the 'Fischof Miscellany, Berlin Autograph 28.'* Ph.D. diss., University of California, Berkeley, 1978 (Ann Arbor, Mich.: University Microfilms, 1979).

Johnson, D. P., A. Tyson, and R. Winter. *Beethoven's Sketchbooks*. Oxford: Clarendon, 1985.

Kalischer, A. C. *The Letters of Ludwig van Beethoven*. Translated by J. S. Shedlock. 2 vols. London: J. M. Dent, 1909.

Kerman, J., and A. Tyson. *The New Grove Beethoven*. London: Macmillan, 1983.

Kerner, D. "Beethovens Krankheiten und sein Tod." *Münchener medizinische Wöchenschrift* 99 (1957): 740–43.

———. *Krankheiten grosser Musiker: Ludwig van Beethoven*. 2 vols. Stuttgart: F. K. Schattauer Verlag, 1973. I: 89–146.

Keynes, M. "Beethoven's Medical History." Letter to the editor. *Journal of Medical Biography* 2 (1994): 59.

Kinsky, G., and H. Halm, eds. *Das Werk Beethovens. Thematisch-Bibliographisches Verzeichnis*. Munich: G. Henle, 1955.

Klapetek, J. "Beethovens letzer Arzt." *Deutsche Medizinische Wöchenschrift* 93 (1963): 368–70.

Klotz-Forest. "La dernière maladie et la mort de Beethoven." *La Chronique Médicale*, in two parts, 13 (1906): 209–18; 241–49.

———. "La surdité de Beethoven." *La Chronique Médicale* 12 (1905): 321–31.

Knight, F. *Beethoven and the Age of Revolution*. London: Lawrence and Wishart, 1973.

Köhler, K-H., G. Herre, and D. Beck, eds. *Ludwig van Beethovens Konversationshefte*. 9 vols. Leipzig: VEB Deutscher Verlag für Musik, 1968–1988.

Krehbiel, H. E., ed. *Alexander Wheelock Thayer's The Life of Ludwig van Beethoven*. 3 vols. London: Centaur Press, 1960.

Krehbiel, H. E., and F. Kerst, eds. *Beethoven: The Man and the Artist as Revealed in His Own Words*. New York: Dover, 1964.

Kubba, A. K., and M. Young. "Ludwig van Beethoven: A Medical Biography." *Lancet* 347 (1996): 167–70.

Landon, H.C.R. *Beethoven: A Documentary Study*. London: Thames and Hudson, 1970.

———. *Mozart and Vienna*. London: Thames and Hudson, 1991.

Landsberger, M. "Beethoven's Medical History." *New York State Journal of Medicine* 78 (1978): 676–79.

Lang, J. *Clinical Anatomy of the Head*. Translated by R. R. Wilson and D. P. Winstanley. Berlin: Springer-Verlag, 1983.

Larkin, E. "Beethoven's Illness: A Likely Diagnosis." *Proceedings of the Royal Society of Medicine London* 64 (1971): 493–96.

———. "Beethoven's Medical History." In *Beethoven: The Last Decade, 1817–1827*, edited by M. Cooper, 439–66. Oxford: Oxford University Press, 1985.

Laskiewicz, A. "Ludwig van Beethovens Tragödie vom audiologischen Standpunkt." *Zeitschr. für Laryngol. Rhinol. Otol. und ihre Grenzgebiete* 43 (1964): 261–70.

Leavesley, J. H. *The Common Touch*. Sydney: William Collins, 1983, 37–44.

Lepel, F. von. "Neues über Beethovens Gehörleiden." *Neues Wien Journ.*, October 10, 1923.

Lesky, E. *The Vienna Medical School of the Nineteenth Century*. Baltimore: Johns Hopkins University Press, 1976.

Ley, S. *Beethovens Leben in authentischen Bildern und Texten*. Berlin: B. Cassirer, 1925.

Loewe-Cannstatt, R. "Beethovens Krankheit und Ende: Eine medizinische Studie." *Die Musik* 19 (1927): 418–24.

London, S. J. "Beethoven: Case Report of a Titan's Last Crisis." *Archives of Internal Medicine* 113 (1964): 442–48.

MacArdle, D. W. *Beethoven Abstracts.* Detroit: Information Coordinators, 1973.

———. *An Index to Beethoven's Conversation Books.* Detroit: Information Service, 1962.

MacArdle, D. W., and L. Misch, eds. *New Beethoven Letters.* Norman: University of Oklahoma Press, 1957.

McCabe, B. F. "Autoimmune Sensorineural Hearing Loss." *Annals of Otology* 88 (1979): 585–89.

———. "Beethoven's Deafness." *Annals of Otology, Rhinology, and Laryngology* 67 (1958): 192–206.

Magenau, C. "Beethovens Gehörleiden und das Heiligenstadter Testament." *Zschr. ärztliche Fortbildung* 34 (1937): 268–71.

Marage, G. "Causes et conséquences de la surdité de Beethoven." *Comptes Rendus Hebdomadaires des Séances de l'Académie des Sciences* 189 (1929): 1036–38.

———. "Nature de la surdité de Beethoven." *Comptes Rendus Hebdomadaires des Séances de l'Académie des Sciences* 186 (1928): 110–12.

———. "Surdité et composition musicale." Comptes Rendus Hebdomadaires des Séances de l'Académie des Sciences 186 (1928): 266–68.

Marek, G. R. *Beethoven: Biography of a Genius.* London: William Kimber, 1974.

Marx, A. B. *Ludwig van Beethoven: Leben und Schaffen.* 2 vols. 2nd ed. Berlin: O. Janke, 1863.

Medici di Marignano, N., and R. Hughes. *A Mozart Pilgrimage: Being the Travel Diaries of Vincent and Mary Novello in the Year 1824.* London: Novello, 1955.

Menier, M. "La surdité de Ludwig van Beethoven." *Archivs Internationales de Laryngologie, D'Otologie et de Rhinologie* 31 (1911): 179–81.

Miller, J. W. "Beethoven's Deafness." Letter to the editor. *Journal of American Medical Association* (JAMA) 213 (1970): 2082.

Möllendorff, W. "Editorial: Zur Beethovens Gehörleiden." *Neue Musik Zeitung* 43 (1922): 349.

Nabarro, D. *Congenital Syphilis.* London: Edward Arnold, 1954.

Nagel, W. "Beethoven's *Heiligenstadter Testament.*" *Die Musik* 1 (1902): 1050–58.

Naiken, V. S. "Beethoven's Deafness." Letter to the editor. *Journal of the American Medical Association* 215 (1971): 1671.

———. "Did Beethoven Have Paget's Disease of Bone?" *Annals of Internal Medicine* 74 (1971): 995–99.

———. "Paget's Disease and Beethoven's Deafness." *Clinical Orthopaedics and Related Research* 89 (1972): 103–5.

Nettl, P. "Beethoven and the Medical Profession." *Ciba Symposium* 14 (1966): 95–103.

———. *Beethoven Encyclopedia.* London: P. Owens, 1957.

Neuman, H. "Surditatea lui Ludwig van Beethoven: 1770–1970." *Oto-Rino-Laringologie* (Bucharest) 15 (1970): 379–87.

Neumann, H. "Beethovens Gehörleiden." *Wiener medizinische Wöchenschrift* 77 (1927): 1015–19.

Neumayr, A. *Music and Medicine: Haydn, Mozart; Beethoven, Schubert.* Translated by Bruce Cooper Clarke. Bloomington, Ind.: Medi-Ed Press, 1994.

Newman, E. *The Unconscious Beethoven.* Rev. ed. London: V. Gollancz, 1968.

Newman, W. S. *Beethoven on Beethoven: Playing His Piano Music His Way*. New York: W. W. Norton, 1988.

―――. *Performance Practices in Beethoven's Piano Sonatas: An Introduction*. London: J. M. Dent, 1972.

Niemack-Charles, J. "Herzschlag und Rhythmus." *Die Musik* 7 (1908): 20–25.

Nohl, Ludwig. *Beethovens Brevier*. Leipzig: E. J. Günther, 1870.

―――. "Beethoven's Death." *Monthly Musical Record* 8 (1878): 145–49.

―――. *Beethovens Leben*. Edited by Paul Sakolowski. 3 vols. Berlin: Schlesische Verlagsanstalt, 1909–1913.

―――. *Beethoven's Letters (1790–1826)*. Translated by Lady Wallace. 2 vols. London: Longmans Green, 1866.

Nohl, Ludwig, ed. *Beethoven Depicted by His Contemporaries*. Translated by E. Hill. London: W. Reeves, 1876.

Nohl, Walther. "Beethoven's and Schubert's Personal Relations."*Music Quarterly* 14 (1928): 553–62.

―――. "Beethoven und sein Arzt Anton Braunhofer." *Die Musik* 30 (1938): 823–28.

Nottebohm, G. *Two Beethoven Sketchbooks*. Translated by J. Katz. London: V. Gollancz, 1979.

―――. *Zweite Beethoveniana*. New York: Johnson Reprint, 1970.

Ober, W. B. "Beethoven: A Medical View." *The Practitioner* 205 (1970): 819–24.

O'Shea, J. G. *Music and Medicine: Medical Profiles of Great Composers*. London: J. M. Dent, 1990.

Ostwald, P., and L. S. Zegans, eds. *The Pleasures and Perils of Genius, Mostly Mozart*. Madison: International University Press, 1993.

Palferman, T. G. "Beethoven: A Medical Biography." *Journal of Medical Biography*. 1 (1993): 35–45.

―――. "Beethoven's Medical History: Themes and Variations." BN 7 (1992): 2–9.

―――. "Beethoven's Nephropathy and Death." Letter to the editor. *Journal of the Royal Society of Medicine* 87 (1994): 247.

―――. "Classical Notes: Beethoven's Medical History: Variations on a Rheumatologic Theme." *Journal of the Royal Society of Medicine* 83 (1990): 640–45.

―――. "Letter to the Editor." *Journal of the Royal College of Physicians of London* 26 (1992): 112–14.

―――. "Letter to the Editor." *Journal of Medical Biography* 2 (1994): 59–61.

Peyser, A. *Vom Labyrinth aus gesehen*. Zurich, 1942.

Pfuhl, J. "Beethovens Taubheit." *Ciba Ztschr.* (Basel) (1933): 121–22.

Pincher le, B. "Giovanni di Malfatti." *Medical Life* 38 (1938): 698–714.

Piroth, M. "Beethovens letzte Krankheit auf Grund der zeitgenössischen medizinischen Quellen." *Beethoven-Jahrbuch* (1959–60): 7–35.

Politzer, Adam. *History of Otology*. Translated by Stanley Milstein, Collice Portnoff, and Antje Coleman. 2 vols. Phoenix, Ariz.: Columella Press, 1981.

―――. *Politzer's Text-book of the Diseases of the Ear and Adjacent Organs*. 3rd ed. Edited by W. Dalby, Translated by Oscar Dodd. London: Baillière, Tindall and Cox, 1894.

Porter, R., ed. *The Medical History of Waters and Spas*. Medical History, Supplement no. 10. London: Wellcome Institute for the History of Medicine, 1990.

Reading, P. "The Deafness of Beethoven." *Guy's Hospital Gazette* 75 (1961): 176–82.

Richards, A. J. "Beethoven's Illness." Letter to the editor. *JRSM* 87 (1994): 722.

Risse, G. B. "The History of John Brown's Medical System in Germany during the Years 1790–1806." Ph.D. diss., University of Chicago, 1971.

———. "Kant, Schelling and the Early Search for a Philosophical Science of Medicine in Germany." *Journal of the History of Medicine* 27 (1972): 145–58.

———. "Philosophical Medicine in Nineteenth-Century Germany: An Episode in the Relation between Philosophy and Medicine." *Journal of Medicine & Philosophy* 1 (1976): 72–91.

———. "Schelling, 'Naturphilosophie,' and John Brown's System of Medicine." *Bulletin of the History of Medicine* 50 (1976): 321–24.

Rogers, J. F. "The Physical Beethoven." *Popular Science Monthly* 84 (1914): 265–70.

Rolland, R. *Beethoven the Creator.* Translated by Ernest Newman. London: Victor Golancz, 1929.

———. "Beethovens Taubheit." *Das Inselschiff* 11 (1929): 38–48.

Rosen, George. "Biography of Dr. Johann Peter Frank: Written by Himself." In two parts. *Journal of the History of Medicine* 3 (1948): 11–46; 279–314.

Sadie, S., ed. *The New Grove Dictionary of Music and Musicians.* 20 vols. London: Macmillan, 1980.

Sandblom, P. *Creativity and Disease.* 5th ed. Philadelphia: G. B. Lippincott, 1989.

Schachter, M. "Beethoven devant ses maladies et ses médecins." *Journal de Médecine de Lyon* 55 (1974): 1319–27.

Scheidt, W. "Quecksilbervergiftung bei Mozart, Beethoven und Schubert?" *Medizinische Kliniks* 62 (1967): 195–96.

Scherf, H. *Die Krankheit Beethovens.* Munich: Eigenverlag, 1977.

Scherman, T. K., and L. Biancolli, eds. *The Beethoven Companion.* New York: Doubleday, 1972.

Schiedermair, L. *Der junge Beethoven.* Leipzig: Quelle and Meyer, 1925.

Schlosser, J. A. *Beethoven: The First Biography.* Edited by B. Cooper, translated by R. G. Pauly. Portland: Amadeus Press, 1996.

Schmidt, F. A. "Noch einmal: Beethovens Gehörleiden und letzke Krankheit." *Deutsche medizinische Wöchenschrift* 54 (1928): 284.

Schmidt-Görg, J., and H. Schmidt. *Beethoven.* Bonn: Beethoven-Archiv, 1972.

Schultze, F. "Die Krankheiten Beethovens." *Münchener medizinische Wöchenschrift* 75 (1928): 1040–41.

Schünemann, G. *Ludwig van Beethovens Konversationshefte.* 3 vols. Berlin: M. Hesses, 1941–1943.

Schweisheimer, W. "Beethovens Krankheiten." *Münchener medizinische Wöchenschrift* 67 (1920): 1473–75.

———. *Beethovens Leiden.* Munich: Georg Müller, 1922.

———. "Beethoven's Physicians." *Musical Quarterly* 30 (1944): 289–98.

Sellars, S. L. "Beethoven's Deafness." *South African Medical Journal* 48 (1974): 1585–88.

Sellers, L. M. "Beethoven the Immortal: His Deafness and His Music." *Laryngoscope* 73 (1963): 1158–83.

Semenoff, M. "Méditation sur la surdité de Beethoven." *Le Courier Musical* 32 (1930): 735.

Seyfried, I. von. *Louis van Beethoven's Studies in Thorough-Bass, Counterpoint, and the Art of Scientific Composition.* Translated by Henry Hugh Pierson. Leipzig: Schuberth, 1853 (originally published by Wien: Haslinger, 1832).

Sharma, Om. P. "Beethoven's Illness: Whipple's Disease Rather Than Sarcoidosis?" *Journal of the Royal Society of Medicine* 87 (1994): 283–85.

Solomon, M. *Beethoven*. London: Cassell, 1978.

————. *Beethoven Essays*. Cambridge: Harvard University Press, 1988.

Solomon, M., ed. *Beethovens Tagebuch*. Bonn: B-H, 1990.

Sonneck, O. G. *Beethoven Letters in America*. New York: G. Schirmer/The Beethoven Association, 1927.

————. *The Riddle of the Immortal Beloved*. New York: G. Schirmer, 1927.

Sonneck, O. G., ed. *Beethoven: Impressions by His Contemporaries*. New York: Dover, 1967.

Sorsby, M. "Beethoven's Deafness." *Journal of Laryngology and Otology* 45 (1930): 529–44.

Specht, R. *Beethoven As He Lived*. Translated by Alfred Kalisch. New York: Harrison Smith and Robert Haas, 1933.

Springer, B. *Die genialen Syphilitiker*. Berlin: Verlag der Neuen Generation, 1926.

Squire, W. Barclay. "Beethoven's Appearance." ML 8 (1927): 122–25.

Squires, Paul C. "The Problem of Beethoven's Deafness." *Journal of Abnormal Psychology* 32 (1937): 11–62.

Stadlen, Peter. "Schindler's Beethoven Forgeries." MT 118 (1977): 549–52.

Steblin, Rita. "Beethoven's Life Mask Reconsidered." BN 8–9 (1993–1994): 66–70.

Steichen, D. *Beethoven's Beloved*. New York: Doubleday, 1959.

Sterba, E., and R. Sterba. *Beethoven and His Nephew. A Psychoanalytic Study of Their Relationship*. Translated by W. R. Trask. London: D. Dobson, 1957.

Stevens, K. M., and W. G. Hemenway. "Beethoven's Deafness." *Journal of the American Medical Association* 213 (1970): 434–37.

Tellenbach, M-E. *Beethoven und seine "Unsterbliche Geliebte" Josephine Brunswick*. Zurich: Atlantis, 1983.

Teply, I. "Ludwig van Beethoven in the Mirror of Medicine." *Bratsl.lek.Listy* 89 (1988): 854–60.

Tremble, E. "The Deafness of Beethoven." *Canadian Medical Association Journal* 27 (1932): 546–49.

Turner, W. J. *Beethoven: The Search for Reality*. London: J. M. Dent, 1945.

Tyson, A. *The Authentic English Editions of Beethoven*. London: Faber and Faber, 1963.

————. "Beethoven's Heroic Phase." MT 110 (1969): 139–41.

————. "Ferdinand Ries (1784–1838): The History of His Contribution to Beethoven Biography." *Nineteenth Century Music* 7 (1984): 209–21.

Tyson, A., ed. *Beethoven Studies 1*. New York: W. W. Norton, 1973.

————. *Beethoven Studies 2*. London: Oxford University Press, 1977.

————. *Beethoven Studies 3*. Cambridge: Cambridge University Press, 1982.

Unger, M. "Beethovens letzte Briefe und Unterschriften." *Die Musik* 34 (1942): 153–58.

Voorhees, I. W. "Beethoven from an Otologist's Viewpoint." *Bulletin of the New York Academy of Medicine* 12 (1936): 105–18.

Wallace, W. "Beethoven's Deafness." Letter to the editor. *Musical Times* 68 (1927): 538.

Waring, E. J. *Bibliotheca Therapeutica or Bibliography of Therapeutics, Chiefly in Reference to Articles of the Materia Medica*. 2 vols. London: New Sydenham Society, 1878.

Webster's Medical Desk Dictionary. Springfield, Mass.: Merriam-Webster, 1986.

Wegeler, F., and F. Ries. *Remembering Beethoven: The Biographical Notes of Franz Wegeler and Ferdinand Ries*. Translated by F. Bauman and T. Clark. London: A. Deutsch, 1987.

Wentges, R. Th., R. "Beethoven's Deafness." Lecture to the Dutch Society ORL, Nijmegan, 1975.

Werther, Dr. "Seltenere Vorkommnisse bei Syphilis." *Kliniks Wöchenschrift* 10 (1931): 1303–6, cited in Walther Forster, *Beethovens Krankheiten*, p. 68.

Willetts, I. E. "Beethoven's Demise." Letter to the editor. *Journal of the Royal Society of Medicine* 86 (1993): 677–78.

Winter, R., and B. Carr, eds. *Beethoven, Performers, and Critics*. Detroit: Wayne State University Press, 1980.

General Index

abdominal compresses, 28
Adams, George (optician), 200
Adams, L. Ashby, 137
Amenda, Carl (1771–1836), 43, 129
Anschütz, Heinrich, 91, 92
ascites, 181, 233
asthenic, 10, 18
atrophic portal cirrhosis, 177
Auenbrugger, Leopold, Dr. (1722–1809), 6
autopsy: Dr.Horan's translation, 102, 103; Dr.Wagner's post-mortem examination, 100–107; errors in the Pierson-Seyfried translations, 103–4; fate of the temporal bones, 105; original Latin text, 101, 102; original manuscript, 101; retrospective diagnoses, 104, 105

Baden bei Wien, 4, 31, 52, 58, 169, 191, 196, 203
Baillie, Matthew, Dr., 177
Bath, hayseed vapor, 79
Beck, Dagmar, 53
Beer, G.J., Prof., 201
Beethoven: Carl Francis van (1806–1858), nephew, 26, 30, 71, 72, 74, 77, 182

Beethoven, Caspar Anton Carl van (1774–1815), brother, 21, 45, 46
Beethoven, Johann van (1740–1792), father, 68, 181
Beethoven, Johanna van (1786–1868), sister-in-law (Reiss), 126
Beethoven, Ludwig van (1770–1827): alcohol consumption, 165, 179; appearance, 66–69; clothing, 67, 68; death, premonition of, 30, 208; emaciation, 106, 208; estate, 68; funeral, 90–94; gaze, 67; height, 66, 69; hypochondriasis, xiii, 190; illnesses with fever, 168–69; liver nodules, 103, 106, 177; masks and busts, 68, 69, 89, 90, 197; melancholia, 1, 80; nose bleeds, 30, 207; pianos, 53; portraits, 67, 68, 201; renal papillary necrosis, 103, 105, 107, 208–11; smallpox, 1, 68, 69; systemic lupus erythematosis, 69, 178, 180, 191, 195; "typhus" in 1796, 1, 13, 128, 135, 137, 140–42; voice, 68
Beethoven, Nikolaus Johann van (1776–1848), brother, 28, 45, 46, 47, 71, 77, 78, 84, 88, 125, 191, 202
Beethoven, Therese van (1787–1828), sister-in-law (Obermayer), 27, 86, 88, 91

Index of Beethoven's Works in This Volume

About the Author

PETER J. DAVIES is a retired Consultant Physician in Internal Medicine and Gastroenterology. He is the author of *Mozart in Person: His Character and Health* (Greenwood, 1989).

Lightning Source UK Ltd.
Milton Keynes UK
UKOW051255180512

192845UK00006B/19/P